Pediatric Ophthalmology in the Emergency Room

Roman Shinder

Editor

Pediatric Ophthalmology in the Emergency Room

Evaluation and Treatment

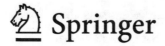 Springer

Editor
Roman Shinder
Professor of Ophthalmology, Otolaryngology
Department of Ophthalmology, Otolaryngology
SUNY Downstate Medical Center
Brooklyn, NY
USA

ISBN 978-3-030-49952-5   ISBN 978-3-030-49950-1   (eBook)
https://doi.org/10.1007/978-3-030-49950-1

This Springer imprint is published by the registered company Springer Nature Switzerland AG
The registered company address is: Gewerbestrasse 11, 6330 Cham, Switzerland

Preface

Thank you for interest in *Pediatric Ophthalmology in the Emergency Room*.

  This text represents 15 years of experience in managing acute ophthalmic problems in children that bring them to the emergency room, and the passion I have in doing so. The chapter authors represent a diverse group of specialists from ophthalmology, emergency medicine, pediatrics, and radiology who offer their expertise in the multidisciplinary team management that I feel yields the best care for children. Many of the authors practice at busy level one trauma centers with a large volume of pediatric visitors.

  This text is intended for a diverse group of healthcare professionals that include anyone who cares for children in an acute setting from initial assessment to final treatment and follow up. This includes pediatricians, emergency room physicians, nurses, physician assistants, trauma surgeons, medical students, residents, fellows, neurologists, neurosurgeons, and ophthalmologists among others.

  The information presented in this text should give the reader a broad insight into the common ophthalmic conditions that may bring a child in for an acute healthcare visit. Each chapter should give a logical approach to the evaluation and management of these various conditions. The text highlights various ways in which children present differently and necessitate different treatment algorithms from adults with similar conditions. With an abundance of clinical and radiographic images, clinicians will be visually aided in their diagnostic care. The important skills of patience and compassion towards children and their parents are highlighted throughout the book, as are the specialized diagnostic and surgical skill needed in caring for pediatric patients. It is my hope that this text serves as a valuable resource in the management of pediatric ophthalmic conditions with the ultimate goal of preserving or improving the vision of our children.

Roman Shinder, MD, FACS
Brooklyn, NY, USA

Contents

IV   Inflammations

V   Ophthalmic Cancer and Masses

Contributors

Richard C. Allen, MD, PhD, FACS   Baylor College of Medicine, Department of Ophthalmology, Houston, TX, USA
richard.allen2@bcm.edu

Jennifer Barger, MD   NYU Grossman School of Medicine, Department of Ophthalmology, New York, NY, USA
Jennifer.Barger@nyulangone.org

Sana Ali Bautista, MD   The Children's Hospital of Philadelphia, Division of Ophthalmology, Philadelphia, PA, USA
sali42388@gmail.com

Frank Cao, MD   Millman-Derr Center for Eye Care, Rochester Hills, MI, USA
caofrank@gmail.com

Christopher B. Chambers, MD, FACS   Department of Ophthalmology, Harborview Eye Institute, University of Washington, Seattle, WA, USA
cbc108@uw.edu

Valerie H. Chen, MD   Lions Eye Institute, Department of Ophthalmology, Albany Medical College, Albany, NY, USA
valeriehchen@gmail.com

Stella Y. Chung, MD, MS   Rutgers New Jersey Medical School, The Institute of Ophthalmology and Visual Science, Newark, NJ, USA
stella.YJC@gmail.com

Liza M. Cohen, MD   Division of Orbital and Ophthalmic Plastic Surgery, Stein and Doheny Eye Institutes, University of California, Los Angeles, Los Angeles, CA, USA
cohenlizam@gmail.com

Lauren A. Dalvin, MD   Wills Eye Hospital, Ocular Oncology Service, Philadelphia, PA, USA

Mayo Clinic, Department of Ophthalmology, Rochester, MN, USA
Dalvin.Lauren@mayo.edu

James A. Deutsch, MD   Department of Ophthalmology, SUNY Downstate Medical Center/Kings Counter Hospital Center, Brooklyn, NY, USA
jadeutschmd@yahoo.com

Levon Djenderedjian, MD   SUNY Downstate Medical Center, Brooklyn, NY, USA
ldjenderedjian@gmail.com

Aslan Efendizade, DO   Department of Diagnostic Radiology, SUNY Downstate Medical Center, Brooklyn, NY, USA
Aslan.efendizade@downstate.edu

Valerie I. Elmalem, MD   New York Eye and Ear Infirmary of Mount Sinai, Department of Ophthalmology, New York, NY, USA
velmalem@nyee.edu

Zerwa Farooq, MBBS   Department of Diagnostic Radiology, SUNY Downstate Medical Center, Brooklyn, NY, USA
ZerwaFarooq@gmail.com

Ekjyot S. Gill, MD   SUNY Downstate Medical Center, Brooklyn, NY, USA
Ekjyot.gill@downstate.edu

Danielle A. S. Holmes, MSc, MD   SUNY Downstate Health Sciences Center, Brooklyn, NY, USA
danielle.holmes@downstate.edu

William Rocamora Katowitz, MD   The Children's Hospital of Philadelphia, Division of Ophthalmology, Philadelphia, PA, USA
billkat@gmail.com

John R. Kroger, MD   Department of Ophthalmology, SUNY Downstate Medical Center, Brooklyn, NY, USA
kroger.johnr@gmail.com

Paul D. Langer, MD, FACS   Rutgers New Jersey Medical School, The Institute of Ophthalmology and Visual Science, Newark, NJ, USA
planger@njms.rutgers.edu

Nicole Lanza, MD, MEd   Department of Ophthalmology, SUNY Downstate Medical Center, Brooklyn, NY, USA
nicole.lanza@downstate.edu

Douglas R. Lazzaro, MD, MBA, FACS   NYU Grossman School of Medicine, Department of Ophthalmology, New York, NY, USA
Douglas.Lazzaro@nyulangone.org

Ilya Leskov, MD, PhD   SUNY Downstate Medical Center, Brooklyn, NY, USA
ilya.leskov@downstate.edu

Li-Anne S. Lim, MBBS   Wills Eye Hospital, Ocular Oncology Service, Philadelphia, PA, USA
lianne@shields.md

Andrei P. Martin, MD, DPBO   Wills Eye Hospital, Ocular Oncology Service, Philadelphia, PA, USA
andrei@shields.md

Charles G. Miller, MD, PhD   Department of Ophthalmology, SUNY Downstate Medical Center, Brooklyn, NY, USA
charlesgmiller@gmail.com

David Mostafavi, MD   Mostafavi Eye Institute, Staten Island, NY, USA
mostafavi.david@gmail.com

Laura Palazzolo, MD   Department of Ophthalmology, SUNY Downstate Medical Center, Brooklyn, NY, USA
laura.palazzolo@downstate.edu

Suraj Patel, MD   Department of Diagnostic Radiology, SUNY Downstate Medical Center, Brooklyn, NY, USA
Suraj.Patel@downstate.edu

Allison E. Rizzuti, MD   Department of Ophthalmology, SUNY Downstate Medical Center, Brooklyn, NY, USA
Allison.Rizzuti@gmail.com

Daniel B. Rootman, MD, MS   Division of Orbital and Ophthalmic Plastic Surgery, Stein and Doheny Eye Institutes, University of California, Los Angeles, Los Angeles, CA, USA
Rootman@jsei.ucla.edu

Duaa Sharfi, MD   New York Eye and Ear Infirmary of Mount Sinai, Department of Ophthalmology, New York, NY, USA
Dsharfi@nyee.edu

Carol L. Shields, MD   Wills Eye Hospital, Ocular Oncology Service, Philadelphia, PA, USA
carol@shields.md

Roman Shinder, MD, FACS   Professor of Ophthalmology, Otolaryngology, Department of Ophthalmology, Otolaryngology, SUNY Downstate Medical Center, Brooklyn, NY, USA
shinder.roman@gmail.com

Eric M. Shrier, MD   SUNY Downstate Medical Center, Brooklyn, NY, USA
eric.shrier@downstate.edu

Nora Siegal, MD, PhD   Department of Ophthalmology, Harborview Eye Institute, University of Washington, Seattle, WA, USA
nsiegal@gmail.com

Adam R. Sweeney, MD   Baylor College of Medicine, Department of Ophthalmology, Houston, TX, USA
Asweeney340@gmail.com

Nizar Tejani, MD   Louisiana State University Health Shreveport, Shreveport, LA, USA
nizartejani91@gmail.com

Nooruddin R. Tejani, MD, FAAP   SUNY Downstate Health Sciences Center, Brooklyn, NY, USA
nooruddin.tejani@downstate.edu

Vinodkumar Velayudhan, DO   State University of New York Downstate Medical Center, Department of Radiology, Brooklyn, NY, USA
Vin.Velayudhan@gmail.com

Daniel Wang, MD   New York Eye and Ear Infirmary of Mount Sinai, Department of Ophthalmology, New York, NY, USA
dwang@nyee.edu

Edward J. Wladis, MD, FACS   Lions Eye Institute, Department of Ophthalmology, Albany Medical College, Albany, NY, USA
tedwladis@gmail.com

Introduction

Contents

Pediatric Patient Encounter in the Emergency Department

Nizar Tejani, Danielle A. S. Holmes, and Nooruddin R. Tejani

Contents

© Springer Nature Switzerland AG 2021
R. Shinder (ed.), *Pediatric Ophthalmology in the Emergency Room*,
https://doi.org/10.1007/978-3-030-49950-1_1

1.1 Introduction

Eye-related visits in the pediatric population represent a small portion of total emergency department visits. In 2010, roughly 2 million, or 1.5%, of emergency department visits received an ophthalmic principle diagnosis. Of these visits, 27.8% were attributed to patients less than 18 years of age [1]. Data from 2006 to 2011 show a similar representation of the pediatric age group at 31.2% [2]. These encounters seem to be increasing – a comparison of data from 2001 to 2007 and 2006 to 2011 suggests a significant rise in the annual number of pediatric eye-related visits to the emergency department [2, 3]. While it is unclear if this increase is proportional to the overall increase in emergency department visits in the United States, this underscores the importance of a strong foundation in evaluating eye-related complaints in this patient population.

Pediatric ophthalmologic complaints in the emergency department include a wide spectrum of emergent and non-emergent conditions that require thorough evaluation. Early diagnosis and management are critical to preserving a child's vision and may be aided by understanding the physiological development of vision in the pediatric population. It is incumbent upon the emergency medicine physician to know when to seek the consultation of the ophthalmologist. This chapter reviews the comprehensive evaluation of a child presenting to the emergency department with an eye complaint.

1.2 Pediatric Eye Anatomy and Visual Development

◘ Figure 1.1 details the ocular anatomy. The eyelids are superficial to the globe and serve three main functions: protection of the eye from trauma through the blink reflex, clearance of foreign bodies, and distribution of tear film across the cornea to provide a clear and undistorted optical surface. The meibomian and Zeis sebaceous glands line the margin of the eyelids and secrete oils which coat the surface of the eye and keep the tears from evaporating too quickly.

Beneath the eyelids is the conjunctiva, a mucus membrane which lines the posterior surface of the lid and extends onto the globe

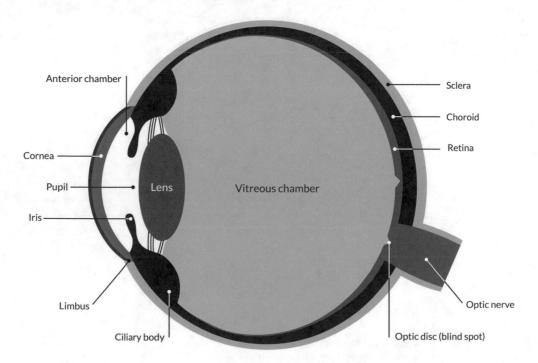

◘ **Fig. 1.1** The ocular anatomy

to the limbus, which represents the peripheral corneal junction. The portion covering the globe is known as the bulbar conjunctiva, and the portion lining the posterior surface of the eyelid is known as the palpebral conjunctiva. The conjunctiva is made of a non-keratinized squamous epithelium containing goblet cells. Beneath the epithelium is the conjunctival stroma also known as the substantia propria, a highly vascularized tissue that is the site of immunologic activity. On exam, the conjunctiva is transparent.

Deep to the conjunctiva lies the sclera, the tough, fibrous white shell of the eye that provides shape and support. Contiguous with the sclera, the transparent cornea is the anterior surface of the globe. Most of the focus power of the eye is from the curvature of the cornea. The cornea is avascular, composed of specialized epithelial cells, and innervated by cranial nerve V, the trigeminal nerve.

The uveal tract has three structures: the choroid, the iris, and the ciliary body. The iris gives the eye its color. The iris' development is completed by the eighth month of gestation developing from the ciliary body [4]. The color which develops throughout the first year of life is determined by the amount of pigment and density of the iris stroma. The iris' function controls the size of the pupil and thus controls the amount of light that falls on the retina. This change in size is an involuntary reflex requiring cranial nerve II, cranial nerve III, and the brain stem connections. Sympathetic stimulation dilates the pupil by causing iris dilator muscles to contract, whereas parasympathetic stimulation causes miosis, or pupillary constriction, by causing the iris sphincter muscles to contract. The ciliary body lies peripherally to the iris and produces aqueous humor. Ciliary muscle fibers adjust the visual focus by releasing tension on the suspensory fibers, or zonules, of the lens which changes the shape and focusing power of the lens. The lens is an avascular, transparent, elliptical structure which further focuses the light rays on the retina. The lens shape is determined by the ciliary muscle contractions. The change in the lens shape is the mechanism by which humans accommodate to clearly see near objects and small print.

There are two chambers in front of the lens – the anterior chamber is the region between the cornea and the iris, and the posterior chamber is between the iris and lens. The anterior and posterior chambers are filled with a clear fluid called aqueous humor. The large space behind the lens is the vitreous body filled with a gel-like fluid called vitreous humor.

The retina is the layer that lies interior to the sclera and choroid. Light stimulates retinal photoreceptors to produce neural signals that the optic nerve carries to the brain. The vascular choroid layer deep to the retina provides the retina with the nutrition it requires. The ophthalmic artery provides most of the blood supply to the orbital structures. It is a branch of the internal carotid artery. The superior and inferior ophthalmic veins drain the orbital tissues into the cavernous sinus.

1.3 Evaluation of Children with Ophthalmic Complaints in the ER

1.3.1 History

The evaluation of a child presenting with an eye complaint begins with a thorough history from both the child and the caregiver present. Chief complaints may include eye pain, discharge, and changes to vision. The history of present illness should identify onset, severity, ameliorating and exacerbating factors, monocular or binocular symptoms, previous ocular history, and associated symptoms. Past medical history encompasses the child's birth history and development as well as the maternal prenatal history. Perinatal infections with ocular sequelae, including toxoplasmosis, rubella, CMV, HSV, and others, are of particular concern. The results of genetic testing may also be pertinent to the child's past medical history. Other important components include past surgical history, contact lens use, allergies to food, environmental substances and medications, vaccination status, family history, and social history. A review of systems can be used to identify any concurrent systemic symptoms.

1

1.3.2 **Physical Exam**

1.3.2.1 Overview

The ophthalmologic physical examination of the child is vital to formulating a diagnosis and management plan and knowing when to involve the ophthalmologist. The challenges to obtaining a comprehensive examination in the emergency department are myriad: the child may be in distress from an injury, the infant or toddler may not be cooperative, and caregivers may not be helpful in comforting their distressed child. This becomes particularly important when the child has a diagnosis of attention deficit hyperactivity disorder or autism.

There are two primary keys to examining a child's eye: speed and distraction. The technique of distraction can be instrumental in examination and can be as simple as using a small toy to test the patient's ability to fix and follow. The fixation reflex is useful to assess vision in young infants or uncooperative patients.

Visual acuity is examined first. The method by which visual acuity is examined depends on the age and mental status of the patient. A letter chart is appropriate to test vision in a child's age 5 years and older, given that they are familiar with the English alphabet. Younger children might use a chart with easily identified pictures. In infants, the ability to perceive light is the most sensitive test for their vision. This is followed by an external examination of the eye looking for any apparent strabismus, ptosis, ocular injection, or other gross abnormalities. Next, extraocular movement is evaluated for any movement limitation, pain, or diplopia. Pupils are assessed for reactivity and symmetry. Using an ophthalmoscope, the red reflex is assessed, and the fundus is examined. The mnemonic VEM PF is often used as a memory aide in recalling the steps of the ophthalmic exam (◘ Table 1.1).

1.3.2.2 Visual Acuity

Visual acuity is the vital sign of the eye and should hold the highest priority in the evaluation of a pediatric patient in the emergency room. A standardized visual acuity exam

◘ **Table 1.1** Eye exam mnemonic: VEM PF

V	Visual acuity
E	External exam
M	Extraocular movements
P	Pupillary response
F	Fundoscopy

allows the consulting ophthalmologist to determine whether the complaint requires an urgent evaluation or a routine follow-up in an outpatient setting.

Visual acuity testing should be modified based on the child's age and development. By 3 months of age, the infant should be able to fixate on and follow an object. In these preverbal children until 3 years of age, the examiner should cover each eye and assess for smooth tracking of the object by the uncovered eye. Patients with decreased visual acuity in one eye will often make a fuss when their better seeing eye is covered.

Vision in verbal children older than 3 years of age should be tested using standardized eye charts. Again, the age of the patient should be considered when interpreting the results of the exam. Children between the ages of 3 and 5 years should have at least 20/40 vision. It is normal for these children to have an acuity difference of one line [5]. Children older than 5 years of age should normally have 20/25 vision or better without any significant difference in vision between both eyes [5]. Eye charts may be chosen based on the child's development. For example, in children who have not learned the English alphabet, the Allen card or Tumbling E chart may be used. In patients who are unable to stand and view diagrams at a distance, the Rosenbaum near vision card or Allen reduced picture card may be placed 14 inches from the child [6]. The Snellen chart is commonly found in most emergency departments and can be used in verbal children who can identify letters. Prior to any eye chart test, the examiner should ensure a standardized exam. Patients should be instructed to wear their corrective glasses or contact lenses and to stand at the recommended distance. The vision of each eye should be tested independently by having the child use an occluder to cover one eye. Children may sometimes try to cheat during this test, particularly when the eye with better visual acuity is occluded. To prevent peeking, the child's guardian can hold the occluder, or an eye patch can be used. When patients are suspected of malingering, a useful exam technique is to ask them to write their name on paper. Typically, children who truly have vision loss will still be able to complete this task. The malingering child may refuse to try to prove to the examiner that vision loss is significant.

The patient may not be able to complete the eye chart exam for many reasons including distress, inadequate pain control, and obstruction of sight due to swelling and compromised vision. Topical analgesia should be administered to patients with pain. However, if unable to complete visual acuity testing using charts, it is important to document vision based on finger counting, detection of motion, and light perception. Start by standing at a distance and asking the patient to cover one eye and to count the number of fingers held up by the examiner. If the patient is unable to do so, move closer to the patient and repeat. If unable to count fingers up close, then inquire if they can detect the waving hand. In the absence of motion detection, shine a light near the patient's eye, and assess for light perception and light projection by asking the patient to identify the presence and position of the light source. In these circumstances, urgent ophthalmologic consultation is imperative as the threat to binocular vision loss remains even if visual acuity in one eye is initially preserved. A delay in referral may increase chances of poor visual outcome and amblyopia.

1.3.2.3 Visual Development

Pediatric visual development is a complex system that requires visual stimulation from both eyes during the first 3–4 months of life to ensure proper development of neuro-ocular pathways. If any disruption of a child's vision occurs during this critical period in visual development, the child will develop a lifelong visual deficit [7]. Hence, the rationale behind the need for urgent ophthalmology consult in conditions like congenital ptosis and strabismus is that it might alter the visual pathway. The rate of vision development remains steep until about 2 years of life, at which time three-dimensional binocular depth perception develops [7]. It is not until 8 years of age that the brain's development of vision is complete.

The macula (area of the retina responsible for central vision) in young infants is not fully developed; therefore, the eyes do not fixate well centrally and do not follow objects until about 3–4 months of age. The quality and duration of fixation can be an indirect measurement of vision – if fixation is steady and maintained, and then visual acuity is assumed to be intact. However, if the fixation is intermittent and poorly maintained, the visual acuity is often found to be compromised. Accommodation (the ability to focus on near objects) develops by 4 months [8].

Visual acuity, like all things in pediatrics, is dependent on the patient's age. Visual acuity for newborns is approximately 20/400; however, a more useful measurement of visual function is assessed by pupillary light responses or by aversion to bright lights [9]. An infant of 6 months should have a visual acuity of 20/60–20/100. A child of 3 years should be able to use the tumbling E chart or recognize common symbols. At this age, they should see at a range of 20/25–20/30. At the age of 5 years, the patient should have a visual acuity of 20/25–20/20, though some variation exists. However, if the visual acuity is less than 20/20 by 8 years of age, the patient should be referred to an ophthalmologist for evaluation.

1.3.2.4 External Exam
Eyelids

The external pediatric eye exam should begin with observation. First, the position, shape, and passive movement of the eyes should be observed. Asymmetry of the lids can give valuable hints to underlying defects in the muscles and nerves that control eyelid function [10]. The eyelid skin should be examined for any lesions such as vesicles associated with a herpes simplex infection or a flesh-colored papule with an umbilicated center characteristic of molluscum contagiosum.

It is essential to look at the eyelid position. Telecanthus refers to widening of the medial canthal distance between each of the eyes. This is often due to a widening of the nasal bridge most commonly secondary to trauma or congenital syndromes. Hypertelorism describes an increased distance between the bony orbits and clinically presents as an increased interpupillary distance. This abnormality can be seen with midline defects or in syndromes such as Down syndrome, fetal alcohol syndrome, cri du chat syndrome, Klinefelter syndrome, Turner syndrome, Ehlers-Danlos syndrome, and Waardenburg syndrome [11].

Eyelid movement is responsible for the distribution of the tear film across the cornea. This provides a clear and undistorted optical surface by evenly distributing the tear film across the eye and clears foreign bodies. On closure, the upper eyelid moves down to cover the cornea, and the lower eyelid only moves up slightly. The muscles responsible for upper lid retraction are the levator palpebrae superioris and Muller muscle [12]. The predominant retractor is the levator palpebrae superioris, which is under voluntary control by the oculomotor nerve (cranial nerve III). The minor retractor is the Muller muscle which is under sympathetic innervation. Dysfunction of either eyelid retractor can result in ptosis or drooping of the upper lid. It is important to remember when evaluating a patient for ptosis that the etiology could be due to disease in the upper lid retractors, oculomotor nerve, sympathetic chain, neuromuscular junction, and birth trauma, among others [13]. Ptosis related to pathology of the sympathetic pathway will be mild (~2 mm), while ptosis related to oculomotor nerve pathology will be significant. Congenital ptosis is frequently diagnosed on a well-child visit because of parental concern about the asymmetry of the eyes. It can be inherited in an autosomal dominant form with variable penetrance and may be either bilateral or unilateral [13]. Ptosis should always be evaluated by an ophthalmologist as amblyopia can develop either from visual deprivation or from induced astigmatism. Other causes of ptosis in children include genetic syndromes such as fetal alcohol syndrome, third nerve palsy, myasthenia gravis, Horner's syndrome, and trauma, among others.

The motion of the eyelids should also be evaluated at rest as the inability to completely close the eyelids is known as lagophthalmos. Most often this is a complication of scarring or fibrosis of the eyelid or facial nerve palsy. Lagophthalmos can result in drying out, infection, or ulceration of the cornea.

Eyelid cilia (eyelashes) emerge from the anterior half of the eyelid margin. Epiblepharon describes a condition in which an excess skin fold is seen just under the lower eyelid margin usually medially and leads to the lower lid lashes being oriented vertically upward [14]. It is most commonly seen in Asian or Hispanic children and is usually asymptomatic and self-limiting and resolves within the first few years of life. Rarely the lashes will rub on the ocular surface and be symptomatic or cause keratopathy in which case surgical correction would be required [14].

There are many small sebaceous glands found in the eyelid that secrete oils that are part of the tear film and prevent the tears from evaporating too quickly [15]. The meibomian glands are found in the tarsal plate, while the glands of Zeis are in close proximity to the eyelash follicles.

Hordeolum and chalazion are the most common acquired eyelid lesions in childhood. A hordeolum, also known as a stye, is an infection of either the meibomian gland (internal hordeolum) or gland of Zeis (external hordeolum) [16]. It presents as an acute, erythematous, tender focal nodule of the eyelid and can at times have purulent discharge. The most common bacterial cause is *Staphylococcus* sp. A Chalazion is a lipogranulomatous inflammation of one of these sebaceous glands. In the acute setting, it is challenging to distinguish a chalazion from a hordeolum, as an acute chalazion can have a similar clinical presentation although will not have any purulent discharge. As the inflammatory process subsides within a few days, a chronic chalazion may remain as a nontender focal subcutaneous nodule.

Nasolacrimal Outflow System

The tears are drained from the eye by the lacrimal outflow system. This network begins with the superior and inferior puncta on the medial lids and courses distally via the canaliculi, lacrimal sac, and eventually the nasolacrimal duct which drains into the nose below the inferior turbinate. It is important to understand that the medial canthal tendon is superior to the lacrimal sac; therefore, pathology of the lacrimal sac or duct will be seen below the medial canthal tendon.

Newborn infants can rarely present with a bluish firm mass in the lacrimal sac fossa called a dacryocele [17]. This requires immediate ophthalmology and otolaryngology consultation given the possibility of infection and, in rare circumstances, sepsis that can develop. In older infants, classically 3–5 weeks after birth, congenital nasolacrimal duct obstruction can become clinically apparent with swelling below the medial canthus and tearing and mucopurulent discharge from the puncta [18]. This can be seen in as many as 30% of newborns [18]. To confirm the diagnosis, apply gentle pressure over the lacrimal sac which may cause reflux of sac contents from the puncta.

Conjunctiva

The conjunctiva is a thin transparent mucous membrane that lines the posterior aspect of the lids and the surface of the globe up to the cornea. The portion covering the globe is known as the bulbar conjunctiva, and the portion covering the lids is known as the palpebral conjunctiva. The conjunctiva is made of non-keratinized squamous epithelium containing goblet cells [19]. These goblet cells produce mucin, which is part of the tear film. Beneath the epithelium is the conjunctival stroma, which is highly vascularized and is the site of immunologic activity.

On exam, the conjunctiva appears transparent, except when inflamed when it appears red because of dilated blood vessels often referred to as conjunctival injection. Subconjunctival hemorrhages will appear as striking bright red discolorations. These hemorrhages might occur spontaneously, with coughing and Valsalva maneuvers, or secondary to trauma. In preverbal children, non-accidental trauma should always be ruled out [20]. Spontaneous resolution, over days to weeks, will occur, but parents should be informed to expect a shift of the blood and a change in color as the blood is reabsorbed.

Conjunctivitis can be from bacterial, viral, or allergic causes. Bacterial conjunctivitis presents with thick mucopurulent discharge often resulting in the lids being stuck together in the morning. The tympanic membranes should also be evaluated when considering bacterial conjunctivitis as frequently there is co-infection of the eustachian tube and middle ear known as unilateral conjunctivitis-otitis media syndrome [21]. Viral conjunctivitis, most commonly caused by adenovirus, presents with tearing and clear discharge and enlarged preauricular lymph nodes [22]. Allergic conjunctivitis presents with bilateral clear and stringy tearing, swelling of the lower eyelids, and intense pruritus [23].

The age of the patient is also important as neonatal conjunctivitis, occurring within 2–4 days after birth, presenting with copious purulent discharge, is classically due to gonorrhea [24]. In this case, there is a possibility of corneal involvement, and if not treated it can result in corneal scarring, thus making it an ophthalmologic emergency. However, if the patient presents after 8–14 days with watery discharge and conjunctivitis, chlamydia trachomatis is the more likely offender. Still, other pathogens must be considered including *Staphylococcus* sp., *Streptococcus* sp., and *Enterococcus* sp.

1.3.2.5 Extraocular Movement

The movement of the eye is controlled by six extraocular muscles that are innervated by the oculomotor, trochlear, and abducens nerves (▪ Table 1.2). Examination of extraocular movement begins with observing the child's gaze at rest. Take note of abnormal head posture as it may signify a compensatory response to ocular misalignment. It is important to understand normal visual development in children and modify the exam accordingly. Infants will fixate but not follow objects until 3–4 months of age. For this age group, the examiner can move the child's head or instruct the caretaker to

1

□ Table 1.2 The extraocular muscles and the name and numerical designation of the cranial nerves that innervate them

Extraocular muscles	Innervation
Superior rectus	Oculomotor (cranial nerve III)
Medial rectus	Oculomotor (cranial nerve III)
Inferior rectus	Oculomotor (cranial nerve III)
Lateral rectus	Abducens (cranial nerve VI)
Superior oblique	Trochlear (cranial nerve IV)
Inferior oblique	Oculomotor (cranial nerve III)

rock the child side to side to evaluate passive motility [25]. Children able to track objects should undergo the traditional exam of following an object in the six cardinal positions of gaze. Toys or other brightly colored objects can be used to maintain the patient's attention.

Strabismus denotes ocular misalignment. This can be congenital or acquired. Misalignment may be normal in newborns as intermittent esotropia or convergence spasm can be seen in infants up to 6 months of age [5]. Pathologic cases of strabismus can have numerous etiologies including stroke, aneurysm, infection, trauma, tumor, or inflammation. Cranial nerve deficits will present with decreased extraocular movements and strabismus. Oculomotor nerve palsy characteristically results in globe that is deviated down and out as supraduction, infraduction, and adduction are limited. The child may also have ptosis and an enlarged pupil. Trochlear nerve palsy leads to hypertropia, or an upward deviation of the eye. Abducens nerve palsy will show esotropia, or inward globe deviation, as the medial rectus muscle loses the antagonistic balance of the lateral rectus muscle which is unable to abduct. It is important to evaluate eye movements in orbital trauma, especially in cases of orbital fracture to assess for any restrictions that may be caused by entrapment of a rectus muscle.

Specific testing can aid in diagnosing strabismus. The first is the Hirschberg test. With the child looking straight, a light is directed at the patient, and the corneal light reflex is observed. If there is asymmetry of the light reflex with one not centered, this reveals a strabismus [26]. The second is the cover-uncover test, which involves placing a cover or patch over one eye. Allow the child to fixate on an object and cover one eye. While doing so, a movement in the uncovered eye points to a strabismus. It is important to differentiate pseudostrabismus from true strabismus. Children with large epicanthal folds may have the appearance of misaligned eyes when in fact no strabismus is present, resulting in pseudoestropia.

1.3.2.6 Pupils

The pupil is an opening in the iris that allows for light to enter the eye and stimulate the retina. Pupillary size is controlled by muscles within the iris, which dilate and constrict in response to light and dark conditions, respectively. Dilation is controlled by sympathetic nerve fibers, while constriction is controlled by parasympathetic fibers. Examination of the pupils begins with assessment of the symmetry, size, and shape of the pupils in ambient light. The child should be instructed to focus on a distant object to prevent any effects of accommodation on the pupil size. Normal pupil size in children ranges from approximately 3 to 6 mm in ambient light [27]. It is important to note that pupil size may be relatively smaller in infants. A stable size discrepancy of less than two millimeters in light and dark environments signifies benign essential anisocoria, a physiologic phenomenon seen in almost 20% of the healthy population [28]. A larger difference in size represents a disruption in the neuromotor pathway prompting the consultation of the ophthalmologist. Causes of pathologic anisocoria include oculomotor nerve palsy, Horner syndrome, tonic pupil, iritis, or trauma. Defects in the shape of the pupil indicate a pathology of the iris. An iris coloboma is a congenital defect where part of the iris is missing, giving an abnormal pupil shape.

Next, the pupils are stimulated with a light source to test the pupillary light reflex. As light enters the eye, the optic nerve is stimulated sending sensory information through afferent nerve fibers through the optic tracts to the visual cortex. Efferent motor nerve fibers from the oculomotor nerve then lead to pupil constriction. Both the direct and consensual response should be noted. The consensual response describes light in one eye leading to constriction of the contralateral pupil. The swinging light test can be used to identify an afferent pupillary defect, commonly known as a Marcus Gunn pupil. When alternating the illumination of both eyes, the abnormal pupil will dilate in response to the light source. Such a finding indicates a disruption of the optic pathway at the retina or optic nerve. Lastly, the near response should be tested; both pupils should briskly constrict when the child is instructed to focus on a central object 1 to 2 centimeters from the face. The acronym PERRLA is often used to indicate a normal pupillary exam when both pupils are found to be equal, round, and reactive to light and accommodation.

1.3.2.7 Fundus

The fundoscopic exam is used to evaluate the posterior structures of the eye, including the retina and optic disc. In the emergency department, ophthalmoscopes are widely available and should be used for this purpose. This part of the exam should be completed in a dark or dimly lit room to allow the pupils to naturally dilate.

The first component of this exam is the red reflex test. This is best evaluated from a distance with the examiner situated at the level of the patient's eyes. As light enters the eye, it is reflected off the retina. This produces the characteristic red-orange color that is seen in healthy children. However, the exact color of the red reflex can vary based on the patient's ethnicity [29]. Each eye should be assessed independently. The Bruckner test looks at both red reflexes simultaneously. The test is considered abnormal if there is absence of the red reflex or asymmetry between the color, intensity, and position of the reflex. This may

be caused by any process that disrupts the normal pathway of light through the eye, including foreign bodies, opacities, ocular misalignment, or malignancy. Leukocoria, or a white reflex, may represent a threat to vision or even life and requires prompt referral to ophthalmology. Bilateral leukocoria is suggestive of congenital cataracts, whereas unilateral leukocoria, particularly in young children, can be associated with retinoblastoma among others.

Dilation of the pupils allows for improved visualization of the fundus. Dilating eye drops are generally considered safe in children. 2.5% phenylephrine and 0.2% cyclopentolate may be used [30]. Internal examination of the fundus begins with identifying the optic disc. The optic disc should have a sharply demarcated border and a yellowish-orange color. Papilledema, or bilateral optic disc swelling, is seen in the setting of increased intracranial pressure. The retina should be inspected next. Beginning at the optic disc, each artery and vein should be traced to the periphery. Veins will appear dark red and large, with minimal light reflection. Conversely, arteries will appear light red and small, with a bright light reflex [19].

1.4 Conclusion

The spectrum of pediatric ophthalmologic complaints arriving at the emergency room ranges from benign, self-limited processes to vision or life-threatening conditions. Like any pediatric exam, the patient's age and underlying behavior can significantly hinder or help in the exam. The physician must employ patience, persistence, and a variety of techniques to elicit important signs and symptoms during the exam. The practitioner must be comfortable and competent with using common equipment during evaluation such as the ophthalmoscope and visual acuity charts. It is the responsibility of practitioners in the pediatric emergency room to be able to efficiently evaluate children with ocular complaints and recognize the situations that necessitate consultation with an ophthalmologist for proper care.

Key Points

- The pediatric ophthalmic examination must be adapted based on the patient's age, visual development, and functional status.
- The ophthalmologic examination of the pediatric patient must include assessment of the visual acuity, external eye, extraocular movement, pupils, and the globe.
- In children unable to provide visual acuity via a chart, it is important to assess visual acuity in other ways such as counting fingers, detecting hand motion, or perceiving a light source.
- Ocular misalignment can be caused by a diverse array of diseases, and failure to evaluate and treat strabismus may result in amblyopia and loss of vision.
- Essential anisocoria is a physiologic phenomenon seen in almost 20% of the healthy population and is defined by a pupil size discrepancy of less than 2 millimeters.
- Dilation of pupils for fundus exam with medications such as phenylephrine and cyclopentolate is considered safe in children.

? Review Questions

1. A 14-year-old male presents to the emergency department with left eye swelling after being hit in the eye by a baseball. Which of the following should be the first physical exam finding to elicit from the patient?
   (a) Upward gaze
   (b) Visual acuity
   (c) Pupillary response
   (d) Proptosis
   (e) Conjunctival injection

2. A 5-year-old female with a history of autism spectrum disorder presents with excessive crying. She appears to have unilateral tearing from the right eye but is uncooperative with the exam. What is the best approach to examining this child in the emergency department?

   (a) Ketamine for sedation
   (b) Tetracaine eye drops
   (c) Lid retractor
   (d) Papoose board
   (e) (b), (c), and (d)
   (f) (a), (c), and (d)

3. What is the vascular supply of the cornea?
   (a) Central retinal artery
   (b) Supraorbital artery
   (c) Anterior ciliary artery
   (d) None of the above

4. The parents bring in their 14-day-old baby very anxious that there is something wrong. They were told after birth that the child had nasolacrimal duct obstruction, but they are worried that it is getting worse. On physical examination, the neonate's left eye is tearing excessively, and the cornea is slightly cloudy when compared to the right eye. The baby is very active, and a red reflex is not elucidated from the left eye. What is the next best step?
   (a) Advise to continue lacrimal sac massage 3–4 times a day.
   (b) Reassure that 90% of cases resolve by the first year of life.
   (c) Refer for immediate evaluation by an ophthalmologist.
   (d) Refer for the next available appointment with an ophthalmologist.

✔ Answer
   1. (b)
   2. (e)
   3. (d)
   4. (c)

References

1. Vaziri K, Schwartz SG, Flynn HW, Kishor KS, Moshfeghi AA. Eye-related emergency department visits in the United States, 2010. Ophthalmology. 2016;123(4):917–9.
2. Channa RS, Zafar SN, Canner JK, Haring RS, Schneider EB, Friedman DS. Epidemiology of eye-related emergency department visits. JAMA Ophthalmol. 2016;134(3):312–9. https://doi.org/10.1001/jamaophthalmol.2015.5778.

3. Armstrong GW, Kim JG, Linakis JG, Mello MJ, Greenberg PB. Pediatric eye injuries presenting to United States emergency departments: 2001-2007. Graefes Arch Clin Exp Ophthalmol. 2013;251: 629–36.

4. Mann IC. The development of the human iris. Br J Ophthalmol. 1925;9(10):495–512. PubMed 18168498.

5. Nye C. A child's vision. Pediatr Clin N Am. 2014;61:495–503.

6. Kircher J, Dixon A. Eye emergencies in infants and children. In: Tintinalli JE, Stapcyznski J, editors. Tintinalli's emergency medicine: a comprehensive study guide. 8th ed. New York: McGraw-Hill; 2016.

7. Loh AR, Chiang MF. Pediatric vision screening. Pediatr Rev. 2018;39:5.

8. Curry DC, Manny RE. The development of accommodation. Vis Res. 1997;37:1525–33.

9. Weinacht S, Kind C, Mounting JS, et al. Visual development in preterm and full-term infants: a prospective masked study. Invest Ophthalmol Vis Sci. 1999;40:346–53.

10. Hodgkins P. Eye pain. In: Hoyt CS, Taylor D, editors. Pediatric ophthalmology and strabismus. 4th ed. London: Elsevier Health Sciences; 2012. p. 1043–6.

11. Stein R. Smith's recognizable patterns of human malformations, 6th ed. Arch Dis Child. 2007;92(6):562.

12. Baldwin HC, Manners RM. Congenital blepharoptosis: a literature review of the histology of levator palpebrae superioris muscle. Ophthal Plast Reconstr Surg. 2002;18:301.

13. Ahmadi AJ, Sires BS. Ptosis in infants and children. Int Ophthalmol Clin. 2002;42:15.

14. Simon JW, Williams KH, Zobal-Ratner JL, Barry GP. Conservative management of lower eyelid epiblepharon in children. J Pediatr Ophthalmol Strabismus. 2017;54(1):15–6.

15. McCulley JP, Shine WE. The lipid layer of tears: dependent on meibomian gland function. Exp Eye Res. 2004;78:361.

16. Lindsley K, Nichols JJ, Dickersin K. Interventions for acute internal hordeolum. Cochran Database Syst Rev. 2012;(4):CD00742.

17. Olitsky SE. Update on congenital nasolacrimal duct obstruction. Int Ophthalmol Clin. 2014;54:1.

18. Schnall BM. Pediatric nasolacrimal duct obstruction. Curr Opin Ophthalmol. 2013;24:421.

19. Bickley LS, Szilagyi PG, Bates B. The head and neck. In: Bates' guide to physical examination and history-taking. 11th ed. Philadelphia: Wolters Kluwer Health/Lippincott Williams & Wilkins; 2013.

20. Richards A, Guzman-Cottrill JA. Conjunctivitis. Pediatr Rev. 2010;31:5.

21. Bodor FF, Marchant CD, Shurin PA, Barenkamp SJ. Bacterial etiology of conjunctivitis-otitis media syndrome. Pediatrics. 1985;76:26–8.

22. Weiss A, Brinser J, Nazar-Stewart V. Acute conjunctivitis in childhood. J Pediatr. 1993;122:10–4.

23. Gigliotti F, Williams WT, Hayden FG, et al. Etiology of acute conjunctivitis in children. J Pediatr. 1981;98:531.

24. Rapoza PA, Chandler JW. Neonatal conjunctivitis: diagnosis and treatment. In: Focal points 1988: clinical modules for ophthalmologists. San Francisco: American Academy of Ophthalmology; 1988. p. 5–6.

25. Prentiss KA, Dorman DH. Pediatric ophthalmology in the emergency department. Emerg Med Clin N Am. 2008;26:181–98.

26. Jung JL, Braverman RS. Eye. In: Hay Jr WW, Levin MJ, editors. Current diagnosis & treatment: pediatrics. 24th ed. New York: McGraw-Hill; 2016.

27. Brown JT, Connelly M, Nickols C, Neville KA. Developmental changes of normal pupil size and reactivity in children. J Ped Ophthal Strabismus. 2015;52(3):147.

28. Spector RH. The pupils. In: Walker HK, Hall WD, Hurst JW, editors. Clinical methods: the history, physical, and laboratory examinations. 3rd ed. Boston: Butterworths; 1990.

29. American Academy of Pediatrics, Section on Ophthalmology, American Association for Pediatric Ophthalmology and Strabismus, American Academy of Ophthalmology, Association of Certified Orthoptists. Red reflex examination in neonates, infants, and children. Pediatrics. 2008;122(6):1401–4. https://doi.org/10.1542/peds.2008-2624.

30. Stout AU. Pediatric eye exam. In: Wright KW, Spiegel PH, editors. Handbook of pediatric strabismus and amblyopia. New York: Springer; 2006.

Ocular Motility in the Pediatric Emergency Room

James A. Deutsch and John R. Kroger

Contents

© Springer Nature Switzerland AG 2021
R. Shinder (ed.), *Pediatric Ophthalmology in the Emergency Room*,
https://doi.org/10.1007/978-3-030-49950-1_2

2.1 Introduction

A child who arrives in the emergency room with eyes that are deviated from the normal, symmetric, straight ahead position can send fear into the heart of the most experienced physician, PA, or consultant ophthalmologist. The goal of this chapter is to offer the panicked provider with the tools and knowledge to work up the child in a calm and thorough manner and review common and uncommon causes of strabismus and ocular motility problems which may cause parents to bring their child to the ER. While most of these conditions outlined below are not dire, some are making it important to appropriately identify, work up, and manage these cases to avoid negative outcomes.

2.2 History

One of the most important tools towards arriving at a correct diagnosis is to determine the course of events which have led to the child's ocular deviation. Try to learn exactly when the problem started. Is the deviation constant or intermittent? Is it getting better or worse? Is there pain? It is important to inquire about birth history as premature infants have a much greater occurrence rate of strabismus. The child's current age and the age of onset are important, because there are typical ages at which common problems present, such as intermittent exotropia, which typically presents between the ages of 2 and 4 years. Learn the overall health of the child; a sick child with a known diagnosis of systemic illness, such as leukemia or developmental abnormalities such as craniosynostosis, may present a different differential from a normal sibling. Try to identify any history of trauma, either to the head, eyes, or orbit. Both sharp and blunt trauma can cause the eyes to deviate. Always be alert to the occurrence of non-accidental trauma, and report it if there is any suspicion for it. Use what has been dubbed, "the retrospectoscope" – old photographs of the child – to try to pinpoint when the problem started. In today's age of smart phones,

use the photos stored within and social media postings to assist in determining when the age of onset of the misalignment. It is important to question about family history. While there is no firm genetic pattern of inheritance for strabismus, it is undeniable that families with a history of strabismus have an increased incidence of ocular deviations, often in similar patterns. Social history can be useful, as intrauterine medication and recreation drug exposure and overuse of smart phones and tablets may contribute to strabismus occurrence.

2.3 The Examination of the Child

In the words of M. Edward Wilson, "…when it comes to the pediatric eye examination, a friendly manner, a little trickery, and a lot of praise can accomplish a great deal" [1]. It is important to establish trust with the child and make the exam as fun as possible. Have a smaller child sit on their parent's lap. Try to be on the level of the child, rather than looming from above. Ask the child for their help in accomplishing the exam. Often, I will say, "Could you help me with this?", and when they agree to help, the exam becomes a game they are participating in, rather than an imposed intervention. When they do something, you wish them to do, praise them with phrases like, "You are very good at this. Did you practice this at home?" The child thus becomes your helper, something they enjoy being. However, realize that you do not have unlimited time for the exam. A child can quickly lose interest, so you must have a plan to extract the information you need quickly and efficiently.

In the evaluation of a child with deviating eyes in the ER, there are several vitally important elements which must be included in the exam.

■■ Vision

You must figure out what the child is able to see and if vision is symmetric between the two eyes. In a child over the age of 3.5 years, it should be possible to document standardized visual acuity on an ABC or picture chart

(Snellen), HOTV letters, or Lea symbols. To test vision in each eye individually, it is important to occlude an eye. Children are experts in cheating when using a standard plastic vision occluder. I recommend using a piece of 2-inch silk surgical tape applied loosely to the brow and hanging inferiorly over the eye. It helps if you tell the child that the tape is only temporary.

■ ■ Recording the Vision

Identifying a large discrepancy in vision between the two eyes may aid in the diagnosis of strabismus. In younger children who cannot read the eye chart, one can still make a good estimate of their ability to see. Use a toy, or any interesting object like keys, and move it through space in front of the child. See if the child's eyes move to keep fixation on the object. If the child is able to do this, it tells you only that at least one of the eyes can see. To determine if there is a difference in visual acuity between the eyes, it will be necessary to occlude one of the eyes. While tape can work as an occluder, in the very young or terrible twos, it can cause undue distress. In these children, it is wise to trick them by using one's thumb as an occluder. You can praise the child while gently touching the top of their head and stating, "Oh what nice hair you have!" Then, stealthily, move your thumb down to occlude one eye while moving the aforementioned shiny object through space (■ Fig. 2.1). If the child does not object to covering either eye and continues to watch the object, the vision can be recorded as roughly equal. A differential response such as objecting to covering one eye by crying or moving the head to avoid occlusion may be a sign that the vision is poor in the non-occluded eye. This can be recorded as "fixes and follows well in one eye, but not in the other." There are several other systems of recording as well (CSM, GSM, etc.), but in the ER fixes and follows should suffice.

■ ■ Amblyopia

Amblyopia represents a decrease in best corrected visual acuity in one or both eyes due to a disruption in normal cortical development

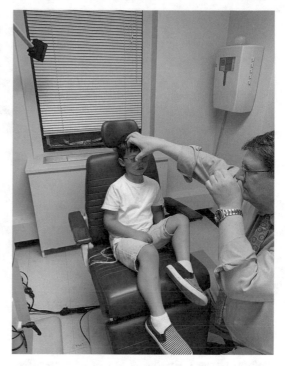

■ **Fig. 2.1** An examiner uses his thumb to sneakily cover an eye, so as to determine if the uncovered eye can fix and follow a moving object

of the visual cortex during childhood. It occurs in 1–5% of children [2–5]. Clinically, amblyopia can result from strabismus. In these cases, the eye which deviates more often has decreased visual acuity due to the brain suppressing images from the deviated eye. A large difference in visual acuity between the eyes in the setting of strabismus suggests long-standing deviation which has resulted in amblyopia. However, decreased vision in a deviated eye can also be seen in neurologic and infectious entities, so a difference in vision should not forestall a complete workup of the patient. It should be remembered that other causes of amblyopia, including asymmetric refractive error, are probably more common than strabismic amblyopia. Treatment including the wearing of appropriate glasses, patching of the better eye, and atropine penalization of the better eye can be employed to correct the "lazy eye." However, the complete evaluation for this is better handled by the ophthalmologist and should not fall on the ER provider (■ Table 2.1).

◻ Table 2.1 Most common underlying causes of amblyopia [34]

Type	Mechanism of amblyopia	Percentage of cases (%)
Anisometropic	Asymmetric refractive error leads to the formation of a poorly focused retinal image in one or both eyes impairing normal visual cortex development	50
Strabismic	Eye misalignment produces non-corresponding cortical images. The visual cortex suppresses the sensory input from the non-dominate eye to prevent cortical confusion and diplopia	19
Mixed	Concurrent anisometropia and strabismus are present (e.g. Accommodative Esotropia)	27
Stimulation deprivation	Media opacity present in the cornea, lens, or vitreous obstructs light from forming visual image of the retina. Lack of a focused retinal image prevents normal visual cortex development	4

■ ■ **Pupils**

Pupil size and light reflex should be noted. Anisocoria or asymmetric pupil size with an enlarged pupil on one side can be a sign of a cranial nerve III palsy. A Marcus Gunn afferent pupillary defect may indicate decreased visual information traveling from the eye to the brain and may suggest more dire problems which affect both movement and vision of the eye.

2.4 Ocular Alignment and Motility Testing

2.4.1 Strabismus

Strabismus or eye crossing represents an issue of ocular misalignment. It is a common problem affecting approximately 4% of children in the USA. Due to this misalignment, one eye will fixate on a target, while the non-fixating eye is deviated inward, outward, upward, or downward. The eye which fixates and the eye which turns may alternate, and eye crossing may be present at all times or only intermittently. To evaluate for the presence of strabismus, the following examination should be undertaken. An observation of how the child's eye move should be made. Do the eyes move smoothly and fully from side to side and up and down, or are there limitations to movement in one or both eyes? Are the eyes still, or

◻ Table 2.2 Classifying strabismus by direction of eye turn

Inward	Eso-
Outward	Exo-
Upward	Hyper-
Outward	Hypo-

is there a rhythmic oscillation back and forth, known as nystagmus? The head position should be observed. Is the head straight, or is there a tilt to one shoulder or a turn to the left or to the right. All these observations aid in diagnosis, direct workup, and determining how best to help the child (◻ Table 2.2).

"The purpose of the motor evaluation of the eyes is threefold: (1) to detect and quantify an eye misalignment, (2) to evaluate the function of each extraocular muscle, (3) to assess control over the deviation" [6]. However, in the emergency room evaluation, the eyes should be examined as they move in the following gaze positions – up, down, left, right, up and inward, and down and inward. The movement of the eye is graded against the movement of the opposite eye in a −4 to +4 scale. Next, the cover test should be done to reveal a turn. Alternately covering one eye and then the other will cause a turned eye to move to pick up fixation, moving in the opposite direction of its initial turn. For example, an inward turned eye (esotropia) will move outward toward the ear to pick up fixation when the other eye is covered. This deviation can be measured by prisms, and the pattern of measurements can pinpoint the cause of an ocular deviation. (This type of detailed measurement will usually be done by the ophthalmic consultant.) The cover test only works when there is sufficient vision in the deviating eye to allow the eye to move to see a target. In the event of a non-seeing eye, measurement of the deviation is better accomplished by the Hirschberg test where a light is shined at the eyes. One eye will usually fixate on the light, and the reflex will land in the center of the pupil. The other eye will show a deviation by the light reflex landing eccentrically on the cornea, either up, down, in, or out. This deviation of the corneal light reflex can be measured using a prism. This is known as the Krimsky method.

An effort should be made to determine whether the deviation measured is constant or intermittent and the child's ability to control the deviation if it is indeed intermittent.

2.4.1.1 Causes of Ocular Motility Disturbance Seen in the Emergency Room

Even though ER visits should be reserved for actual emergencies, parents who are worried about their child do not know whether the observation they have made of a perceived turn is urgent or not. Thus, we will discuss many causes of concern, from benign to extremely worrisome. This chapter is not meant to be an exhaustive review of every esoteric form or cause of ocular motility disturbance; rather it emphasizes the most common and most important entities which present to the ER. We start with an examination of comitant deviations – deviations with nearly the same amount of turn in all gaze positions.

2.4.1.2 Intermittent, Small Angle Strabismus of Infancy

Chronologically, the earliest manifestation of strabismus is the intermittent, variable, small angle turn of infancy. Up to 20% of normal infants have eyes with slight inward or outward measuring less than 10 ° of a

turn. These deviations can be present at birth and typically resolve by 3–4 months of age. These babies usually end up with straight, normally functioning eyes. In the absence of other signs of illness, no further workup is needed, and re-assurance should be given. Should a turn still be present after the age of 4 months, consultation is warranted [7].

2.4.2 Pseudostrabismus

Pseudoesotropia, the illusion of an inward eye turn is a common referral to pediatric ophthalmology clinics. This optical illusion is caused by the presence of epicanthal lid folds and a wide nasal bridge, which cover up the nasal sclera in one eye, and give the appearance of crossing when none is there. Alternate cover testing with no refixation movement, and a light reflex centered in the pupils confirms that the eyes are straight, and that pseudoesotropia exists (◻ Fig. 2.2)

2.4.2.1 Infantile (Congenital) Esotropia

Parents will often bring their child for evaluation of crossed eyes. Early childhood esotropia can interrupt eye contact, an important element of creating the bond between parent and child, and so this becomes an emergency to the parents. Although formerly called "congenital" esotropia, this crossing is rarely seen at birth, typically presenting by 6 months of age. Unlike the transient turn of early

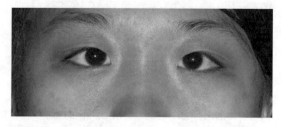

◻ **Fig. 2.2** Pseudostrabismus (pseudoesotropia). Although on first glance the eyes appear crossed, the pupils are centered and symmetric, and so the eyes are in fact straight. A wide nasal bridge and epicanthal lid folds can be misleading for parents and physicians. (Image provided by Roman Shinder, MD)

2

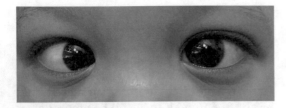

◻ **Fig. 2.3** Congenital (infantile) esotropia. Note that one eye looks straight ahead, while the other deviates inward. Treatment for the condition is surgical repair before age 2 years

infancy, the crossing of infantile esotropia is large (greater than 30 prism diopters), stable in size, and present constantly. Cover testing reveals an outward movement as the previously covered eye move to pick up fixation. Vision is often good in each eye, and patients can exhibit "cross-fixation," where the child views objects on the left side with the right eye and objects on the right side with the left eye. Imaging studies are not indicated in this condition. While infantile esotropia is not a true emergency, prompt referral to a pediatric ophthalmology is essential, because surgical realignment prior to 2 years of age results in better fusional ability and binocular vision [8] though there is ongoing debate about the timing of this surgery [9, 10] (◻ Fig. 2.3).

2.4.2.2 Accommodative Esotropia

A second surge in the incidence of crossed eyes occurs between the ages of 12–18 months and reaches its peak between 2 and 4 years of age due to the onset of accommodative esotropia. Accommodative esotropia is initially present intermittently and is associated with variable turn size that increases in amplitude when the child fixates on near targets. This entity is most commonly seen in farsighted children whose eyes deviate inward (converge) in a response to accommodative focusing effort [11]. A healthy child, with the above presentation, needs no further ER workup, but does need a prompt referral to a pediatric ophthalmologist. Treatment of this condition usually consists of the prescribing hyperopic correcting glasses which often completely corrects the turn when the glasses are worn. Occasionally bifocal or progressive glasses may be needed. Delayed treatment of accom-

modative esotropia can lead to tightening of the extraocular muscles, which may require strabismus surgery in addition to glasses to correct. Parents must be advised that the glasses work to straighten the eyes only when they are being worn and that the turn will return with the glasses off!

2.4.2.3 Acute Acquired Esotropia

A sudden onset of constant esotropia, which measures the same amount in all gaze positions, in an older child (or adult) is unusual and raises concern for intracranial pathology. Concomitant neurological symptoms, headache, nausea, vomiting, gait disturbance, and tinnitus, increase the likelihood of underlying intracranial malignancy. If a sudden acquired esotropia is intermittent, it is more likely that it is the result of decompensation of previously controlled fusional mechanisms; however, imaging and workup for underlying illness is still recommended.

2.4.3 Exotropia

2.4.3.1 Intermittent Exotropia

By far and away, the most common type of outward turn of the eyes in children is intermittent exotropia. In this form of strabismus, the eyes may demonstrate good alignment with only occasional episodes of outward deviation. Children are not born with this problem – most cases present between the ages of 8 months and 4 years of age, although older presentation is common. Children do not typically report diplopia, because the deviating eye is suppressed when it moves outward. The deviation is typically worse when looking in the distance and when the child is outdoors with parents often reporting that the child closes their non-dominant eye when in bright sunlight. This sensitivity to light is termed "photalgia." It is thought that this closure is an attempt to avoid double vision [12]. Many patients deteriorate in terms of how frequently the eye drifts and in how much it drifts (◻ Fig. 2.4). Imaging studies are not required in typical cases that present to the ER; however, a prompt referral to the

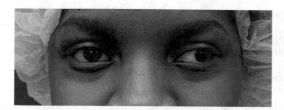

■ **Fig. 2.4** Exotropia in a young boy. Note that the left eye is deviated outward

■ **Table 2.3** Characteristics of the primary types of strabismus

Type	Age of onset	Size (ΔPD)
Intermittent small angle strabismus of infancy	0–4 months	<10 ΔPD
Infantile esotropia	>6 months	>30 ΔPD
Accommodative esotropia	12–48 months	Variable with larger angle esotropia with fixation at a near relative to distance target
Infantile exotropia	0–12 months	>35–90 ΔPD
Intermittent exotropia	8–48 months	Variable with equal or larger angle of exotropia with fixation at distance relative to near

pediatric ophthalmologist for evaluation and treatment is important. Both surgery and non-surgical methods such as glasses and patching can be used to restore control of this condition.

2.4.3.2 Congenital or Infantile Exotropia

This condition is a large angle (35–90 PD), constant exotropia which is present at birth or in early infancy. It is rare, occurring in only 1 in 300,000 births [13]. Amblyopia in one eye is common and may be resistant to patching therapy. Surgery is needed to correct the turn, with the goal to have straight eyes before age 24 months. Reoperations are common [13] (■ Table 2.3).

2.4.3.3 Incomitant Strabismus

For the common types of childhood comitant strabismus described above, the ultimate cause for the turn is unknown. However, in the following incomitant strabismus conditions, there is often an identifiable underlying cause. It is important to recognize the patterns that they occur in and to know how to proceed in the workup.

2.4.4 Cranial Nerve Palsies

2.4.4.1 Third Cranial Nerve Palsy

The third cranial nerve carries impulses to four of the six extraocular muscles – the medial, inferior, and superior rectus muscles, as well as the inferior oblique. It supplies innervation to the levator muscle in the eyelid, causing it to rise. Additionally, parasympathetic nerve fibers travel to the pupil causing constriction. Thus, a complete third cranial nerve palsy will cause the eye to be depressed and abducted (down and out) secondary to the unopposed action of the intact lateral rectus (sixth nerve) and superior oblique (fourth nerve). The pupil will be fixed and dilated, and the eyelid will be ptotic (droopy). A lesion to the third nerve nucleus results in bilateral ptosis in addition to the above clinical findings. While a complete third nerve palsy is easy to recognize, partial or slowly progressive palsies can be difficult to diagnose, and chronic or congenital palsies can result in aberrant regeneration with bizarre patterns of eye movement. While microvascular third nerve palsies are common in adults [14], they are rare in children [15, 16]. The most common causes in pediatric surveys are congenital, trauma, tumors, vascular (including migraines), and infection (viral and bacterial meningitis, encephalitis, and post-infectious encephalomyelitis) [15–17]. Imaging studies are necessary. Treatment is aimed at the underlying cause of the palsy. This may involve neurosurgery to remove tumors or

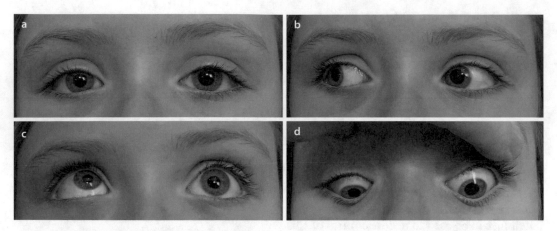

Fig. 2.5 Third cranial nerve palsy in the left eye, partial. Note the following signs: ptosis, deviation of the eye laterally, and downward, dilated, non-reactive pupil. The palsy in this young girl was caused by an arachnoid cyst of the nerve. **a** Primary gaze – note the anisocoria with a larger pupil in the left eye, with mild left lid ptosis. **b** Right gaze – note the mild limitation of adduction in the left eye. **c** Upgaze – limitation of left supraduction. **d** Downgaze – limitation of left infraduction

vascular treatments to ameliorate aneurysms. Management of resultant strabismus is complex and is best handled by a pediatric ophthalmologist (■ Fig. 2.5).

2.4.4.2 Fourth Cranial Nerve Palsy

Cranial nerve IV, the trochlear nerve, innervates the superior oblique muscle. Nerve fibers originate in the midbrain, cross the midline, and innervate the contralateral superior oblique. That muscle acts to depress, abduct, and rotate the eye inward toward the nose (incyclotorsion). The affected eye will be higher than the unaffected with worsening subjective diplopia and increased misalignment in inward gaze. Individuals with fourth nerve palsies usually present with a head tilt to the opposite shoulder. This positioning compensates for the decreased action of the superior oblique muscle, maintains binocular vision, and avoids double vision. The most common cause of fourth nerve palsy is congenital, accounting for 84% of cases in children [18]. Acute palsies can be caused by blunt trauma, increased intracranial pressure, and tumors. MRI imaging should be done in acute cases. Chronic cases do not need urgent workup, and old photos may confirm a head tilt present many years previous. Prism glasses can be used to correct for small angle turns, but strabismus surgery is necessary to correct severe, large angle palsies.

2.4.4.3 Sixth Cranial Nerve Palsies

An inward turn (esotropia), worse in side gaze, and often worse in the distance and better controlled at near, is the hallmark of a bilateral sixth cranial nerve palsy. These nerves innervate the lateral rectus muscles, which pull the eyes outward. Their weakness causes an inward turning. A unilateral sixth nerve palsy can result in a head turn away from the affected lateral rectus with fusion in the gaze position away from the weakness, but it can also present with diplopia when there is no position where the eyes can align for fusion. The sixth nerve has a long course from its nucleus in the pons to the lateral rectus [19]; thus it is particularly susceptible to injury from trauma along that course. A high percentage of sixth cranial nerve palsy in children are secondary to intracranial pathology, and a full neurologic and MRI evaluation is needed at the time of presentation. Common causes of adult palsies, such as microvascular diabetic, are rarely seen in children. Rather, trauma, neoplasm, intracranial hypertension, and aneurysm are more common causes of CN VI palsy in the pediatric population. Infections, such as an abscess along the nerve's path, Gradenigo syndrome (otitis media, trigeminal pain, and fourth nerve palsy), varicella zoster, meningitis, Lyme disease, cytomegalovirus, and Epstein-Barr, have all been implicated. A relatively common post-viral syndrome can produce sixth nerve palsy in children. This condition typically resolves by itself but can recur, often involving the opposite eye.

Duane retraction syndrome is often misdiagnosed for sixth nerve palsy. This congenital problem results from the failure of the sixth nerve nucleus to form embryologically. In the absence of CN VI, CN III innervates the lateral rectus muscle. This results in the eyes generally being straight in primary position, with inability to abduct the eye, and inward retraction of the globe on attempted abduction. Again, this condition is present at birth, and should not be a cause of urgent presentation.

Treatment for sixth nerve palsy is available. In the initial 6 months, the goal is to avoid double vision and allow patients to function as normally as possible in their life. Occlusion of one eye with a patch or tape over one lens of the glasses may be of help initially. Prisms, often in the form of Fresnel Press-On prisms, can be applied to glasses to improve alignment in primary gaze and lessen diplopia. Botulinum toxin treatment of the opposing medial rectus to decrease diplopia has been done [20]. After 6 months, multiple surgical techniques are available to straighten the eye and reduce diplopia in primary gaze. Following strabismus repair, these patients will continue to experience diplopia in lateral gaze due to the lateral rectus palsy (◘ Table 2.4).

◘ **Table 2.4** Anticipated strabismus secondary to cranial nerve palsy

Oculomotor (CN III)	Concurrent: Exotropia – loss of innervation medial rectus Hypotropia – loss of innervation to superior rectus and inferior oblique
Trochlear (CN IV)	Excyclotorsion (patient may have compensatory contralateral head tilt) Hypertropia
Abducens (CN VI)	Esotropia

2.4.5 Supranuclear Gaze Palsies

There are several gaze abnormalities or palsies which result from cortical centers which provide input and feedback to the cranial nerve nuclei responsible for extraocular motility. These conditions are rare in children and are rarely encountered in the emergency room.

2.4.5.1 Dorsal Midbrain Syndrome (Induced Convergence Retraction)

Lesions of the posterior commissure in the dorsal rostral midbrain can be from many causes and may produce problems with vertical gaze, eyelid control, pupils, and fixation. In a typical case, the child will have limitation of up gaze, often with convergence spasm or nystagmus on attempted up gaze. Causes in children include pineal tumors, hydrocephalus, ventricular shunt malposition, and demyelinating diseases such as multiple sclerosis. Prognosis depends on the underlying causation. Radiologic evaluation is needed [21, 22].

2.4.5.2 Internuclear Ophthalmoplegia

Internuclear ophthalmoplegia represents the inability to move inward from primary gaze (adduction), and the contralateral eye moves outward (abducts) with a nystagmoid movement. This entity is caused by damage to the interneurons which connect the sixth and third cranial nerves. The most common cause in young people is from demyelinating disease, but it can also be caused by trauma and tumor. Microvascular disease is a common cause of INO in adults but is rare in the pediatric population [23, 24]. Prognosis depends on the underlying etiology. MRI scan is needed.

2.4.6 Skew Deviation

Skew deviation is a strange acquired hyperdeviation in which there is an alternating ipsilateral hypertropia, resulting from disruption of the supranuclear input from the otoliths in the inner ear. Skew deviation is caused by brain lesions in the posterior fossa, most commonly tumors and vascular disease. This condition is differentiated from fourth cranial nerve palsies by the absence of excyclotropia on fundus torsion or double Maddox rod testing, as well as a lessening of the hypertropia when the patient is lying down, which does not occur in fourth nerve palsies [25].

2.4.6.1 Chronic Progressive External Ophthalmoplegia (CPEO)

Chronic progressive external ophthalmoplegia is a slowly progressive weakness of the ocular muscles including the orbicularis oculi. This disease is caused by a mitochondrial DNA deletion disease and can be associated with systemic problems including cardiac conductive abnormalities. Due to the slow progressive nature of symptoms, this disease entity is unlikely to cause presentation to the ER.

2.4.7 Nystagmus

Nystagmus is the uncontrollable, rhythmic oscillations of one or both eyes. To the examiner it appears as the constant, to and fro motion of the eye(s). The most common forms of nystagmus are infantile nystagmus, fusion maldevelopment syndrome, and idiopathic nystagmus (congenital motor nystagmus) [26]. It is important to differentiate the "benign" forms of infantile nystagmus from later acquired forms as the later acquired forms are often associated with neurological and drug-related causations.

Infantile nystagmus syndrome starts in early infancy. It can occur as a primary entity or secondary to defects in the visual system, such as albinism, inherited retinal disease, optic nerve hypoplasia, congenital cataracts, corneal opacities, and aniridia. Due to onset early in infancy, affected individuals rarely experience oscillopsia, the perception of objects in the world moving to and fro.

Fusion maldevelopment nystagmus (latent nystagmus) presents or becomes manifest when an observer covers one eye. It is commonly seen in individuals with pre-existing strabismus, such as esotropia. Neither INS nor FMNS requires emergent imaging or in-depth workup in the absence of other neurologic or toxic findings.

A third type of early childhood nystagmus is spasmus nutans. Here there is a triad of clinical findings: a fine, extremely fast pendular oscillation (a flag snapping back and forth in a brisk wind), head nodding, and a head tilt [27]. True spasmus nutans usually resolves within 2 years, but an identical triad of symptoms is seen in intracranial tumors of the diencephalon. Imaging studies are needed but can be deferred in favor of an urgent outpatient workup if the child is otherwise well and does not have any evidence of neurologic or developmental deficits.

Nystagmus which develops after the first 3–9 months of age is more concerning to the ER practitioner. Drugs use, both licit and illicit, can cause new onset of nystagmus. Causative agents include almost all anticonvulsants, including phenobarbital, phenytoin, and carbamazepine. Sedatives, hypnotics, lithium, ethambutol, dextromethorphan cough suppressant, quinine drugs including chloroquine, loop diuretics including furosemide, aminoglycoside antibiotics including gentamicin, several chemotherapy agents including carboplatin and cisplatin, aspirin, and alcohol can cause nystagmus. Illicit drugs such as PCP (phencyclidine), LSD, and marijuana have been implicated. Additionally, exposure to environmental toxins such as butyl nitrite, carbon disulfide, hexane, lead, manganese, mercury, styrene, tin, toluene, trichloroethylene, and xylene can cause nystagmus. A teenager who presents with new-onset nystagmus certainly deserves a drug and toxicology screening blood test. Intracranial disease, including trauma, inflammation, cerebral malformation, and mass can cause nystagmus, but there are usually other signs and symptoms present to guide the workup in these cases [28, 29].

Finally, there are common benign forms of nystagmus that do not warrant further workup. End-gaze nystagmus, where the eyes oscillate in far lateral gaze, is a normal finding. Voluntary nystagmus of the eyes, where a talented person can intentionally cause the eyes to rapidly flutter back and forth, is present in 7–15% of the population and is a popular party trick.

2.5 Strabismus Following Trauma to the Extraocular Muscles

The authors are indebted to the excellent review of this topic by Andrea Molinari as published in the Knights Templar Eye Foundation Pediatric Ophthalmology Education Center of the AAO.

A child can present to the ER after trauma that directly affects the extraocular muscles, rather than the cranial nerves or supranuclear structures. According to Molinari, there are "three basic mechanisms that can affect the extraocular muscles in the event of trauma to produce strabismus:

1. Muscle involvement in orbital wall fractures
2. Muscle contusion
3. Traumatic disinsertion or laceration of the extraocular muscle [30]"

Injuries to extraocular muscles from orbital wall fracture can result from two mechanisms: muscle entrapment in the orbital fracture and a flap tear of a rectus muscle [31]. Orbital fractures usually affect the medial and inferior walls, which are the thinnest and most likely to fracture. The muscles most likely to be entrapped in a fracture are the inferior rectus, medial rectus, and superior oblique. More than one muscle can be affected. In adults, orbital fractures typically produce large comminuted fractures ("blow out fracture") which may result in enophthalmos. Conversely, in children, the bone is elastic, and when it snaps and bends, a "trapdoor" is created which entraps a muscle or the adnexa attached to the muscle. Ischemia of the muscle is common in children, and orbital surgeons may not be able to wait for swelling to go down before repair is done. A special type of trapdoor fracture, known as the "white-eyed floor fracture" [32]. Here, there is little external evidence of injury, but on extraocular motility exam, there is restricted up gaze, and often, there is triggering of the oculocardiac reflex with nausea/vomiting, syncope, and bradycardia. Here the fracture must be repaired quickly to avoid cardiovascular compromise (❏ Table 2.1).

A second type of rectus muscle injury caused by orbital trauma is the flap tear. Here, traction of the orbital tissue causes a tearing away of the outer layer of the muscle from the inner layer. As opposed to the restriction of an entrapped muscle which limits movement away from the muscle, in a flap tear, this injury produces limitation toward the affect muscle. In either injury, the patient may adopt an abnormal head position adopted to maintain binocular vision, away from the restricted or limited muscle.

2.5.1 Muscle Contusion

According to Molinari, a muscle contusion is formed by the impact of an "object on the surface of the muscle without perforating any structure in the eye or surrounding tissues" [31]. A hematoma results which prevents the muscle from functioning normally. The hallmark of this injury is spontaneous improvement as the blood resorbs and muscle contractility improves. Both restrictions away from the injured muscle and decreased movement in the field of action of the muscle can be seen. Both improve as again the blood resorbs.

2.5.2 Traumatic Disinsertion or Laceration of the Extraocular Muscles

Traumatic disinsertion results from a blunt object impact injury that goes through the conjunctiva to sever the connection of the muscle to the globe, at a point 5–7 mm back from the limbus. While the muscle may retract, intermuscular membranes usually prevent the full retraction into the deep orbit, and some muscle function may be preserved [33].

Laceration of a muscle is usually caused by a sharp object which transects the muscle.

2

Laceration injuries are typically deeper than the disinsertions. Repair can be done for both types of muscle disinsertions, but it is technically difficult and often requires coordination between a strabismologist, the orbital plastic surgeon, and occasionally an ENT endoscopic surgeon to locate and repair the muscles. Orbital imaging is crucial for the diagnosis and treatment of these patients. The best imaging modalities for assessing orbital fracture are CT scan of the orbits with slices of 1–2 mm and MRI with fat suppression. In the ER the best way to proceed with these injuries is to apply cool compresses to the affected eye to reduce swelling and to urgently consult oculoplastic surgery for assistance in management.

Case Presentation

A 14-year old girl is brought to the emergency department by her mother, who is concerned that the eyes appear to cross inward, especially when she looks to the side. She states that the condition has been present since birth. She is concerned that her daughter may have a brain tumor, since she read on the Internet that that is a common cause of crossed eyes. A careful exam reveals a wide nasal bridge and epicanthal lid folds. Light reflex testing shows a symmetric light reflex centered in the pupil in each eye (◘ Fig. 2.6). The diagnosis of pseudoesotropia, the false appearance of crossed eyes when the eyes are in fact straight, is made. No further diagnostic tests were performed. The mother is reassured but is urged to follow up with a pediatric ophthalmologist for confirmation of the condition.

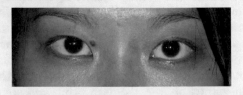

◘ **Fig. 2.6** Clinical photograph of pseudostrabismus related to epicanthal folds. (Image provided by Roman Shinder, MD)

Key Points

- Ocular motility can be daunting for emergency department personnel, but calm, systematic exam of the child can reveal the etiology of strabismus.
- Esotropia, a true inward turn of the eyes, must be differentiated from pseudoesotropia, the false appearance of crossed eyes caused by epicanthal lid folds.
- Exotropia is a common form of strabismus and is commonly seen intermittently in the second to third year of life.
- Cranial nerve palsies must be suspected in incomitant strabismus, where the deviation varies in different gaze positions. Trauma, congenital, and inflammatory causes must be ruled out.
- Nystagmus, the rhythmic oscillation of the eyes, can be a benign congenital problem; however, newly developing nystagmus in later childhood can be associated with neoplastic or toxic causations. Drugs, alcohol, and toxins should be suspected in any teenager with new nystagmus.
- Direct trauma to the extraocular muscles can result in acute strabismus. Various mechanisms can cause different patterns of strabismus. Surgical repair may be needed.

❓ Review Questions

1. A 1-year old presents with a new-onset rapidly beating nystagmus which resembles a flag ripping back and forth in a strong wind. What diagnosis is most likely?
   (a) Acute alcohol intoxication
   (b) Multiple sclerosis
   (c) Spasmus nutans, requiring MRI to rule out chiasmal tumor
   (d) Voluntary "party trick" nystagmus

2. A 3-month-old girl is brought to the ER by her concerned parents. She is observed to have a very large angle exotropia which is constantly present and

which appears to be the same measurement in all gaze positions. The most likely diagnosis and therapy is:

   (a) Intermittent exotropia – observe

   (b) Acute alcohol intoxication –send to rehab

   (c) Congenital esotropia – eye muscle exercises

   (d) Congenital exotropia – early strabismus repair

3. A 6-year-old girl presents to the ER with a sudden onset of a head turn to the right shoulder. Motility testing reveals failure of the left eye to fully move laterally past midline. There is no sign of trauma. The parents state that their daughter recently recovered from a severe viral upper respiratory illness. What is the most likely diagnosis and workup?

   (a) Third cranial nerve palsy – MRI scan.

   (b) Fourth cranial nerve palsy – MRI scan.

   (c) Post viral Sixth cranial nerve palsy – MRI scan and blood tests; observe for spontaneous improvement.

   (d) Traumatic laceration of the lateral rectus – repair in the OR.

✅ **Answer**

   1. (c)

   2. (d)

   3. (c)

References

1. Wilson ME, Saunders RA, Trivedi RH. Pediatric ophthalmology: current thought and a practical guide. Berlin: Springer; 2009.
2. Aldebasi Y. Prevalence of amblyopia in primary school children in Qassim province, Kingdom of Saudi Arabia. Middle East Afr J Ophthalmol. 2015;22(1):86–91.
3. Fu J, Li SM, Liu LR, Zhu BD, Yang Z, Li JL, et al. Prevalence of amblyopia and strabismus in a population of 7th-grade junior high school students in Central China: the Anyang Childhood Eye Study (ACES). Ophthalmic Epidemiol. 2014;21(3):197–203.
4. Ganekal S, Jhanji V, Liang Y, Dorairaj S. Prevalence and etiology of amblyopia in Southern India: results from screening of school children aged 5–15 years. Ophthalmic Epidemiol. 2013;20(4):228–31.
5. Oscar A, Cherninkova S, Haykin V, Aroyo A, Levi A, Marinov N, et al. Amblyopia screening in Bulgaria. J Pediatr Ophthalmol Strabismus. 2014;51(5):284–8.
6. Arnoldi K. Orthoptic evaluation and treatment. In: Wilson ME, Saunders RA, Trivedi RH, editors. Pediatric ophthalmology: current thought and a practical guide. Berlin, Heidelberg: Springer; 2009. p. 113–4.
7. Archer SM. Strabismus in infancy. Ophthalmology. 1989;96(1):133–7.
8. Ing M, Costenbader FD, Parks MM, Albert DG. Early surgery for congenital esotropia. Am J Ophthalmol. 1966;61(6):1419–27.
9. Ing MR. Early surgical alignment for congenital esotropia. Trans Am Ophthalmol Soc. 1981;79:625–63.
10. Wright KW, Edelman PM, McVey JH. High-grade stereo acuity after early surgery for congenital esotropia. Arch Ophthalmol. 1994;112(7):913–9.
11. Raab EL. Etiologic factors in accommodative esodeviation. Trans Am Ophthalmol Soc. 1982;80:657–94.
12. Wang FM, Chryssanthou G. Monocular eye closure in intermittent exotropia. Arch Ophthalmol. 1988;106(7):941–2.
13. Beidner B, Marcus M, David R. Congenital constant exotropia: surgical results in 6 patients. Binocular Vis Eye Muscle Surg. 1993;8:137–40.
14. Keane JR. Third nerve palsy: analysis of 1400 personally-examined inpatients. Can J Neurol Sci. 2010;37(5):662–70.
15. Ng YS, Lyons CJ. Oculomotor nerve palsy in childhood. Can J Ophthalmol. 2005;40(5):645–53.
16. Schumacher-Feero LA, Yoo K, Solari FM, Biglan AW. Third cranial nerve palsy in children. Am J Ophthalmol. 1999;128(2):216–21.
17. Harley RD. Paralytic strabismus in children. Etiologic incidence and management of the third, fourth, and sixth nerve palsies. Ophthalmology. 1980;87(1):24–43.
18. Dosunmu EO, Hatt SR, Leske DA, Hodge DO, Holmes JM. Incidence and etiology of presumed fourth cranial nerve palsy: a population-based study. Am J Ophthalmol. 2018;185:110–4.
19. Clark RA. Strabismus: sixth nerve palsy. Knights Templar Eye Foundation Pediatric Ophthalmology Education Center [Internet]. 2015 Oct 14. [cited 5 Sep 2019].
20. Dutton JJ, Fowler AM. Botulinum toxin in ophthalmology. Surv Ophthalmol. 2007;52(1):13–31.
21. Eggenberger ER. Supranuclear eye movement abnormalities. Continuum (Minneap Minn). 2014;20(pt 4 Neuro-ophthalmology):981–92.

22. Shallat RF, Pawl RP, Jerva MJ. Significance of upward gaze palsy (Parinaud's syndrome) in hydrocephalus due to shunt malfunction. J Neurosurg. 1973;38(6):717–21.

23. Muthukumar N, Veerarajkumar N, Madeswaran K. Bilateral Internuclear Ophthalmoplegia following mild head injury. Childs Nerv Syst. 2001;17(6):366–9.

24. Smith JW, Cogan DG. Internuclear ophthalmoplegia; a review of fifty-eight cases. AMA Arch Ophthalmol. 1959;61(5):687–94.

25. Donahue SP, Lavin PJ, Hamed LM. Tonic ocular tilt reaction simulating a superior oblique palsy. Arch Ophthalmol. 1999;117(3):347–52.

26. Nash DL, Diehl NN, Mohney BG. Incidence and types of pediatric nystagmus. J AAPOS. 2016;182: 31–4.

27. Gottlob I, Wizov S, Reinecke R. Spasmus nutans. A long-term follow-up. Invest Ophthalmol Vis Sci. 1995;36(13):2768–71.

28. Leigh RJ, Ramat S. Neuropharmacologic aspects of the ocular motor system and the treatment of abnormal eye movements. Curr Opin Neurol. 1999;12(1):21–7.

29. Bartlett JD, Jaanus SD. Ocular adverse drug reactions to systemic medications. In: Fiscella RG, Holdeman NR, Prokopich CL, editors. Clinical ocular pharmacology. St. Louis: Butterworth-Heinemann; 2007. p. 701–60.

30. Molinari AD. Strabismus following extraocular muscle trauma. Ophthalmology [Internet]. 2018 Jun 18. [cited 1 Sep 2019]. Available from: https://www.aao.org/disease-review/strabismus-following-extraocular-muscle-trauma.

31. Ludwig IH, Brown MS. Strabismus due to flap tear of a rectus muscle. Trans Am Ophthalmol Soc. 2001;99:53–63.

32. Jordan DR, Allen LH, White J, Harvey J, Pashby R, Esmaeli B. Intervention within days for some orbital floor fractures. Ophthalmic Plast Reconstr Surg. 1998;14(6):379–90.

33. Krarup J, De Decker W. Kompendium der direkten Augenmuskelverletzungen. Klin Monatsbl Anhilkd. 1982;181(12):437–43.

34. Kanonidou E. Amblyopia: a mini review of the literature. Int Ophthalmol. 2011;31(3):249–56.

Imaging the Pediatric Patient

Aslan Efendizade, Suraj Patel, Zerwa Farooq, and Vinodkumar Velayudhan

Contents

© Springer Nature Switzerland AG 2021
R. Shinder (ed.), *Pediatric Ophthalmology in the Emergency Room*,
https://doi.org/10.1007/978-3-030-49950-1_3

3.1 Introduction

Orbital anatomy is complex. In the setting of ophthalmic emergencies, the ideal imaging modality is one that can provide a fast and high-resolution view of orbital anatomy without the risk of exacerbating an acute pathology. By understanding the advantages and disadvantages of the different imaging techniques that are available, one can choose the best examination for each clinical scenario. The main options for imaging in the emergent setting are digital radiography (DR), ultrasound (US), computed tomography (CT), and magnetic resonance imaging (MRI).

3.2 Digital Radiography

DR (plain-film) evaluation represents the most basic of tests in radiology. DR is widely available and has a lower radiation dose when compared to CT. However, plain films no longer play a significant role in evaluating the central nervous system and orbits as their sensitivity is extremely limited compared to MRI and CT. The sensitivity of DR is relatively low for detection of orbital fractures, ranging from 64% to 78% in some series [1]. Importantly, the orbital soft tissues (e.g., the globes, extraocular muscles, and optic nerves) are not visualized on plain radiographs. Orbital foreign bodies are also not optimally detected by DR, with one recent study reporting an overall sensitivity of only approximately 72% in detecting metallic foreign bodies of varying sizes [2]. For these reasons, CT has largely supplanted DR for evaluating the orbits in the acute setting.

3.3 Ultrasound

Ultrasound (US) has long been utilized by ophthalmologists and has emerged as a rapid bedside screening tool in the ED for evaluating intraocular pathology. In a study in 2002 by Blaivas et al. evaluating the diagnostic performance of US compared to the gold standard of CT in patients presenting to the ED

with acute visual changes or ocular trauma, 60 out of 61 patients had sonographic findings that were confirmed on CT [3]. US provides excellent soft tissue contrast resolution, particularly around fluid-filled spaces [4, 5]. Since the anterior and posterior segments are largely composed of fluid, the globe provides an excellent medium for transmission of sound waves and is thus amenable to producing high-quality images of the eye.

US uses sound waves for creation of an image instead of ionizing radiation, making it particularly useful for the pediatric population, where exposure to radiation is always a concern. In addition, US is noninvasive, widely available, fast, and allows for dynamic imaging in real time. However, US is largely operator dependent and thus is limited in its reproducibility. Other limitations of ultrasound imaging include limited spatial resolution (relatively small field of view), poor evaluation of osseous structures, and inability to evaluate adjacent structures outside the bony confines of the orbit as the sound waves are blocked by the bones.

> Ultrasound evaluation is contraindicated in cases of suspected globe rupture or recent surgery, as pressure applied to the globe during the exam can lead to extrusion of intraocular contents [6].

US evaluation of the eye, like other superficial structures, utilizes high-frequency (7–10 MHz) linear probes. Ultrasound gel is applied to the eyelids while the eye is closed. The probe is then placed in close contact with the eyelid overlying the gel [3, 7]. Starting the exam with the normal eye will give a better idea of the expected anatomy and will highlight abnormalities in the symptomatic eye. US of the eye in the ED is typically performed using the B-scan, which produces grayscale cross-sectional images. The eye should be scanned in at least two planes, usually axial, sagittal, and oblique orientations. Compression will limit visualization of the anterior chamber and is thus avoided for anterior chamber evaluation.

US has shown great value in diagnosing emergent conditions of the eye, such as retinal detachment, lens dislocation and subluxation, endophthalmitis, and intraocular and retrobulbar hemorrhage with high accuracy in the emergency setting [3]. It is critical to distinguish between these entities as their relative urgency, treatment, and prognosis differ considerably. US is also very helpful and accurate in the evaluation of an orbital foreign body (when globe rupture is not expected) and is especially useful in identifying non-radiopaque foreign bodies that can be missed on DR and CT, such as wood. US becomes particularly relevant in conditions such as dense cataract, hyphema, or vitreous hemorrhage, where fundoscopic examination is limited or impossible. Lastly, sonography avoids the need for pupillary dilatation and sedation in pediatric patients.

The use of spectral and color Doppler imaging can determine blood flow to a lesion [6–8] and may be useful in identifying an orbital varix, arteriovenous fistula, or flow in other vascular and venolymphatic malformations. While US produces no radiation, Doppler imaging is believed to expose the patient to greater mechanical and thermal energy than routine grayscale B-scan images. As such, power and pulsed Doppler scanning duration should be limited to only what is necessary for diagnosis [9].

3.4 Computed Tomography

CT is the preferred initial imaging modality to evaluate the orbits for trauma, infection, and most other acute pathology. It is widely accessible, fast (usually not requiring sedation), cost-effective and easily detects fractures, calcifications, and most foreign bodies [10–12].

While less sensitive than MRI, CT still offers exquisite soft tissue detail and can accurately diagnose soft tissue injuries, including extraocular muscle entrapment and retrobulbar hemorrhage, assess the integrity of the globe and its contents, and evaluate for proptosis and orbital compartment syndrome [10–15]. Additionally, CT does not require the special positioning needed for radiographs and can evaluate the entire patient in one sitting, an important advantage in complex trauma and other pathology requiring imaging of different parts of the body. While there are many advantages, CT comes at the cost of exposing the patient to ionizing radiation.

3.4.1 Image Acquisition

CT technology has significantly evolved over time with each newer generation of scanners designed to reduce scan time and increase image quality. Images are generated by rapid rotation of an x-ray tube around the patient while delivering ionizing radiation in slices that are measured by an array of detectors that surrounds the body part being scanned. The amount of radiation that passes through the tissue and into the detectors varies depending on its density. The data acquired by the detectors is then converted into grayscale units and reconstructed into images. On CT, density (attenuation, or ability to absorb x-rays) is measured in Hounsfield units (HU), with air having the lowest HU value (and seen as darkest), followed by fat, water, soft tissue, bone, and finally metal having the highest HU value and brightness.

Multidetector CT (MDCT) scanners can produce multiple slices per rotation with most current scanners in the 16–256-slice range. Once a volume of tissue has been scanned using thin-section images, they can be reconstructed into any plane and into soft tissue and bone algorithm images. 256-, 128-, and 64-slice MDCT scanners can image the entirety of the orbits in one rotation, depending on patient size and selected slice thickness. This is particularly advantageous for children as it allows for rapid imaging with shorter scan times, which results in reduced opportunity for motion artifact, less need to repeat scans (resulting in lower radiation dose), and better image quality.

3.4.2 CT Contrast

Intravenous contrast significantly aids in delineating vascular lesions, inflammation, infections, and masses and should be administered whenever possible to evaluate for these diseases [13, 16]. CT contrast contains iodine with varying osmolality and viscosity. Only nonionic iso-osmolar or hypo-osmolar contrast should be used as they are safer. CT contrast dose is determined by the patient's weight (typically 2.0 mL/kg up to 100 mL) and can easily be calculated before the scan. Because younger pediatric patients often have IV access via small-gauge angiocatheters (e.g., 24 gauge), in tenuous locations, such as the hand or foot, it is important to use a lower injection rate and pressure (e.g., 1.5 mL/sec and 150 psi) or even hand inject contrast in those situations to prevent catheter failure or vascular injury [17].

Because iodinated contrast is excreted by the kidneys, all patients with risk factors such as preexisting renal dysfunction, proteinuria, and hypertension should be screened to identify impaired renal function as a predisposing factor for contrast induced nephropathy [17]. Allergic and other adverse reactions to contrast are exceedingly rare in children, particularly in younger children. However, infants and younger children should still be closely monitored after receiving IV contrast as they may not be able to verbalize symptoms of an adverse reaction.

3.4.3 Radiation Safety and Dose Reduction Techniques

Radiation exposure should always be a consideration when imaging pediatric patients, who have a greater likelihood of developing radiation-associated diseases, including cataracts and malignancy. This is due to different factors, including having more actively proliferative tissues, a different distribution of tissue compared to adults (e.g., more active, cellular red marrow compared to fatty marrow in adults), and a longer life expectancy over which to develop cancer. This is especially significant in younger children, with the estimated lifetime cancer risk for a 1-year old child from a single head CT estimated at 0.07% [18]. Although fast, widely accessible, and convenient, CT has been found to account for approximately two thirds of the collective medical radiation dose [19]. This has continued to increase over the past two decades due to greater utilization of CT, particularly in the emergent setting. As such, there has been increased regulation and public awareness of the risks of radiation exposure in recent years with campaigns to "image gently" in children and "image wisely" in adults in order to follow the principle of keeping radiation exposure "as low as reasonably achievable" (the ALARA principle) [20]. While dose reduction techniques can reduce image resolution and may not be suitable in all situations (e.g., a head CT to evaluate for early brain parenchymal changes in acute ischemia), low-dose CT has been shown to produce more than adequate images when evaluating the orbits and facial bones for fractures and soft tissue changes due to inflammation [21, 22].

The goal of an orbital CT protocol is a balance of good image quality with minimized radiation exposure. ◻ Table 3.1 lists specific guidelines to limit CT radiation dose in pediatric patients. The voltage (kilovolt peak, kVp) and tube current (milliamperes, mA) are major determinants of the amount of energy and radiation the patient is exposed to. Modification of the scanning mode, kVp, mA, exposure time, pitch (ratio of table movement per rotation/beam thickness), slice thickness, and reconstruction algorithms all allow reduction of radiation dose while maintaining image quality. While these parameters vary between institutions, it is imperative to optimize them in an effort to keep radiation doses as low as possible. Orbital CT images are obtained from the level of the frontal sinuses to the hard palate with a field of view extending from the orbital soft tissues anteriorly through the cavernous sinuses. Parameters are typically set to 120 kVp, 100 mAs, 0.625–1.25 mm slice thickness with 1.25 mm intervals, and a pitch of roughly 1 [14, 15]. Using a low-dose CT protocol with lower kVp and mAs (e.g., 80 kVp and 20 mAs or less) can

◻ Table 3.1 Guidelines to limit radiation dose for pediatric CT
1. Only perform CT if it will affect management and consider alternatives
Can evaluation be performed without radiation using US or MRI or with less radiation using DR?
2. Properly prepare the patient
Take measures to limit anxiety and pain
Involve parents and staff members experienced with interacting with children
Place IV lines well in advance of scanning, if possible
Consider sedation, if necessary
3. Optimize scan parameters and protocol to reduce radiation dose
Pediatric patients are typically smaller and require less radiation for the same scan as an adult
Decrease tube current (mAs) and voltage (kVp) accordingly
Limit size of scout view and tighten field of view of CT scan to area of interest
Use the maximal slice thickness appropriate for obtaining a specific diagnosis
Scan with pitch >1 to avoid redundant radiation
4. Precontrast images rarely provide additional information to postcontrast scans and should be avoided
5. Use shielding (e.g., lens, thyroid, breast, and gonadal shields) to reduce dose to radiosensitive organs
6. Use dose modulating software (automatic exposure and voltage control) and consider using iterative reconstruction algorithms

significantly lower the effective dose to the patient, with one study demonstrating that low-dose sinus CT in children can have similar effective dose as two radiographic views of the paranasal sinuses [22]. Modern MDCT scanners also have automatic exposure and voltage control systems (AEC and AVC, respectively) that modulate tube current and voltage (mAs and kVp, respectively) based on patient size

and other parameters to substantially decrease radiation dose. In addition, using a processing technique known as iterative reconstruction can reduce artifacts from hardware and foreign bodies and minimize radiation exposure while preserving and sometimes improving image quality [23]. Lastly, with the lens being the most radiation sensitive part of the body, special lens protection devices worn similar to eyeglasses can decrease the effective radiation dose to the eyes by approximately 50% [21]. Thus, by adjusting scan parameters, using dose modulating software, and shielding of the lens and other radiosensitive organs, high-quality images can be obtained while minimizing radiation exposure.

Modern CT scanners automatically record the CT dose for each study, and these values are often included with the images sent for clinical review (◻ Fig. 3.1). Standard parameters used to describe CT radiation dose include the volume computed tomography dose index (CTDI-vol) and the dose length product (DLP). CTDI (expressed in milligrays, mGy) is an estimate of the average x-ray tube output from an acquired set of CT images. DLP (expressed in milligray-centimeters, mGy-cm) is an estimate of the total x-ray tube output for an entire scan and is obtained by multiplying the CTDI-vol by the length of the patient that was scanned. DLP closely parallels the effective dose, the best parameter to estimate the biological impact of radiation, and should be closely monitored by physicians and technologists [24].

3.4.4 Specific Indications for CT in the Emergent Setting

3.4.4.1 Trauma

Thin-section non-contrast CT is the best initial imaging modality for trauma. CT can easily detect fractures of the orbit and skull base, characterize displaced fracture fragments, and evaluate involvement of the skull base and orbital apex foramina, including the optic canals (◻ Fig. 3.2). CT detects radiopaque foreign bodies with a high degree of sensitivity and is the best modality to exclude metallic foreign bodies [2, 25]. CT can also determine

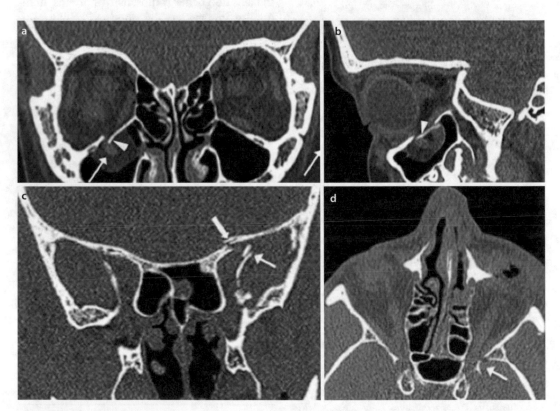

Exam Description: Orbits CT- w/Contrast

			Dose Report		
Series	Type	Scan Range (mm)	CTDIvol (mGy)	DLP (mGy-cm)	Phantom cm
1	Scout	-	-	-	-
2	Helical	153.000-11.125	4.21	29.17	Head 16
			Total Exam DLP:	29.17	

Fig. 3.1 Orbit CT dose report. Standard parameters used to describe CT radiation dose include the volume computed tomography dose index (CTDI-vol) and the dose length product (DLP). The DLP estimates the total x-ray tube output for the entire scan and most closely parallels the effective dose, the best parameter to estimate the biological impact of radiation

Fig. 3.2 Trapdoor (**a** coronal, **b** sagittal) and orbital apex (**c** coronal, **d** axial) fractures. CT clearly demonstrates a minimally depressed right orbital floor fracture (arrowhead, **a** and **b**) and herniation of the inferior rectus muscle through the defect with entrapment (arrow, **a**). CT clearly depicts a fracture through the left orbital apex with fragments impinging upon the superior orbital fissure (arrows, **c** and **d**)

if there is evidence of entrapment and orbital hemorrhage and aid in predicting the development of enophthalmos based on the degree and pattern of bony fracture involvement [10, 26] (**Figs. 3.2 and 3.3). Three-dimensional reconstructions are also useful for characterizing fractures for surgical planning [26] (**Fig. 3.3c). When the mechanism of injury is severe or if fractures with a high risk of concomitant intracranial injuries are present (e.g., orbital roof fractures), a non-contrast head CT should also be obtained [27].

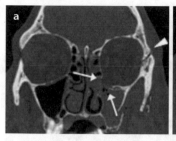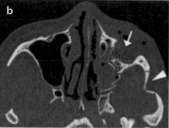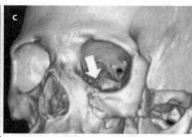

Fig. 3.3 Characterization of zygomaticomaxillary complex (ZMC) fracture. Coronal **a**, axial **b**, and 3-D reconstruction CT **c** demonstrate a ZMC fracture, including depressed fractures of the left orbital floor and inferior orbital rim (arrows), lateral orbital wall and rim (arrowhead, **a**), and the left zygomatic arch (arrowhead, **b**). Severely displaced left maxillary sinus lateral and anterior wall fractures are also seen

3.4.4.2 Orbital Infection and Inflammatory Diseases

In patients with suspected orbital cellulitis, contrast-enhanced CT is usually the initial imaging modality performed to confirm the diagnosis, delineate the pattern and degree of paranasal sinus disease, and screen for complications that may require surgery, such as orbital and subperiosteal abscess. Vascular complications of orbital and sinus infection, such as cavernous sinus and superior ophthalmic vein thrombosis, can also be assessed with CT utilizing intravenous contrast. Images should be carefully evaluated with the Chandler criteria in mind when evaluating for orbital complications of sinusitis [28] (▪ Table 3.2, ▪ Figs. 3.4 and 3.5).

> Non-contrast CT images almost never contribute any additional information to post-contrast images in the setting of acute nontraumatic orbital inflammation and should be avoided to prevent unnecessary radiation [27]. Alternatively, if iodinated contrast cannot be administered, non-contrast CT will still provide valuable information about post-septal infection and sinus disease.

MRI may be complimentary to CT and should be considered if more detailed assessment of orbital or intracranial involvement of infection is clinically warranted [27].

Contrast-enhanced CT can also aid in the diagnosis of inflammatory diseases that can mimic infection, such as idiopathic orbital

▪ Table 3.2 Chandler classification

Group I: Preseptal (periorbital) cellulitis

Group II: Orbital cellulitis

Group III: Subperiosteal abscess

Group IV: Orbital abscess

Group V: Cavernous sinus thrombosis

The Chandler classification system of orbital complications of sinusitis divides complications by subsite. This classification does not represent progression of disease as each category can have different causes and occur independently.

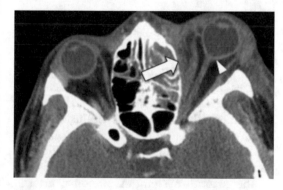

▪ Fig. 3.4 Orbital compartment syndrome. Axial CT demonstrates left ethmoid sinusitis with extension through the medial orbital wall causing an orbital cellulitis adjacent to the left lamina papyracea (arrow), left proptosis, and tenting of the posterior globe margin (arrowhead) consistent with orbital compartment syndrome

inflammatory syndrome (IOIS), IgG4-related orbital disease, and other inflammatory and granulomatous disease entities. Lastly, the

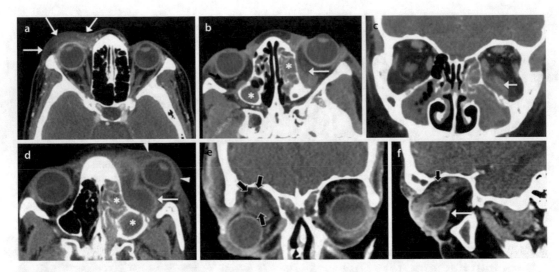

◘ Fig. 3.5 Orbital infections (Chandler groups I–IV). **a** Contrast-enhanced axial CT (CECT) demonstrates preseptal cellulitis with marked inflammatory change involving the eyelid and preseptal tissues. The postseptal tissues are spared **b**. Axial CT in a patient with ethmoid and sphenoid sinusitis (asterisks) demonstrating extensive infiltration of the left retrobulbar fat adjacent to the lamina papyracea consistent with orbital cellulitis. (**c** Coronal, **d** Axial) CECT demonstrates extensive left ethmoid (asterisk), maxillary, and sphenoid (asterisk) sinusitis and large rim enhancing fluid collection adjacent to lamina papyracea consistent with subperiosteal abscess causing globe compression (arrow). Left preseptal cellulitis is also noted (arrowheads). (**e** Coronal, **f** sagittal) CECT shows large orbital abscess (black arrows) causing hypoglobus with a clear fat plane separating it from adjacent bone superiorly. Marked tenting of the posterior globe (white arrow) consistent with orbital compartment syndrome

optic nerves are poorly evaluated with CT; if there is strong clinical concern for optic neuritis and demyelinating disease, contrast-enhanced MRI remains the gold standard [27].

3.4.4.3 Vascular Lesions

CT angiography (CTA) may be indicated in cases where vascular abnormalities and/or injuries are suspected, such as aneurysm, carotid-cavernous fistulas (CCF), dissection, or intracranial large vessel occlusion. CTA involves administration of a bolus of iodinated contrast through a large-gauge IV catheter with images acquired while contrast is still in the arterial system. A standard arterial delay time or bolus tracking software can be used to determine the optimal time to begin image acquisition after contrast injection.

CTA has been shown to reliably detect aneurysms 3 mm or larger with a sensitivity approaching the gold standard of catheter angiography [29] and has been shown to be as useful as angiography for detecting CCF [27, 30]. CTA also depicts the relationship of aneurysms to bony structures (such as the anterior clinoid process) much better than MRA but is less sensitive for cavernous and petrous internal carotid artery aneurysms. Lastly, CTA can depict intracranial large vessel occlusions and stenosis of greater than 50% with virtually 100% sensitivity [31].

While cerebral venous structures are often visualized on CTA, dedicated CT venography (CTV) using delayed images gives the best depiction of the cerebral venous system, superior ophthalmic veins, and, specifically, the cavernous sinuses. CTV can detect cerebral venous and cavernous sinus thrombosis with approximately 95% sensitivity, though contrast-enhanced MRV and MRI are felt to be slightly superior (◘ Fig. 3.6) [32–34].

In general, CTA and CTV provide excellent images of the intracranial and orbital vasculature. However, both have a relatively high radiation dose and provide poorer images when dose reduction techniques are employed. Further, CTA and CTV always require administration of contrast, while MRA and MRV can be performed without contrast, though at

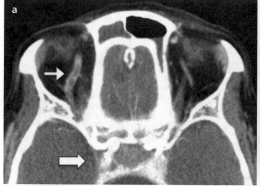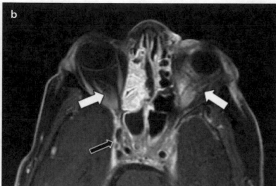

Fig. 3.6 Cavernous sinus and superior ophthalmic vein thrombosis (Chandler Group V). **a** Axial CECT demonstrates lack of enhancement of the right cavernous sinus (wide arrow) with an enlarged, thrombosed right superior ophthalmic vein (SOV) containing filling defects (narrow arrow). Note normal appearing left SOV. **b** Axial T1 MRI with contrast demonstrates ethmoid and sphenoid sinusitis with filling defects (black arrow) due to thrombosis of the right cavernous sinus and bilateral retrobulbar enhancement due to orbital cellulitis (white arrows)

the cost of reduced accuracy. Aside from the setting of acute trauma and when clinically feasible, MRI, MRA, and MRV should be considered prior to performing CT in pediatric patients, even if sedation is required.

3.5 Magnetic Resonance Imaging

MRI provides the best visualization of the orbital soft tissues. MRI is performed using powerful magnetic fields to manipulate hydrogen protons in the patient. When the protons return to their resting state, they emit energy that can be measured and reconstructed into images for diagnostic information. Unlike CT, MRI involves no ionizing radiation, which is a major benefit in the pediatric population.

Despite these major advantages, MRI has several limitations, including lack of widespread availability, long scan times, and the need for sedation in many pediatric patients, which requires MRI-compatible equipment.

MRI also lacks fine bony detail and is contraindicated in patients with ferromagnetic intraorbital foreign bodies (IOFB) and certain implanted medical devices. Screening must always be performed to ensure that no MR-incompatible devices or foreign bodies are present for patient safety. These limitations make it difficult to perform MRI in the emergent setting and make CT the first choice for trauma and other orbital emergencies.

However, CT and MRI are often complementary with MRI providing better ability to detect and characterize infectious and inflammatory orbital diseases and the best evaluation of the optic nerves, chiasm and tracts, cavernous sinuses, and brain [27]. MRI can also detect subtle traumatic ocular pathology not seen on CT [27]. Table 3.3 lists advantages and disadvantages of CT and MRI.

Strict screening must be performed prior to scanning to ensure no ferromagnetic foreign bodies or MR-incompatible implanted medical devices are present. Prior operative notes, information cards, and imaging must be reviewed to know the exact type of device and if it is MRI-compatible. Physical examination can also be performed to screen for scars from prior trauma or surgery, and, if necessary, plain films or CT can be obtained to screen for implanted devices, bullet fragments, and other metallic foreign bodies. Lastly, ferromagnetic detection devices are also available that can detect even extremely small ferromagnetic objects and differentiate between ferromagnetic and nonferromagnetic materials. These devices supplement, but do

Table 3.3 Comparison of advantages and disadvantages of computed tomography and magnetic resonance imaging

	CT	MRI
Advantages	1. Widely available 2. Rapid imaging with less possibility for motion and need for repeat scanning 3. No associated safety issues with ferromagnetic devices and foreign bodies 4. Imaging modality of choice for orbital trauma and foreign bodies 5. Excellent evaluation of bony destruction and calcification in soft tissue masses	1. No exposure to ionizing radiation 2. Excellent evaluation of orbital soft tissues 3. Best modality for imaging the entire optic nerve, sella, and parasellar regions 4. Most sensitive modality to exclude coexisting brain, posterior fossa, and spinal cord lesions 5. More accurate and sensitive than CT for intracranial and orbital collections and inflammation
Disadvantages	1. Ionizing radiation 2. Poor evaluation of fine detail of optic nerves 3. Limited evaluation of intracranial lesions (especially posterior fossa) 4. Poor evaluation of spinal cord	1. Ferromagnetic foreign bodies and certain implanted medical devices are contraindicated 2. Requires MRI compatible support and monitoring equipment in some patients 3. Long scan times and safety issues make MRI less feasible for emergencies 4. Many patients may need sedation

not replace a thorough MR safety screening process. Dental braces are not a contraindication to MRI but may result in significant image distortion, especially on fat saturated images. Table 3.4 lists important contraindications to MRI.

3.5.1 Sedation

Once contraindications are excluded, the most critical consideration when performing an MRI on a pediatric patient is if they will be able to cooperate for the study. This may prove difficult as orbital emergencies often present themselves in a child who is in pain and distress. High-quality MRI examinations require significantly greater time than CT. If a child is not able to lie still for a prolonged period of time and follow careful instructions, the MRI will be motion degraded and of either limited utility or nondiagnostic. Anesthesia may therefore be needed to ensure that the MRI is diagnostic and avoid having to repeat scanning.

The degree of sedation required may range from minimal sedation/anxiolysis to

Table 3.4 Contraindications to MRI

1. Metallic orbital foreign bodies, which can dislodge or heat up and injure the eye, optic nerve, and other orbital contents

2. MRI incompatible cardiac pacemakers and implanted cardiac defibrillators (AICD). Heating and torqueing of the device and changes to its electronic function, such as failure to pace may occur

Newer MRI compatible pacemakers and AICDs are available, but require monitoring before, after, and during the scan

3. MRI incompatible aneurysm clips, which may dislodge or heat

4. Cochlear, otologic, and ear implants

5. Metallic tension wire fixation for mandible fracture

6. Some external or implanted medication pumps and neurostimulator devices

7. Metallic bullet fragments and shrapnel are potential contraindications depending on location (e.g., in the eye or lung)

A thorough screening process is needed for ferromagnetic foreign bodies and MRI incompatible devices. Several important contraindications to MRI are listed here

general anesthesia, depending on the type of imaging study and patient specific factors. Moderate sedation is usually successful when performing MRI. However, general anesthesia has been reported to significantly improve the chances of obtaining a good-quality study in selected patients [35]. General anesthesia may be the best choice for MRI in patients who are neurologically impaired and have global developmental delay and severe disturbances in behavior and when the MRI is likely to be a long examination [35, 36]. Imaging with sedation is most successful when performed by a dedicated anesthesiology team [36].

Anesthesia is not without risks, and each patient must be evaluated prior to sedation to limit adverse events. Imaging with sedation that is unlikely to change management should be avoided [37]. In 2016, the FDA issued a communication stating that the use of anesthesia for longer than 3 hours or repeat use of anesthesia in pregnancy or children under the age of 3 years may affect brain development [38]. However, more recent data published in 2019 from a multicenter study indicates that brief general anesthesia administered to infants for approximately an hour is safe and does not affect IQ and neurocognitive development later in life [39]. When the clinical context demands the use of sedation for imaging purposes, it is recommended that physiologic monitoring must be performed during and after the procedure in all infants and children [37]. Monitoring devices must be MRI compatible and "flexible" enough to maintain their integrity and function in a narrow magnet bore.

■ ■ *Alternatives to Sedation*
When imaging neonates, alternatives to sedation are available. For example, neonates can be successfully scanned if they are fed, kept warm, and provided with a barrier to reduce the perceived noise level within the magnet (termed a "feed and wrap"). More recently, the development of neonatal incubators which are MR-compatible and packaged with radiofrequency coils has also reduced the need for sedation [40]. However, the success rate of these techniques begins to drop off

once patients reach the age of 2 months and develop increased awareness of their surroundings. Another technique for children aged 3–10 years involves the use of an audiovisual system during the exam to engage their attention [41, 42].

3.5.2 MRI Contrast

Gadolinium-based contrast agents (GBCA) can significantly improve visualization of certain disease entities, including neoplasms, inflammatory diseases, and infection. GBCA are considered extremely safe when administered at recommended doses based on weight. Adverse events and allergic reactions to gadolinium are exceedingly rare—far less common than iodinated contrast agents used for CT, recently reported to be <0.0002% [43]. Two major concerns regarding GBCA include nephrogenic systemic fibrosis (NSF, seen in patients with impaired renal function) and gadolinium deposition in deep brain structures [44]. Gadolinium is contraindicated in patients with acute, severe, and dialysis-dependent renal failure due to the risk of developing NSF, a disease where free gadolinium leads to deposits of collagen and scarring throughout the body [17, 45]. If risk factors are present, one should screen for reduced renal function by obtaining an estimated glomerular filtration rate (eGFR) prior to administering gadolinium [17, 45]. Gadolinium deposition in the brain is a more recently described phenomenon that occurs in patients who have had multiple exposures to GBCA [44]. Thus, it is important to limit the number of contrast-enhanced MRI examinations a patient undergoes to only those that are necessary for management.

3.5.3 Basic MR Imaging Sequences and Protocols

Physics of MR imaging can be quite confusing even for radiologists, but the pulse sequences that are used can be understood as follows:

3

- *T1-weighted images (T1WI)* result in high signal intensity from tissue with high fat content. The normal high signal orbital fat provides excellent intrinsic contrast that outlines the orbital soft tissues. Protein, melanin, methemoglobin (a subacute blood product), and gadolinium are other substances that also have bright signal on T1WI. Simple fluids, such as CSF and vitreous and aqueous humor, are dark on T1WI (▢ Fig. 3.7).
- *T2-weighting images (T2WI)* result in high signal originating from both simple fluid (such as water, CSF, and vitreous and aqueous humor) and areas of abnormal fluid (e.g., edema and collections).

- *Heavily T2WI* include what are known as steady-state free precession sequences (SSFP), such as fast imaging employing steady-state acquisition (FIESTA), constructive interference in steady state (CISS), and driven equilibrium (DRIVE) images. SSFP uses thin-section images that produce very bright CSF signal that allows one to trace the course of vessels and cranial nerves (which appear dark) in the cisterns intracranially and delineates the anatomy of the optic nerve sheath complex (▢ Fig. 3.8).
- *Fluid-attenuated inversion recovery (FLAIR)* is a technique that nulls the signal from "normal" fluid. It is normally used for brain imaging to suppress the signal from CSF

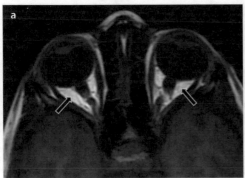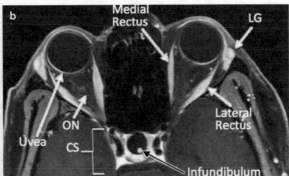

▢ **Fig. 3.7** Non-contrast axial T1-weighted MR image **a** demonstrates abundant, high-signal intraorbital fat (arrows). Note the dark signal of the aqueous and vitreous chambers of the globes. Post-contrast, fat-suppressed T1WI demonstrates normal enhancement of the uvea/choroid, lacrimal glands (LG), extraocular muscles, cavernous sinuses (CS), and other venous structures and the infundibulum **b**. (ON optic nerve)

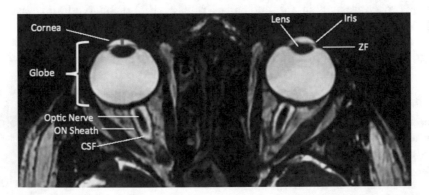

▢ **Fig. 3.8** Heavily T2-weighted MR images depicting normal anatomy. Axial FIESTA image demonstrates the globes with cornea projecting anteriorly. The lens is an ovoid anterior structure. Zonular fibers (ZF) extend lateral to the lens and attach to the ciliary body. The iris is visualized as a hypointense line anterior to the lens. The optic nerve is seen centrally with low signal surrounded by bright cerebrospinal fluid and low signal of the dura of the optic nerve sheath. The posterior segment includes the vitreous fluid behind the lens. The anterior segment contains aqueous fluid and is divided into anterior and posterior chambers by the iris. Anterior chamber depth (blue line) should be relatively symmetric and not exceed 2–3.5 mm

and make pathologic fluid outside the brain (such as hemorrhage or pus) and diseases within the brain parenchyma (such as edema and demyelination) more conspicuous (◼ Fig. 3.9).

– *Short-tau inversion recovery (STIR)* is a technique similar to T2WI in which fluid is bright and substances with similar MR characteristics to fat are suppressed. STIR is helpful when evaluating for infections, collections, and masses in the head and neck, optic nerve swelling in demyelination, and marrow edema.

– *Fat suppression* is a special technique used to remove the normal high signal from the fat within the orbit (◼ Fig. 3.7b). Fat normally has high signal on T1WI and also on T2WI performed using modern MR techniques. Post-contrast images should always be performed with fat suppression to remove the normal high T1 signal of fat and make enhancing lesions more conspicuous. Fat suppression should also be employed on T2WI of the orbits to make masses, collections, and edema more conspicuous.

– *Diffusion-weighted imaging (DWI)* is an important sequence that measures Brownian motion of water molecules. Pathologic processes that result in decreased free motion of water (termed *restricted diffusion*) result in bright signal on DWI and corresponding dark signal on an apparent diffusion coefficient (ADC) map. DWI is the most sensitive sequence for brain ischemia and can also show

restricted diffusion in abscesses, densely cellular tumors, and acute demyelination (◼ Fig. 3.10).

– *Gradient echo (GRE) and susceptibility weighted imaging (SWI)* are sequences used to detect hemorrhage and areas of mineralization in the brain, both of which typically appear dark. SWI is much more sensitive than the older GRE technique.

– Contrast-enhanced images are obtained with T1WI and fat suppression to reveal abnormal enhancement patterns due to inflammatory diseases and neoplasm. Venous structures, including the cavernous sinuses, may also show filling defects or absent enhancement due to thrombosis. The extraocular muscles, lacrimal glands, superior ophthalmic veins, and uvea/choroid all normally enhance and should not be confused for pathology, unless there is abnormal morphology (◼ Fig. 3.7b).

Typical MR imaging protocol of the orbits includes the following:

– Thin-section axial and coronal images of the orbits with 3 mm slice thickness or less

– A field of view including the periorbital soft tissues anteriorly through the cavernous sinuses posteriorly

– T1WI, STIR, or fat-suppressed T2WI, post-contrast T1WI with fat suppression, and SSFP (e.g., FIESTA) sequences

– Routine brain MR sequences, including DWI, FLAIR, T2WI, and pre- and post-contrast T1WI

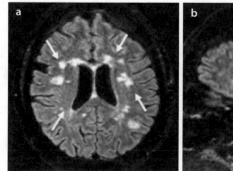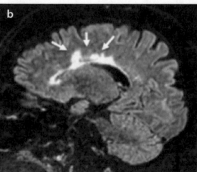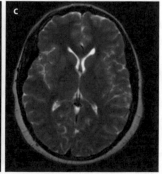

◼ **Fig. 3.9** Axial and sagittal FLAIR images demonstrate periventricular white matter lesions (arrows, **a**) extending toward the corpus callosum (arrows, **b**) in a patient with multiple sclerosis. Normal axial T2 for comparison, **c**

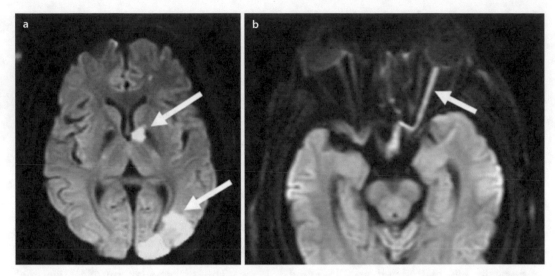

Fig. 3.10 Axial diffusion-weighted images demonstrate areas of restriction consistent with acute ischemic infarcts involving the left occipital lobe and left internal capsule (arrows, **a**) and infarction of the entire left optic nerve (arrow, **b**) in a patient with invasive fungal sinusitis and involvement of the left cavernous sinus and internal carotid artery

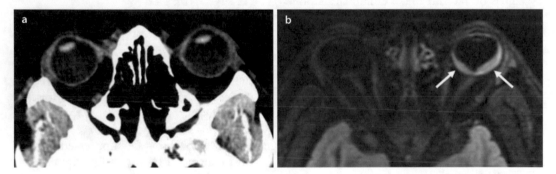

Fig. 3.11 Greater sensitivity of MRI for intraocular pathology. Axial CT **a** demonstrates subtle left intraocular pathologic finding. Axial FLAIR MRI image **b** more clearly demonstrates a left retinal detachment (arrows)

Additional sequences can be added depending on suspected pathology (see specific clinical scenarios below). For example, MR venography can be performed if there is concern for cerebral venous thrombosis, or MR angiography can be performed in the case of a suspected aneurysm resulting in third nerve palsy, vascular malformations, and arteriovenous fistulas or to detect large vessel occlusion in suspected stroke. Ultimately, the ideal series of sequences will be determined by careful discussion with the radiologist as it pertains to the clinical context.

3.5.4 Specific Indications

3.5.4.1 Trauma

CT is the first-line imaging modality for orbital trauma. MRI may have a complementary role to better depict optic nerve injury and avulsion and subtle abnormalities of the globe such as small retinal or choroidal detachments and intraocular hemorrhage (Fig. 3.11). Metallic IOFB must be excluded prior to MRI. Contrast is not needed to evaluate orbital trauma.

3.5.4.2 Orbital Inflammation and Infection

MRI of the orbits is complimentary to CT when evaluating orbital infection, including ocular infection (e.g., endophthalmitis), orbital cellulitis, and abscess. Both CT and MRI adequately demonstrate inflammatory changes, though CT offers better depiction of bony changes, while MRI has greater soft-tissue characterization [27]. Non-contrast images can demonstrate orbital inflammatory changes well, though contrast-enhanced images with fat suppression delineate abscesses much better. If there is additional concern for intracranial spread of infection, a contrast-enhanced brain MRI offers greater sensitivity than CT for meningitis, abscess, and empyema [17, 45]. DWI is also useful for demonstrating pus within the paranasal sinuses and orbits. Contrast-enhanced MRI and MRV are more accurate than CT for cavernous sinus and cerebral venous thrombosis.

3.5.4.3 Optic Neuritis

MRI is the best modality to evaluate demyelination in the CNS and diseases of the optic nerves in general. Optic neuritis is best visualized using fat-suppressed post-contrast T1WI and either STIR or fat-suppressed T2WI through the orbits. Optic neuritis is often seen as the initial manifestation in patients with multiple sclerosis but can also be secondary to neuromyelitis optica (NMO) spectrum disorders and infectious and inflammatory diseases.

MRI of the brain should be performed in conjunction with orbit MRI as optic neuritis has a high association with MS. Those with optic neuritis and concomitant brain lesions on MRI have a markedly increased likelihood of having MS. MRI of the spine can be performed if there is clinical suspicion of coexisting cord lesions or to screen for cord lesions that may help confirm the diagnosis of demyelination when the orbit and brain MRI are abnormal, but nonspecific. Demyelinating lesions in the brain are seen best on FLAIR images (◘ Fig. 3.9), while in the posterior fossa, T2WI often outperforms FLAIR. Spinal cord lesions are best seen on STIR and T2WI (◘ Fig. 3.12). Active areas of demyelination in the brain and spinal cord enhance on post-contrast T1WI and may demonstrate restricted diffusion on DWI.

3.5.4.4 Tumor

Contrast-enhanced MRI is the most accurate modality to evaluate the soft tissues within and around the orbits for masses, including the sellar and parasellar regions. In patients with monocular vision loss and concern for a mass involving the globe (such as retinoblastoma), a lesion intrinsic to the optic nerve (such as a glioma), or extrinsically compressing it (such as an optic nerve sheath meningioma), contrast-enhanced MRI of the orbits provides the best soft tissue evaluation.

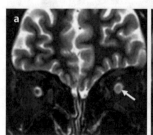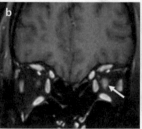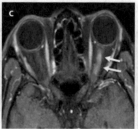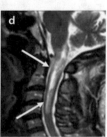

◘ **Fig. 3.12** Optic neuritis in a patient with neuromyelitis optica (NMO). Coronal **a** STIR and coronal **b** and axial **c** post-contrast T1WI MRI demonstrate high signal in the left optic nerve (arrow, **a**) and diffuse enhancement of the optic nerve sheath (arrows, **b** and **c**). **d** Sagittal T2WI MRI demonstrates a longitudinally extensive lesion involving the caudal brainstem and cervical cord (arrows)

In patients with junctional scotoma or bitemporal hemianopia, and suspected mass effect upon the optic chiasm, a contrast-enhanced brain MRI with thin-section images through the sella provides excellent assessment of the optic chiasm and its relationship to an underlying mass, such as a pituitary adenoma or craniopharyngioma. Patients with homonymous hemianopia or quadrantanopia are best evaluated with a contrast-enhanced brain MRI to evaluate for a post-chiasmatic lesion. CT is complementary to evaluate for calcifications in soft tissue masses (such as in optic nerve sheath meningioma, retinoblastoma, or craniopharyngioma).

3.5.4.5 Ischemia and Vascular Lesions

Acute homonymous vision loss with post-chiasmatic deficits may be secondary to ischemic and hemorrhagic stroke that are best evaluated with brain imaging. DWI is the gold standard to assess for acute brain ischemia. Acute parenchymal hemorrhage is easily seen on CT but can also be seen on MRI using GRE or SWI. Because homonymous vision loss is most likely post-chiasmatic, a dedicated orbit MRI is likely to be low yield [27].

MRA and CTA are both sensitive for excluding large vessel occlusions in cases of ischemic stroke. MRA and CTA are complementary and may both be used to evaluate for aneurysms, vascular malformations, and arteriovenous fistulas (◘ Fig. 3.13). Time-resolved CTA and contrast-enhanced MRA can be performed to evaluate for early venous filling in cases of arteriovenous malformations and fistulas. MRV is useful to evaluate patients with papilledema and those with hemorrhagic infarcts to exclude cerebral venous thrombosis and is best when performed with IV contrast.

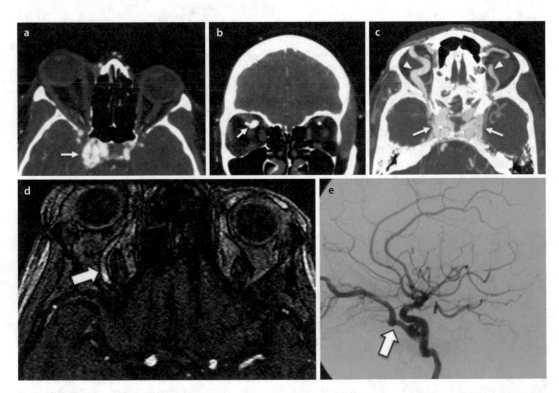

◘ **Fig. 3.13** Direct carotid cavernous fistula. Axial **a** and coronal **b** CTA images demonstrate an enlarged right cavernous sinus (arrow, **a**) with early venous enhancement and a dilated right SOV (arrow, **b**). **c** Axial MIP image demonstrates dilated CS bilaterally (arrows) with early enhancement and dilated SOVs bilaterally (arrowheads). **d** Axial MRA demonstrates abnormal flow in the right SOV (arrow). **e** Lateral view from a conventional angiogram demonstrates early filling of the cavernous sinus and a dilated SOV (arrow)

3.5.4.6 Ophthalmoplegia and Diplopia

The differential diagnosis of ophthalmoplegia and diplopia is broad and may be caused by pathology involving the globes (for diplopia), extraocular muscles, neuromuscular junction, and cranial nerves III, IV, and/or VI (including their courses in the subarachnoid space, cavernous sinuses, orbital apex, and orbits) and their nuclei and connecting tracts within the brainstem. These structures can be assessed using a contrast-enhanced orbit MRI and brain MRI with additional high-resolution T2WI through the posterior fossa to evaluate for skull base and brainstem lesions and thin-section SSFP sequences (e.g., FIESTA) through the cranial nerves to evaluate for primary lesions arising from or extrinsically compressing the cranial nerves.

The pattern of involvement, age, and acuity can aid in localization and predicting the lesion and best sequences:

- Acute intranuclear ophthalmoplegia may be due to demyelination in young patients or possibly ischemia that can be seen on brain MRI.
- Pupil-involving CN III palsy suggests extrinsic compression of the oculomotor nerve, for which an MRA may also be obtained to exclude an aneurysm.
- When multiple ipsilateral cranial nerve palsies are present involving cranial nerves III, IV, and VI, a lesion affecting the cavernous sinuses (such as thrombosis) or basal cisterns (such as meningitis, leptomeningeal carcinomatosis, and inflammatory diseases) may be best seen on post-contrast images.
- In the setting of trauma, CT can be performed to look for orbital fractures and skull base injuries that may affect cranial nerves.

❓ Review Questions

1. A 17-year-old male presents following trauma to the left orbit. The patient reports inability to move the left globe and monocular blindness, and clinical examination is concerning for an open globe injury. Which of the following is the next best step for imaging this patient?
   - (A) Obtain an MRI immediately to evaluate the ophthalmoplegia
   - (B) Immediately perform ultrasound of the globe to avoid radiation
   - (C) Screen the patient for contraindications for MRI
   - (D) Obtain an orbit CT

2. What sequence is the gold standard for detecting acute infarcts?
   - (A) Diffusion-weighted images (DWI)
   - (B) Fluid-attenuated inversion recovery (FLAIR)
   - (C) T2-weighted images
   - (D) Contrast-enhanced, fat-suppressed T1WI

3. Which of the following is true regarding cavernous sinus thrombosis?
   - (A) Non-contrast CT is sufficient for diagnosis
   - (B) Non-contrast MRI is sufficient for diagnosis
   - (C) Non-contrast MRV is sufficient for diagnosis
   - (D) CT or MRI with IV contrast is needed to confirm cavernous sinus thrombosis

✅ Answer

1. (D)
2. (A)
3. (D)

Key Points

1. Digital radiography has a very limited role in modern orbital imaging. CT is far more sensitive for bony and soft tissue abnormalities and foreign bodies.
2. US is a useful bedside tool for the evaluation of pathology of the globe with no radiation. However, US is contraindicated in patients with suspected open globe injury.
3. Non-contrast CT is the best initial examination for orbital trauma.

4. Contrast-enhanced CT and MRI are complementary in assessing orbital inflammation, infection, and masses, with CT often performed first in the emergent setting for practicality.

5. When possible, CT dose reduction techniques and shielding should be used to minimize radiation.

6. Contraindications to MRI (e.g., metallic IOFB and medical devices that are not safe for MRI) should be excluded before scanning.

7. Optic neuritis and vision loss related to lesions at the optic chiasm or post-chiasm (e.g., masses, ischemia, and demyelination) are best identified with MRI.

8. Homonymous vision loss is usually due to a post-chiasmatic lesion and typically only requires imaging of the brain.

9. CTA and MRA are useful for excluding aneurysms, vascular malformations, and AV fistulas. Time-resolved contrast-enhanced MRA and CTA have increased sensitivity in detecting vascular malformations and fistulas.

10. MRV is useful to exclude cerebral venous thrombosis in patients with papilledema and/or findings suspicious for venous infarcts on brain imaging and is more accurate with IV contrast. Cavernous sinus thrombosis cannot be excluded without IV contrast.

11. Sedation is usually needed in younger children to obtain a high-quality MRI and is best performed in conjunction with anesthesiology.

References

1. Iinuma T, Hirota Y, Ishio K. Orbital wall fractures. Conventional views and CT. Rhinology. 1994;32:81.
2. Momoniat HT, England A. An investigation into the accuracy of orbital X-rays, when using CR, in detecting ferromagnetic intraocular foreign bodies. Radiography. 2017. https://doi.org/10.1016/j.radi.2016.09.006.
3. Blaivas M, Theodoro D, Sierzenski PR. A study of bedside ocular ultrasonography in the emergency department. Acad Emerg Med. 2002. https://doi.org/10.1197/aemj.9.8.791.
4. Shung KK. High frequency ultrasonic imaging. J Med Ultrasound. 2009. https://doi.org/10.1016/S0929-6441(09)60012-6.
5. Byrne S, Green R. Ultrasound of the eye and orbit. 2nd ed. Philadelphia: Mosby; 2002.
6. Berrocal T, De Orbe A, Prieto C, Al-Assir I, Izquierdo C, Pastor I, Abelairas J. US and color doppler imaging of ocular and orbital disease in the pediatric age group. Radiographics. 1996. https://doi.org/10.1148/radiographics.16.2.8966285.
7. McNicholas MMJ, Brophy DP, Power WJ, Griffin JF. Ocular sonography. Am J Roentgenol. 1994. https://doi.org/10.2214/ajr.163.4.8092036.
8. Bedi DG, Gombos DS, Ng CS, Singh S. Sonography of the eye. Am J Roentgenol. 2006. https://doi.org/10.2214/AJR.04.1842.
9. Martin K. The acoustic safety of new ultrasound technologies. Ultrasound. 2010. https://doi.org/10.1258/ult.2010.010024.
10. Betts AM, O'Brien WT, Davies BW, Youssef OH. A systematic approach to CT evaluation of orbital trauma. Emerg Radiol. 2014;21:511–31.
11. Winegar BA, Gutierrez JE. Imaging of orbital trauma and emergent non-traumatic conditions. Neuroimaging Clin N Am. 2015. https://doi.org/10.1016/j.nic.2015.05.007.
12. Nguyen VD, Singh AK, Altmeyer WB, Tantiwongkosi B. Demystifying orbital emergencies: a pictorial review. Radiographics. 2017;37:947–62.
13. LeBedis CA, Sakai O. Nontraumatic orbital conditions: diagnosis with CT and MR imaging in the emergent setting. Radiographics. 2008. https://doi.org/10.1148/rg.286085515.
14. Kubal WS. Imaging of orbital trauma. Radiographics. 2008;28:1729–39.
15. Sung EK, Nadgir RN, Fujita A, Siegel C, Ghafouri RH, Traband A, Sakai O. Injuries of the globe: what can the radiologist offer? Radiographics. 2014. https://doi.org/10.1148/rg.343135120.
16. Nguyen M, Koshy JC, Hollier LH. Pearls of naso-orbitoethmoid trauma management. Semin Plast Surg. 2010;24:383–8.
17. Committee on Drugs and Contrast Media A. ACR Manual on Contrast Media, 10.3. American College of Radiology. 2017.
18. Brenner DJ, Elliston CD, Hall EJ, Berdon WE. Estimated risks of radiation-induced fatal cancer from pediatric CT. Am J Roentgenol. 2001. https://doi.org/10.2214/ajr.176.2.1760289.
19. Linton OW, Mettler FA. National conference on dose reduction in CT, with an emphasis on pediatric patients. Am J Roentgenol. 2003. https://doi.org/10.2214/ajr.181.2.1810321.
20. Goske MJ, Applegate KE, Bulas D, et al. Image gently 5 years later: what goals remain to be accomplished in radiation protection for children? Am J Roentgenol. 2012. https://doi.org/10.2214/AJR.12.9655.

21. Wang JW, Tang C, Pan BR. Data analysis of low dose multislice helical CT scan in orbital trauma. Int J Ophthalmol. 2012. https://doi.org/10.3980/j.issn.2222-3959.2012.03.22.

22. Mulkens TH, Broers C, Fieuws S, Termote JL, Bellnick P. Comparison of effective doses for low-dose MDCT and radiographic examination of sinuses in children. Am J Roentgenol. 2005. https://doi.org/10.2214/ajr.184.5.01841611.

23. Boudabbous S, Arditi D, Paulin E, Syrogiannopoulou A, Becker C, Montet X. Model-based iterative reconstruction (MBIR) for the reduction of metal artifacts on ct. Am J Roentgenol. 2015. https://doi.org/10.2214/AJR.14.13334.

24. Vock P. CT dose reduction in children. Eur Radiol. 2005. https://doi.org/10.1007/s00330-005-2856-0.

25. Saeed A, Cassidy L, Malone DE, Beatty S. Plain X-ray and computed tomography of the orbit in cases and suspected cases of intraocular foreign body. Eye. 2008. https://doi.org/10.1038/sj.eye.6702876.

26. Dreizin D, Nam AJ, Diaconu SC, Bernstein MP, Bodanapally UK, Munera F. Multidetector CT of midfacial fractures: classification systems, principles of reduction, and common complications. Radiographics. 2018;38:248–74.

27. Kennedy TA, Corey AS, Policeni B, et al. ACR appropriateness criteria ® orbits vision and visual loss. J Am Coll Radiol. 2018. https://doi.org/10.1016/j.jacr.2018.03.023.

28. Botting AM, McIntosh D, Mahadevan M. Paediatric pre- and post-septal peri-orbital infections are different diseases. A retrospective review of 262 cases. Int J Pediatr Otorhinolaryngol. 2008. https://doi.org/10.1016/j.ijporl.2007.11.013.

29. Hiratsuka Y, Miki H, Kiriyama I, Kikuchi K, Takahashi S, Matsubara I, Sadamoto K, Mochizuki T. Diagnosis of unruptured intracranial aneurysms: 3T MR angiography versus 64-channel multidetector row CT angiography. Magn Reson Med Sci. 2008. https://doi.org/10.2463/mrms.7.169.

30. Chen CCC, Chang PCT, Shy CG, Chen WS, Hung HC. CT angiography and MR angiography in the evaluation of carotid cavernous sinus fistula prior to embolization: a comparison of techniques. Am J Neuroradiol. 2005;26:2349.

31. Nguyen-Huynh MN, Wintermark M, English J, Lam J, Vittinghoff E, Smith WS, Johnston SC. How accurate is CT angiography in evaluating intracranial atherosclerotic disease? Stroke. 2008. https://doi.org/10.1161/STROKEAHA.107.502906.

32. Rodallec MH, Krainik A, Feydy A, Hélias A, Colombani J-M, Jullès M-C, Marteau V, Zins M. Cerebral venous thrombosis and multidetector CT angiography: tips and tricks. Radiographics. 2006;26 Suppl 1:S5–18; discussion S42–3.

33. Mahmoud M, Elbeblawy M. The role of multidetector CT venography in diagnosis of cerebral venous sinus thrombosis, 4th ed. Research J Med Med Sci. 2009;4:284.

34. Meckel S, Reisinger C, Bremerich J, Damm D, Wolbers M, Engelter S, Scheffler K, Wetzel SG. Cerebral venous thrombosis: diagnostic accuracy of combined, dynamic and static, contrast-enhanced 4D MR venography. Am J Neuroradiol. 2010. https://doi.org/10.3174/ajnr.A1869.

35. Malviya S, Voepel-Lewis T, Eldevik OP, Rockwell DT, Wong JH, Tait AR. Sedation and general anaesthesia in children undergoing MRI and CT: adverse events and outcomes. Br J Anaesth. 2000. https://doi.org/10.1093/oxfordjournals.bja.a013586.

36. Arlachov Y, Ganatra RH. Sedation/anaesthesia in paediatric radiology. Br J Radiol. 2012. https://doi.org/10.1259/bjr/28871143.

37. Coté CJ, Wilson S, Casamassimo P, Crumrine P, Gorman RL, Hegenbarth M, Koteras RJ. Guidelines for monitoring and management of pediatric patients during and after sedation for diagnostic and therapeutic procedures: an update. Pediatrics. 2006. https://doi.org/10.1542/peds.2006-2780.

38. Woodcock J. FDA drug safety communications. In: Cent. Drug Eval Res. 2018. www.fda.gov/drugs/drug-safety-and-availability/fda-drug-safety-communication-fda-review-results-new-warnings-about-using-general-anesthetics-and. Accessed 6 Dec 2019.

39. McCann ME, Berde C, Soriano S, et al. Neurodevelopmental outcome at 5 years of age after general anaesthesia or awake-regional anaesthesia in infancy (GAS): an international, multicentre, randomised, controlled equivalence trial. Lancet. 2019. https://doi.org/10.1016/S0140-6736(18)32485-1.

40. Blüml S, Friedlich P, Erberich S, Wood JC, Seri I, Nelson MD. MR imaging of newborns by using an MR-compatible incubator with integrated radiofrequency coils: initial experience. Radiology. 2004. https://doi.org/10.1148/radiol.2312030166.

41. Törnqvist E, Månsson Å, Hallström I. Children having magnetic resonance imaging. J Child Heal Care. 2015;19:359–69.

42. Harned RK, Strain JD. MRI-compatible audio/visual system: impact on pediatric sedation. Pediatr Radiol. 2001. https://doi.org/10.1007/s002470100426.

43. McDonald JS, Hunt CH, Kolbe AB, Schmitz JJ, Hartman RP, Maddox DE, Kallmes DF, McDonald RJ. Acute adverse events following gadolinium-based contrast agent administration: a single-center retrospective study of 281 945 injections. Radiology. 2019. https://doi.org/10.1148/radiol.2019182834.

44. Kanda T, Ishii K, Kawaguchi H, Kitajima K, Takenaka D. High signal intensity in the dentate nucleus and globus pallidus on unenhanced T1-weighted MR images: relationship with increasing cumulative dose of a gadolinium-based contrast material. Radiology. 2014. https://doi.org/10.1148/radiol.13131669.

45. Committee on Drugs and Contrast Media A. ACR Manual on Contrast Media, 10.3. Reston: American College of Radiology; 2017.

Ophthalmic Trauma

Contents

Orbital Trauma

Stella Y. Chung and Paul D. Langer

Contents

© Springer Nature Switzerland AG 2021
R. Shinder (ed.), *Pediatric Ophthalmology in the Emergency Room*,
https://doi.org/10.1007/978-3-030-49950-1_4

4.1 Introduction

Children who sustain midfacial trauma may suffer a variety of orbital complications that present to the emergency room for management; of these, orbital fractures are by the far the most common, sometimes requiring fairly urgent surgical intervention. Vision-threatening orbital hemorrhage as well as orbital foreign bodies may also result from periocular trauma, and, in many instances, these conditions may also require prompt management and sometimes surgical intervention.

4.2 Epidemiology

The periorbital area is the third most commonly involved region of all facial fractures, accounting for up to 45% of all facial fractures in children [1–7]. Motor vehicle collision, violence, and falls constitute the most common mechanisms of facial injury in the United States [8]. Orbital fractures occur more frequently in boys than in girls, with a ratio ranging from 1.1:1 to 8.5:1, although studies report that there is no gender difference in very young children [1, 2, 4, 6, 9–16].

Fractures of the orbital floor are relatively uncommon in children younger than 5 years old, since maxillary sinus pneumatization occurs primarily from 6 to 12 years of age, and the orbital floor is more susceptible to fractures when it overlies an aerated sinus [17–19]. Orbital floor fractures in small children therefore occur less frequently than fractures of the orbital roof, whereas the frequency of these injuries is reversed in older children and adults.

4.3 Assessment

Ophthalmic evaluation is often overlooked in the trauma setting [20, 21]. As occult ophthalmic injuries occur in approximately 20% of patients with blunt facial trauma [21], ophthalmology consultation must be sought in all cases of midfacial and/or orbital fractures to detect serious ocular injury. Visual acuity determination, ocular motility evaluation, pupillary function testing, slit lamp examination, and a dilated funduscopic examination should all be performed in the acute setting if possible and globe injury ruled out. In the presence of vision-threatening injuries, such as a ruptured globe or retinal detachment, orbital and periorbital repair should be delayed until the ocular pathology is managed and sufficient time is allowed for recovery [22]. Note that this approach may inevitably delay orbital surgery several weeks or more [22].

Signs and symptoms suggestive of an orbital floor fracture in children with a history of midface trauma include infraorbital anesthesia, limited and sometimes painful extraocular movements, enophthalmos, and subcutaneous emphysema. A common presentation of a so-called "trapdoor" orbital floor fracture (see below) is the oculocardiac reflex, which includes nausea and vomiting, bradycardia, and syncope upon attempted eye movement. These symptoms were shown to have a positive predictive value of 75% for a trapdoor fracture and 83.3% for the presence of inferior rectus herniation on imaging [23]. The presence of an oculocardiac reflex in the setting of an orbital floor fracture is an indication for immediate surgical repair [24–26]. Forced duction testing, in which the examiner grasps the eye and forcibly moves it to determine if restriction is present, is rarely if ever required in an awake patient with any type of orbital wall fracture. It is inadvisable to perform as part of the routine evaluation of orbital fractures, though it occasionally may be informative in unresponsive patients in an ICU setting [22].

Lateral orbital wall fractures are most commonly seen as part of a larger zygomaticomaxillary complex fracture. Patients with ZMC fractures may present with a flattened malar eminence, lateral canthal dystopia, and trismus in addition to signs and symptoms of other orbital wall fractures.

> — Common presentation of orbital floor fracture:
>   — Infraorbital anesthesia/hypoesthesia
>   — Limited and sometimes painful extraocular movements, diplopia
>   — Enophthalmos
>   — Subcutaneous emphysema
> — Signs and symptoms of trapdoor fracture:
>   — Nausea and vomiting
>   — Bradycardia or syncope associated with extraocular movements

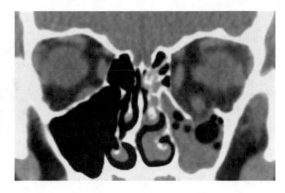

◘ Fig. 4.1 A. Classic coronal CT appearance of a left orbital blowout fracture where the fracture line runs over the infraorbital groove

4.4 Imaging

Computed tomography (CT) is the imaging gold standard for the detection of orbital fractures. A dedicated, thin cut (1.0–1.5 mm slices) orbital CT scan with coronal and sagittal reconstructions is recommended. Reconstruction of images (as opposed to direct coronal imaging) is preferred as it limits radiation exposure and avoids potential artifact caused by dental amalgam. If there are clinical signs of soft tissue entrapment suggesting an orbital fracture, such as diplopia or pain on eye movement, and no tissue herniation is seen on CT imaging (or if there is concern for radiation exposure), MRI may be considered, though its usefulness in the evaluation of midfacial fractures remains very limited [27]. While some past reports suggested using the size of an isolated orbital floor defect on imaging as a guide in determining surgical candidacy, the ability to precisely measure the size of such defects is suspect, and it is not possible to predict from imaging which patients will develop permanent clinical sequelae requiring surgery. It is advisable therefore to use clinical criteria alone when deciding if

repair of an orbital floor fracture should be undertaken [22, 28].

4.4.1 Orbital Floor Blowout Fractures

An indirect orbital floor fracture, also known as an orbital "blowout" fracture, is a fracture of the orbital floor in which the orbital rim remains intact. This type of fracture most commonly occurs above, or just medial to, the roof of the infraorbital groove, the thinnest bone of the orbit [29] (◘ Fig. 4.1). Blowout fractures may result in herniation of orbital tissue into the maxillary sinus, sometimes restricting the motility of the inferior rectus muscle, and can thus lead to clinically significant diplopia, especially in vertical gaze. Additionally, the increase in the orbital volume that results from a depressed fragment of the orbital floor can lead to cosmetically significant enophthalmos or hypoglobus (inferior displacement of the globe) (◘ Fig. 4.2). Either of these problems may be severe enough to warrant surgical repair. Children with orbital floor fractures are much more likely to require surgical repair than children with orbital roof fractures [20].

Trapdoor fractures are an anatomic subtype of orbital floor fracture seen almost

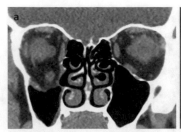
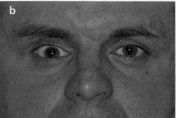
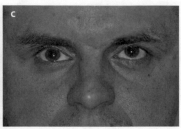

Fig. 4.2 **a** Coronal CT image demonstrating a very large right orbital blowout fracture with herniation of orbital tissue into the maxillary sinus, resulting in **b** enophthalmos, hypoglobus and **c** impaired upgaze of the right eye

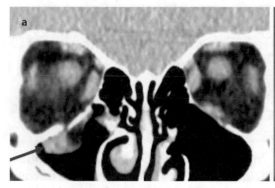
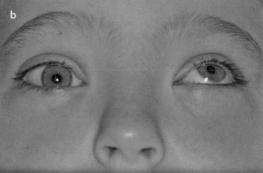

Fig. 4.3 **a** Coronal CT image demonstrating a right orbital "trapdoor" fracture in which the size of the orbital tissue herniating into the maxillary sinus is much smaller than the hole in the orbital floor. The inferior rectus muscle lies beneath the plane of the orbital floor (red arrow). **b** Marked restriction in upgaze results

exclusively in children. In these fractures, a segment of the orbital floor breaks, becomes transiently displaced inferiorly while hinged at the junction of the medial and inferior orbital walls, and then rebounds superiorly close to its original position [30]. During the transient, momentary period of bony displacement, orbital tissue may herniate into the maxillary sinus and become incarcerated when the bony fragment returns close to its original position with minimal displacement. In some cases, herniation and entrapment of a significant amount of soft tissue and muscle within the maxillary sinus may ensue despite a very small or even radiologically imperceptible fracture (□ Fig. 4.3). Trapdoor fractures are seen primarily in children because their bones are more elastic than in adults, which allows the attached bone fragment to open and recoil like a trapdoor [31], resulting in restrictive strabismus, pain on extraocular movement, and, if repair is not prompt, isch-

emia and early tissue necrosis [30]. Jordan et al. first coined these medially hinged trapdoor fractures "white-eyed blowout fractures" [32]. The term emphasizes the fact that these patients may frequently present with mild to no signs of periocular injury, such as periocular ecchymosis and edema, despite the presence of severe motility restriction.

4.4.2 Medial Wall Fractures

Medial orbital wall fractures can occur in isolation ("medial orbital wall blowout fracture"), in conjunction with other orbital fractures (most commonly the orbital floor), or can be a part of more extensive naso-orbito-ethmoid (NOE) fractures. Due to their proximity to the ethmoid sinus and nose, medial orbital fractures commonly cause orbital emphysema, which rarely can be severe enough to cause a compartment syndrome

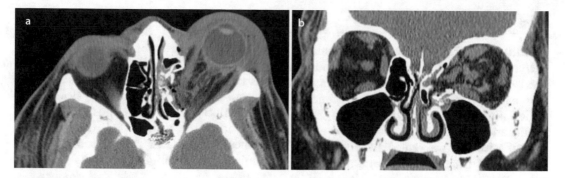

◼ **Fig. 4.4** **a** Axial and **b** coronal CT images of a left orbital medial wall fracture with herniation of the medial rectus muscle into the defect

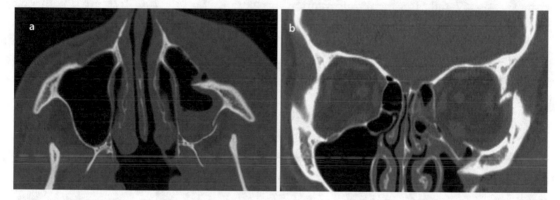

◼ **Fig. 4.5**   Left zygomaticomaxillary complex fracture with posterior and medial displacement of the malar eminence of the zygoma viewed on axial **a** and coronal **b** images

[33]. Patients with isolated medial orbital wall fractures may show limited abduction or adduction of the involved eye, diplopia on horizontal gazes, or even pseudo-Duane retraction syndrome (in which the eye recesses into the orbit on attempted abduction) [34] (◼ Fig. 4.4). Medial rectus muscle entrapment with an oculocardiac reflex as a result of a medial wall fracture is rare, but like its orbital floor counterpart (the trapdoor fracture), it requires emergent surgical repair [5, 35–41]. Most cases of isolated medial wall fractures can be managed conservatively without surgical intervention.

4.4.3 Lateral Orbital Wall Fractures

The lateral orbital wall is the strongest of the orbital walls. Lateral orbital wall fracture is rare in children and is typically associated with additional orbital wall and/or zygomaticomax-illary complex fractures [42, 43] (◼ Fig. 4.5). Entrapment of the lateral rectus muscle or enophthalmos is extremely uncommon [43, 44]. Inferiorly displaced zygomatic fractures can lead to a laterally downward slanting of the palpebral aperture (lateral canthal dystopia) since the lateral canthal tendon is attached to the zygoma [33]. Severe pediatric zygomatic fractures can cause complications such as globe dystopia, trismus, sensory deficits in the infraorbital nerve (V2) distribution, enophthalmos, and malar flattening [45]. Most cases of minimally displaced or nondisplaced lateral wall fractures can be managed conservatively without surgery [2, 7, 20, 44, 46–51]. In general, the decision as to whether or not a ZMC fracture should be repaired depends upon the clinical deficits produced by the fracture and not by the appearance of the fractures on imaging studies alone. Many displaced ZMC fractures without aesthetic or functional compromise can be observed without surgery.

4.4.4 Orbital Roof Fractures

Orbital roof fractures in younger children are commonly nondisplaced linear fractures [2, 4, 43, 52–55]. Orbital roof fractures are associated with a high incidence of neurologic injuries such as cerebral edema, hematoma, and herniation [2, 56]. Neurosurgical consultation is warranted in all cases of orbital roof fracture to rule out and manage any associated intracranial injury [53]. Superior orbital fissure syndrome or orbital apex syndrome may occur, but it is extremely rare [2, 49, 57–60]. Emergent intervention may be required for optic canal or optic nerve compression, orbital apex syndrome, or orbital compartment syndrome [61]. Coon et al. reported that linear orbital roof fractures smaller than 2 cm without a significant frontal bone injury are unlikely to develop encephalocele or globe malposition and recommended observation [56]. Overall, management of pediatric orbital roof fractures requires a multidisciplinary approach (◘ Fig. 4.6), though the vast majority is managed conservatively without surgery. From an ophthalmic standpoint, surgical repair of an orbital roof fracture is indicated

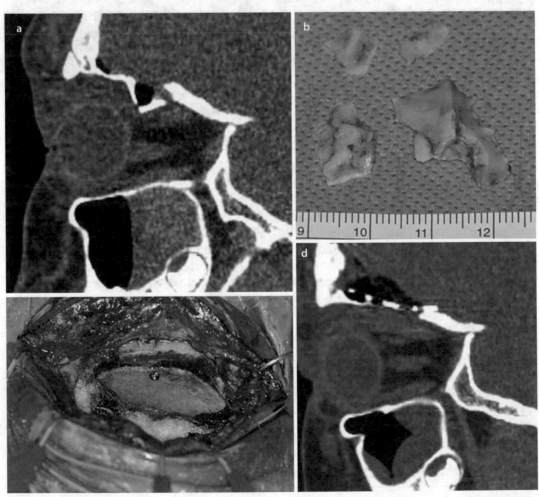

◘ **Fig. 4.6**   **a** Sagittal CT image of a right orbital roof fracture with bony fragments impinging on the superior rectus muscle, causing marked restriction of supraduction of the right eye; **b** Bony fragments removed from the superior orbit through a craniotomy approach; **c** A porous polyethylene implant is positioned through the craniotomy exposure to cover the orbital defect and screwed in place; **d** A sagittal postoperative CT image reveals the implant (visible due to titanium strips within it) covering the bony defect

only in the presence of cosmetically apparent globe displacement (hypoglobus from a depressed bony fragment) or clinically significant diplopia, which when present usually occurs on upgaze.

4.5 Indications and Timing of Surgery

In children with midfacial trauma, a high index of suspicion must be maintained for a trapdoor orbital floor fracture with an incarcerated inferior rectus muscle. Patients presenting with strong clinical signs of tight tissue incarceration, such as an oculocardiac reflex and/or severe limitation in upgaze should undergo surgical exploration and repair [23, 25, 27, 32, 35, 62–64]. Repair is indicated in these circumstances even if there is minimal radiographic evidence of a fracture. Repairing these fractures within 24–48 hours of presentation is strongly recommended and considered by most to be associated with better outcomes, such as improved motility [5, 25, 27, 32, 35, 39, 40, 63, 65]. In patients presenting with severe oculocardiac reflex and hemodynamic instability, early stabilization and repair would therefore seem ideal [2].

The indications and timing of surgical intervention for non-trapdoor orbital blowout fractures has long been a subject of controversy. Most of the current recommendations for management in the pediatric population are extrapolated from studies on adults. Orbital fractures, including large-sized defects, with minimal to no enophthalmos and without clinically significant diplopia, can be managed conservatively without adverse consequences [66]. Repair is only required to address either disfiguring enophthalmos or persistent diplopia.

Evaluation of extraocular movements at the time of presentation is important in determining which patients with orbital wall fractures will require repair. In patients with non-trapdoor fractures who exhibit normal extraocular movements on initial examination, diplopia will not develop, and if diplopia is present it will not worsen over time. Diplopia present on initial examination will improve significantly or resolve completely over the span of several weeks without any surgical repair in the majority of cases [67]. On the other hand, the degree of enophthalmos either remains the same or worsens over time as orbital swelling resolves over the subsequent weeks or months after the injury. The size of the orbital floor defect in children is only poorly associated with the subsequent amount of enophthalmos [68]. Commonly accepted indications for surgical repair of non-trapdoor orbital wall blowout fractures are non-resolving clinically significant diplopia and cosmetically unacceptable enophthalmos [25, 27, 32, 36]. An operative window of 2 weeks following the injury has often been reflexively advocated in the literature [5, 7, 35, 63, 69], but retrospective studies have shown that non-trapdoor fracture repair performed more than 2 weeks after injury produces results equivalent to surgery performed prior to 2 weeks [70, 71]. A conservative approach to the repair of orbital wall fractures is therefore appropriate [22]. Patients without severe motility restriction at presentation can be safely followed, on a weekly or biweekly basis, to monitor the resolution in diplopia as orbital edema resolves. Once the diplopia is ascertained to be no longer improving, the patient, parents, and surgeon can then determine if any residual double vision is clinically significant and if surgical correction is then warranted. A similar approach can be taken in the management of non-trapdoor fracture patients with respect to the development of enophthalmos, regardless of the size of the fracture defect. The injured child can be followed conservatively for several weeks and surgery only performed if noticeable enophthalmos is bothersome to the parents and patient. Early surgical repair of a large orbital floor fracture to prevent the development of enophthalmos should be discouraged, since the ultimate degree of enophthalmos cannot be reliably predicted from the CT images and unnecessary surgical intervention can thus be avoided [22].

To re-emphasize, "watchful waiting" in the treatment algorithm for repairing isolated

4

orbital wall fractures does not apply to patients with severe incarceration of tissue and marked limitation of ocular motility. In children with these trapdoor fractures, in which there is severe restriction of ocular movement and an oculocardiac reflex, urgent repair within 24–48 hours of diagnosis is strongly recommended. Non-trapdoor fractures can be followed conservatively to determine if cosmetically unacceptable enophthalmos develops, or if disabling diplopia does not resolve, over a several week period. Successful surgical outcomes can be obtained repairing non-trapdoor fractures many weeks after the injury, and many patients can avoid surgery altogether by delaying the surgery by several weeks.

4.6 Surgical Technique

The two most common surgical approaches to the orbital floor are the transconjunctival and the subciliary (transcutaneous) incisions. The transconjunctival approach avoids a cutaneous scar and is associated with a lower incidence of eyelid malposition [58, 59] and thus is the preferred approach by the great majority of experienced surgeons. Specifically, a subciliary incision results in a higher rate of cicatricial lower eyelid retraction [72, 73], the correction of which is frequently challenging. The transconjunctival approach yields excellent exposure even without an associated lateral canthotomy and cantholysis [26, 61, 74–76] (◻ Fig. 4.7). The surgeon should aim to (1) reposition all herniated tissue back into the orbit with the bony edges of the fracture visible for 360 ° after reduction and (2) place an implant to cover the defect, ensuring that the posterior aspect of the implant rests on the posterior bony ledge of the fracture (◻ Fig. 4.8). In trapdoor fractures especially, repositioning adhered herniated tissue may pose a challenge requiring aggressive lysis of adhesions and rarely necessitating enlarging the bony defect. Correct positioning of the implant is crucial. The most common reason a patient seeks secondary repair of a previously repaired orbital floor fracture is an improp-

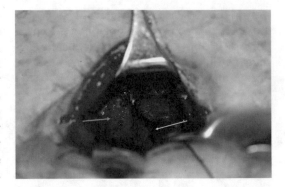

◻ **Fig. 4.7** Surgeon's view of a left orbital floor defect during surgical repair, demonstrating the excellent exposure provided by the inferior transconjunctival approach. The infraorbital neurovascular bundle (blue arrow) is visible just adjacent to the large hole (yellow arrow)

erly placed orbital floor implant, usually incorrectly placed under the posterior bony ledge [21].

The indications for repair of medial orbital wall blowout fractures mirror those for repair of orbital floor fractures: in the absence of evidence of a trapdoor fracture or oculocardiac reflex, surgery can be postponed for several weeks to determine if cosmetically apparent enophthalmos develops or disabling diplopia persists. When surgery is indicated, operative exposure of the medial orbital wall is best accomplished through a transcaruncular approach [77], which can be an extension of an inferior transconjunctival incision when both the medial and inferior orbital walls require repair. The goals of medial orbital wall fracture repair are the same as orbital floor fracture repair: lysis of adhesions, repositioning of herniated tissue, and placement of an implant that rests on the posterior bony ledge of the fracture.

A lateral canthotomy, transconjunctival approach can be used to access the lateral orbit [78–80]. In symptomatic children with large and displaced zygomatic fractures, open reduction of the fractures with stabilization with titanium plates and screws using 2-point (frontozygomatic suture, infraorbital rim) or 3-point (frontozygomatic suture, infraorbital rim, zygomaticomaxillary buttress) fixation is adequate, depending on the type and location of the fracture [10, 45, 81]. Unlike orbital blowout

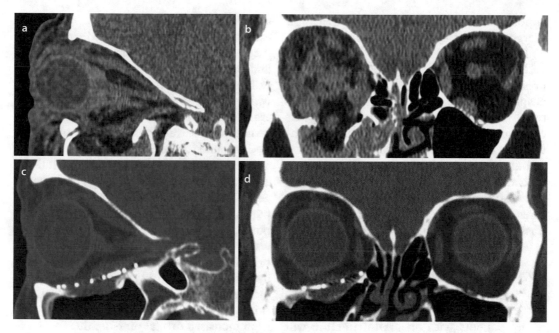

Fig. 4.8 The goal of surgical repair of an orbital floor fracture is complete coverage of the defect, with the implant resting securely on the posterior bony ledge of the defect. **a, b** Sagittal and axial CT images of a right orbital blowout fracture. **c, d** Sagittal and axial postop- erative CT images demonstrating the orbital implant resting on the bony edges of the fracture to inure there is complete separation between the sinus cavity and the orbit

fractures, repair of lateral wall and ZMC frac- tures should be undertaken within a 3–4 weeks period, prior to ossification of the displaced fragments that would necessitate osteotomies or secondary implants for successful repair.

In patients with large, displaced fractures of the orbital roof, surgical intervention often requires a multidisciplinary team approach. A coronal flap with craniotomy is usually neces- sary to repair symptomatic fractures of the orbital roof. In cases of isolated, inferiorly displaced, symptomatic orbital roof fractures with relatively little comminution, an anterior orbitotomy through an upper eyelid crease incision and reduction of the bony fragment can sometimes be utilized [56].

Alloplastic implants are most commonly used in the repair of orbital wall fractures, as they avoid a second incision and the need for tissue harvesting. Porous polyethylene is fre- quently favored as it eventually becomes incorporated with native fibrovascular tissue [22]. Each technique and implant has its own advantages and disadvantages [27]. Ultimately, the surgeon should decide which technique

and implant to use at his or her discretion and comfort. Success of the operation more cru- cially depends upon the complete reposition- ing of the herniated orbital tissue, adequate lysis of adhesions, and correct placement of the implant.

4.7 Outcome/Complications

Most cases of preoperative diplopia following surgical repair of both trapdoor and non- trapdoor orbital blowout fractures recover completely over time [82]. Persistent diplopia may be a result of direct inferior rectus muscle injury, fibrosis, or cranial nerve palsy [83]. Children with repaired trapdoor fractures may experience a higher rate of extraocular motility restriction and persistent diplopia, as these patients are more likely to be misdiag- nosed and undergo delayed orbital imaging in the emergency department and delayed surgi- cal repair. Children with trapdoor fractures are also less likely to be seen urgently by an ophthalmologist and are given follow-up

4

appointments with an ophthalmologist an average of 4–5 days later than those children with non-trapdoor orbital floor fractures [64].

Some degree of enophthalmos may be present after repair of an orbital wall fracture, despite complete repositioning of prolapsed tissue and proper placement of the implant over the defect. Development of late enophthalmos may occur due to delayed orbital tissue atrophy [84–86]. Surgical technique is a crucial element in avoiding a poor postoperative result in the repair of orbital wall fractures. Inadequate repair may lead to persistent postoperative diplopia and/or enophthalmos.

4.7.1 Orbital Hemorrhage and Compartment Syndrome

Many patients with an orbital fracture will have some degree of intraorbital hemorrhage on imaging studies, and most require no treatment. However, the constellation of proptosis, subconjunctival hemorrhage, periorbital ecchymosis, markedly elevated intraocular pressure (IOP), an afferent pupillary defect, and unilateral loss of vision indicate a clinically significant retrobulbar hemorrhage for which urgent surgical decompression via lateral canthotomy and inferior cantholysis may be needed to salvage vision [61] (◘ Fig. 4.9).

Profound decrease in visual acuity, an afferent pupillary defect, and elevated IOP are especially helpful diagnostic signs in the emergency room. In narcotic-induced miotic pupils, in which the detection of an afferent pupillary defect is difficult, decreased color vision in the setting of a clinically significant orbital hemorrhage may reveal optic nerve dysfunction. An asymmetric, markedly increased IOP measured by portable applanation tonometer may indicate a "tight" orbit from increased orbital pressure due to significant orbital hemorrhage. Retinal perfusion abnormalities can be assessed using indirect ophthalmoscopy.

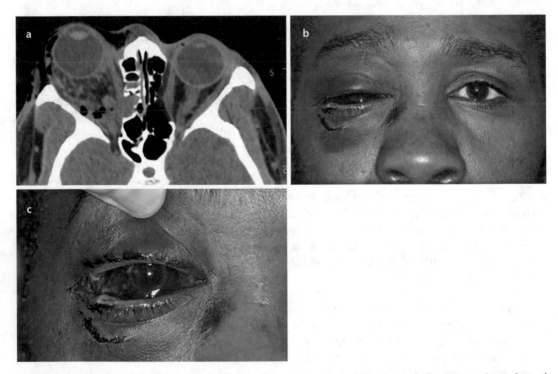

◘ **Fig. 4.9** **a** Axial CT image of a right orbital medial wall fracture presenting with **b** right proptosis, no light perception vision, and subconjunctival hemorrhage in the setting of acute retrobulbar hemorrhage. Lateral canthotomy and cantholysis **c** resulted in rapid return of vision to the 20/60 range

Imaging is often not necessary prior to performing canthotomy/inferior cantholysis in severe, acute cases. (Imaging may sometimes be appropriate in the acute setting, and though MRI is more sensitive in visualizing intraorbital hemorrhage [87–90], CT scanning is more rapid and will permit earlier intervention). The IOP is virtually always elevated in this scenario, and following lateral canthal decompression, the IOP should fall markedly. If the IOP remains elevated, further reduction in IOP should be accomplished with topical ocular antihypertensive drops and even intravenous acetazolamide or mannitol. Intravenous steroids are also typically given to reduce orbital edema, decreasing the pressure on the compromised optic nerve and/or retinal circulation [85]. Even an eye with no light perception vision due to an acute orbital hemorrhage can have full restoration of vision following prompt canthotomy/inferior cantholysis and other pressure-lowering interventions. In some patients, surgical evacuation of the hemorrhage may be necessary if efforts to relieve the pressure on the nerve or retinal circulation otherwise fail.

4.7.2 Orbital Foreign Body

Traumatic intraorbital foreign bodies in pediatric patients are managed similarly as in adult patients, and in the appropriate clinical scenario (i.e., fever, persistent orbital inflammation, elevated white count), their presence must be suspected until proven otherwise [91, 92]. The presence of an intraorbital foreign

body can be easily overlooked, especially in asymptomatic patients, and therefore clinicians must carefully examine the periorbital skin and conjunctiva, especially the conjunctival fornices, for entrance wounds. Reactive intraorbital foreign bodies made of iron and copper and organic foreign bodies made of wood and vegetative material are frequently associated with a severe, persistent inflammatory reaction, fistula development, and abscess formation and require urgent surgical removal [93]. Inert intraorbital foreign bodies (such as those made of glass, gold, silver, platinum, porcelain, plastic, sand, cilia, or rubber) can be treated conservatively with close observation in asymptomatic patients.

CT scan is the most reliable method for identifying intraorbital foreign bodies compared to clinical examination and B-scan echography, regardless of location within the orbit [22, 87, 90]. Intraorbital wooden foreign bodies present a particular diagnostic challenge to physicians, as they are frequently mistaken for air on CT scans, and are often difficult to distinguish from adjacent soft tissue or fat; widening the window settings on CT imaging can be helpful in detection [94–98] (◘ Fig. 4.10). Trauma patients with orbital infection refractory to antibiotics and those who develop chronic inflammation, fistula, or abscess formation should be suspected as having a retained intraorbital wooden foreign body.

Systemic broad spectrum antibiotic coverage should be given to all patients with an orbital foreign body, and extracted foreign

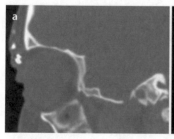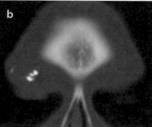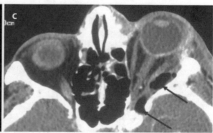

◘ **Fig. 4.10** **a** Sagittal and **b** coronal CT images of of multiple periorbital glass foreign bodies implanted during a motor vehicle collision. While glass is always visible on a CT scan, wood foreign bodies in the orbit can be mistakenly interpreted as intraorbital air (arrows), as demonstrated on this axial CT image **c**

bodies should be cultured and sent for antibiotic sensitivity. Whenever possible, extracting an orbital foreign body through an upper eyelid crease incision or inferior transconjunctival incision will minimize any additional trauma to adjacent orbital structures. Multiple explorations may be required to retrieve an intraorbital foreign body if the intraorbital foreign body is located in an area that is difficult to access surgically [99].

Case Presentation

A 10-year-old boy presented to the emergency room with impaired right supraduction, intermittently associated with nausea, following a fall (◘ Fig. 4.11a). A CT scan of the orbits revealed a "trapdoor" right orbital floor fracture in which the fracture segment recoiled to trap orbital tissue in the maxillary sinus (◘ Fig. 4.11b). Following transconjunctival surgical repair, the right eye motility returned to normal (◘ Fig. 4.11c).

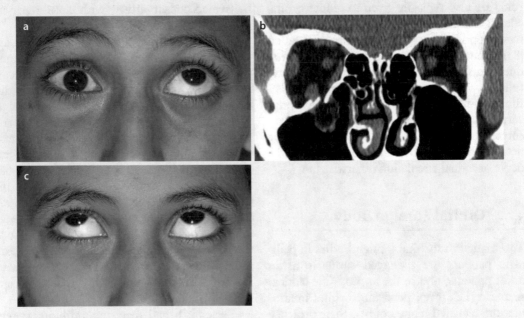

◘ **Fig. 4.11**   **a** Impaired right supraduction; **b** "Trapdoor" right orbital floor fracture; **c** Right eye motility returned to normal

Key Points

- Ophthalmology consultation is imperative in all midfacial and/or orbital fractures to rule out serious ophthalmic injury.
- Children displaying severe ocular motility restriction and/or an oculocardiac reflex following periorbital trauma should be suspected as having a trapdoor fracture, an indication for urgent repair (within 24 hours of diagnosis).
- Most isolated orbital floor fractures can be followed conservatively for several weeks, and the decision to ultimately undergo surgical repair is based solely on clinical findings (disfiguring enophthalmos or persistent diplopia) that are monitored during serial examinations.

- Complete repositioning of the herniated orbital tissue, adequate lysis of adhesions, and correct placement of the orbital implant are crucial to the success of orbital fracture repair. The transconjunctival approach is associated with a lower incidence of postoperative lower eyelid malposition.
- Profound decrease in visual acuity, an afferent pupillary defect, subconjunctival hemorrhage, decreased ocular motility, and elevated IOP are especially helpful diagnostic clues in the emergency room to the presence of orbital compartment syndrome, usually due to an orbital hemorrhage. Urgent canthotomy and inferior cantholysis are indicated and can often salvage vision.
- Trauma patients with orbital infection refractory to antibiotics, and those who develop chronic inflammation, fistula, or abscess, should be suspected as having a retained, undiagnosed intraorbital foreign body, especially one composed of wood.

❓ Review Questions

1. A 9-year-old girl sustained forceful blunt trauma to her right periorbital area while playing baseball. Examination of the right eye reveals vision loss, proptosis, subconjunctival hemorrhage, a relative afferent pupillary defect, decreased ocular motility, and significantly elevated right intraocular pressure. Examination of the left eye is within normal limits. This constellation of findings is concerning for which diagnosis?
   (a) Orbital floor fracture with entrapment
   (b) Orbital hemorrhage and compartment syndrome
   (c) Traumatic retinal detachment
   (d) LeFort II fracture

2. In the case above, what is the most appropriate next step?
   (a) CT imaging
   (b) Analgesics and antiemetics
   (c) Ice pack and close outpatient follow-up
   (d) Urgent canthotomy and cantholysis

3. Which one of the following symptoms associated with orbital floor fractures requires urgent repair (within 24–48 hours)?
   (a) Diplopia
   (b) Enophthalmos
   (c) Bradycardia or nausea/vomiting with attempted extraocular movement
   (d) Decreased extraocular motility

✅ Answer

1. (b)
2. (d)
3. (c)

References

1. Alcalá-Galiano A, Arribas-García IJ, Martín-Pérez MA, et al. Pediatric facial fractures: children are not just small adults. Radiographics. 2008;28:441–61.
2. Koltai PJ, Amjad I, Meyer D, et al. Orbital fractures in children. Arch Otolaryngol Head Neck Surg. 1995;121:1375–9.
3. Koltai PJ, Rabkin D. Management of facial trauma in children. Pediatr Clin N Am. 1996;43:1253–75.
4. Zimmermann CE, Troulis MJ, Kaban LB. Pediatric facial fractures: recent advances in prevention, diagnosis and management. Int J Oral Maxillofac Surg. 2006;35:2–13.
5. Chandler DB, Rubin PA. Developments in the understanding and management of pediatric orbital fractures. Int Ophthalmol Clin. 2001;41:87–104.
6. Hatef DA, Cole PD, Hollier LH Jr. Contemporary management of pediatric facial trauma. Curr Opin Otolaryngol Head Neck Surg. 2009;17:308–14.
7. Hatton MP, Watkins LM, Rubin PA. Orbital fractures in children. Ophthal Plast Reconstr Surg. 2001;17:174–9.
8. Imahara SD, Hopper RA, Wang J, et al. Patterns and outcomes of pediatric facial fractures in the United States: a survey of the National Trauma Data Bank. J Am Coll Surg. 2008;207:710–6.

4

9. Eggensperger Wymann NM, Hölzle A, Zachariou Z, et al. Pediatric craniofacial trauma. J Oral Maxillofac Surg. 2008;66:58–64.

10. Ferreira PC, Amarante JM, Silva PN, et al. Retrospective study of 1251 maxillofacial fractures in children and adolescents. Plast Reconstr Surg. 2005;115:1500–8.

11. Gassner R, Tuli T, Hächl O, et al. Craniomaxillofacial trauma in children: a review of 3,385 cases with 6,060 injuries in 10 years. J Oral Maxillofac Surg. 2004;62:399–407.

12. Holland AJ, Broome C, Steinberg A, et al. Facial fractures in children. Pediatr Emerg Care. 2001;17:157–60.

13. Losee JE, Afifi A, Jiang S, et al. Pediatric orbital fractures: classification, management, and early follow-up. Plast Reconstr Surg. 2008;122:886–97.

14. Li Z, Li ZB. Characteristic changes of pediatric maxillofacial fractures in China during the past 20 years. J Oral Maxillofac Surg. 2008;66:2239–42.

15. Nowinski D, Di Rocco F, Roujeau T, et al. Complex pediatric orbital fractures combined with traumatic brain injury: treatment and follow-up. J Craniofac Surg. 2010;21:1054–9.

16. Vyas RM, Dickinson BP, Wasson KL, et al. Pediatric facial fractures: current national incidence, distribution, and health care resource use. J Craniofac Surg. 2008;19:339–49; discussion 350.

17. Smith B, Regan WF Jr. Blow-out fracture of the orbit; mechanism and correction of internal orbital fracture. Am J Ophthalmol. 1957;44:733–9.

18. de Haan AB, Willekens B, Klooster J, et al. The prenatal development of the human orbit. Strabismus. 2006;14:51–6.

19. Haas A, Weiglein A, Faschinger C, Müllner K. Fetal development of the human orbit. Graefes Arch Clin Exp Ophthalmol. 1993;231:217–20.

20. Hink EM, Wei LA, Durairaj VD. Clinical features and treatment of pediatric orbit fractures. Ophthal Plast Reconstr Surg. 2014;30:124–31.

21. Kim JS, Lee BW, Scawn RL, Korn BS, Kikkawa DO. Secondary orbital reconstruction in patients with prior orbital fracture repair. Ophthal Plast Reconstr Surg. 2016;32(6):447–51.

22. Chung SY, Langer PD. Pediatric orbital blowout fractures. Curr Opin Ophthalmol. 2017;28:470–6.

23. Cohen SM, Garrett CG. Pediatric orbital floor fractures: nausea/vomiting as signs of entrapment. Otolaryngol Head Neck Surg. 2003;129:43–7.

24. Kim J, Lee H, Chi M, Park M, Lee J, Baek S. Endoscope-assisted repair of pediatric trapdoor fractures of the orbital floor: characterization and management. J Craniofac Surg. 2010;21:101–5.

25. Sires BS, Stanley RB, Levine LM. Oculocardiac reflex caused by orbital floor trapdoor fracture: an indication for urgent repair. Arch Ophthalmol. 1998;116:955–6.

26. Cobb A, Murthy R, Manisali M, et al. Oculovagal reflex in paediatric orbital floor fractures mimicking head injury. Emerg Med J. 2009;26:351–3.

27. Wei LA, Durairaj VD. Pediatric orbital floor fractures. J AAPOS. 2011;15(2):173–80.

28. Vicinanzo MG, McGwin G Jr, Allamneni C, Long JA. Interreader variability of computed tomography for orbital floor fracture. JAMA Ophthalmol. 2015;133(12):1393–7.

29. Jones DE, Evans JN. "Blow-out" fractures of the orbit: an investigation into their anatomical basis. J Laryngol Otol. 1967;81(10):1109–20.

30. Meyer DR. Orbital fractures. In: Tasman W, Jaeger EA, editors. Duane's clinical ophthalmology, revised edition. Philadelphia: Lippincott-Raven; 1996; chap. 48.

31. Phan LT, Jordan Piluek W, McCulley TJ. Orbital trapdoor fractures. Saudi J Ophthalmol. 2012;26(3):277–82.

32. Jordan DR, Allen LH, White J, Harvey J, Pashby R, Esmaeli B. Intervention within days for some orbital floor fractures: the white-eyed blowout. Ophthal Plast Reconstr Surg. 1998;14:379–90.

33. Segrest DR, Dortzbach RK. Medial orbital wall fractures: complications and management. Ophthal Plast Reconstr Surg. 1989;5:75–80.

34. Duane TD, Schatz NJ. Pseudo-Duane's retraction syndrome. Trans Am Ophthalmol. 1976;79:122.

35. Bansagi ZC, Meyer DR. Internal orbital fractures in the pediatric age group: characterization and management. Ophthalmology. 2000;107:829–36.

36. Burnstine MA. Clinical recommendations for repair of isolated orbital floor fractures: an evidence-based analysis. Ophthalmology. 2002;109:1207.

37. Kosaka M, Sakamoto T, Yamamichi K, Yamashiro Y. Different onset pattern of oculocardiac reflex in pediatric medial wall blowout fractures. J Craniofac Surg. 2014;25:247–52.

38. Egbert JE, May K, Kersten RC, et al. Pediatric orbital floor fracture: direct extraocular muscle involvement. Ophthalmology. 2000;107:1875–9.

39. Grant JH 3rd, Patrinely JR, Weiss AH, et al. Trapdoor fracture of the orbit in a pediatric population. Plast Reconstr Surg. 2002;109:482–9; 490–495.

40. Tse R, Allen L, Matic D. The white-eyed medial blowout fracture. Plast Reconstr Surg. 2007;119:277–86.

41. Jurdy L, Malhotra R. White-eyed medial wall blowout fracture mimicking head injury due to persistent oculocardiac reflex. J Craniofac Surg. 2011;22:1977–9.

42. Oppenheimer A, Monson LA, Buchman SR. Pediatric orbital fractures. Craniomaxillofac Trauma Reconstr. 2013;6:9–20.

43. Hink EM, Durairaj VD. Evaluation and treatment of pediatric orbital fractures. Int Ophthalmol Clin. 2013;53(3):103–15.

44. McInnes AW, Burnstine MA. White-eyed medial wall orbital blowout fracture. Ophthal Plast Reconstr Surg. 2010;26(1):44–6.

45. DeFazio MV, Fan KL, Avashia YJ, Danton GH, Thaller SR. Fractures of the pediatric zygoma: a review of the clinical trends, management strategies,

and outcomes associatedwith zygomatic fractures in children. J Craniofac Surg. 2013;24(6):1891–7.

46. Lin KY, Bartlett SP, Yaremchuk MJ, Grossman RF, Udupa JK, Whitaker LA. An experimental study on the effect of rigid fixation on the developing craniofacial skeleton. Plast Reconstr Surg. 1991;87:229–35.

47. Costantino P, Wolpoe M. Short-and long-term outcome of facial plating following trauma in the pediatric population. Facial Plast Surg. 1999;7:231–42.

48. Haug RH, Foss J. Maxillofacial injuries in the pediatric patient. Oral Surg Oral Med Oral Pathol Oral Radiol Endod. 2000;90:126–34.

49. Gussack GS, Luterman A, Powell RW, Rodgers K, Ramenofsky ML. Pediatric maxillofacial trauma: unique features in diagnosis and treatment. Laryngoscope. 1987;97:925–30.

50. Schliephake H, Berten JL, Neukam FW, Bothe KJ, Hausamen JE. Growth disorders following fractures of the midface in children (in German). Dtsch Zahnarztl Z. 1990;45:819–22.

51. Luck JD, Lopez J, Faateh M, et al. Pediatric zygomaticomaxillary complex fracture repair: location and number of fixation sites in growing children. Plast Reconstr Surg. 2018;142:51e–60e.

52. Alcala-Galiano A, Arribas-Garcia I, Martin-Perez MA, et al. Pediatric facial fractures: children are not just small adults. Radiographics. 2008;28:441–61.

53. Fulcher TP, Sullivan TJ. Orbital roof fractures: management of ophthalmic complications. Ophthal Plast Reconstr Surg. 2003;29:359–63.

54. Whatley WS, Allison DW, Chandra RK, et al. Frontal sinus fractures in children. Larygoscope. 2005;115:1741–5.

55. Greenwald MJ, Boston D, Pensler JM, et al. Orbital roof fractures in childhood. Ophthalmology. 1989;96:491–6.

56. Coon D, Yuan N, Jones D, Howell LK, Grant MP, Redett RJ. Defining pediatric orbital roof fractures: patterns, sequelae, and indications for operation. Plast Reconstr Surg. 2014;134:442e–8e.

57. Rowe NL. Fractures of the facial skeleton in children. J Oral Surg. 1968;26:505–15.

58. McGraw BL, Cole RR. Pediatric maxillofacial trauma: age-related variations in injury. Arch Otolaryngol Head Neck Surg. 1990;116:41.

59. Thaller SR, Huang V. Midfacial fractures in the pediatric population. Ann Plast Surg. 1992;29:348.

60. Posnick JC, Wells M, Pron GE. Pediatric facial fractures: evolving patterns of treatment. J Oral Maxillofac Surg. 1993;51:836–44.

61. Stotland MA, Do NK. Pediatric orbital fractures. J Craniofac Surg. 2011;22:1230–5.

62. Baek SH, Lee EY. Clinical analysis of internal orbital fractures in children. Korean J Ophthalmol. 2003;17:44–9.

63. Carroll SC, Ng SG. Outcomes of orbital blowout fracture surgery in children and adolescents. Br J Ophthalmol. 2010;94:736–7.

64. Lane K, Penne RB, Bilyk JR. Evaluation and management of pediatric orbital fractures in a primary care setting. Orbit. 2007;26:183–91.

65. Criden MR, Ellis FJ. Linear nondisplaced orbital fractures with muscle entrapment. J AAPOS. 2007;11:142–7.

66. Putterman AM, Stevens T, Urist MJ. Nonsurgical management of blow-out fractures of the orbital floor. Am J Ophthalmol. 1974;77(2):232–9.

67. Nishida Y, Hayashi O, Miyake T, et al. Quantitative evaluation of ocular motility in blow-out fractures for selection of nonsurgically managed cases. Am J Ophthalmol. 2004;137(4):777–9.

68. Broyles JM, Jones D, Bellamy J, et al. Pediatric orbital floor fractures: outcome analysis of 72 children with orbital floor fractures. Plast Reconstr Surg. 2015;136(4):822–8.

69. de Man K, Wijngaarde R, Hes J, et al. Influence of age on the management of blow-out fractures of the orbital floor. Int J Oral Maxillofac Surg. 1991;20:330–6.

70. Simon GJ, Syed HM, McCann JD, Goldberg RA. Early versus late repair of orbital blowout fractures. Ophthalmic Surg Lasers Imaging. 2009;40(2):141–8.

71. Dal Canto AJ, Linberg JV. Comparison of orbital fracture repair performed within 14 days versus 15 to 29 days after trauma. Ophthalmic Plast Reconstr Surg. 2008;24(6):437–43.

72. Appling WD, Patrinely JR, Salzer TA. Transconjunctival approach vs subciliary skin-muscle flap approach for orbital fracture repair. Arch Otolaryngol Head Neck Surg. 1993;19(9):1000–7.

73. Patel PC, Sobota BT, Patel NM, Greene JS, Millman B. Comparison of transconjunctival versus subciliary approaches for orbital fractures: a review of 60 cases. J Craniomaxillofac Trauma. 1998;4(1):17–21.

74. Waite PD, Carr DD. The transconjunctival approach for treating orbital trauma. J Oral Maxillofac Surg. 1991;49:499–503.

75. Bernardini FP, Nerad J, Fay A, Zambelli A, Cruz AA. The revised direct transconjunctival approach to the orbital floor. Ophthal Plast Reconstr Surg. 2016;33(2):93–100.

76. Murchison AP, Matthews AE, Bilyk JR. Specific issues in pediatric periocular trauma. 3rd ed. New York: Springer-Verlag; 2012.

77. Shorr N, Baylis HI, Goldberg RA, Perry JD. Transcaruncular approach to the medial orbit and orbital apex. Ophthalmology. 2000;107: 1459–63.

78. Tessier P. The conjunctival approach to the orbital floor and maxilla in congenital malformation and trauma. J Maxillofac Surg. 1973;1:3–8.

79. Converse JM, Firmin F, Wood-Smith D, Friedland JA. The conjunctival approach in orbital fractures. Plast Reconstr Surg. 1973;52:656–7.

80. Nunery WR. Lateral canthal approach to repair of trimalar fractures of the zygoma. Ophthal Plast Reconstr Surg. 1985;1:175–83.

81. Foncesca RJ. Oral and maxillofacial trauma, vol. 3. Elsevier Saunders: St Louis; 2005.

82. Su Y, Shen Q, Lin M, Fan X. Predictive factors for residual diplopia after surgical repair in pediatric

patients with orbital blowout fracture. J Craniomaxillofac Surg. 2016;44(9):1463–8.

83. Yu DY, Chen CH, Tsay PK, et al. Surgical timing and fracture type on the outcome of diplopia after orbital fracture repair. Ann Plast Surg. 2016;76:91–5.

84. Kim SM, Jeong YS, Lee IJ, Park MC, Park DH. Prediction of the development of late enophthalmos in pure blowout fractures: delayed orbital tissue atrophy plays a major role. Eur J Ophthalmol. 2017;27(1):104–8.

85. Gagnon MR, Yeatts RP, Williams Z, et al. Delayed enophthalmos following a minimally displaced orbital floor fracture. Ophthal Plast Reconstr Surg. 2004;20:241–3.

86. Harris GJ, Garcia GH, Logani SC, Murphy ML. Correlation of preoperative computed tomography and postoperative ocular motility in orbital blowout fractures. Ophthal Plast Reconstr Surg. 2000;16(3):179–87.

87. McGuckin JF Jr, Akhtar N, Ho VT, Smergel EM, Kubacki EJ, Villafanna T. CT and MR evaluation of a wooden foreign body in a vitro model of the orbit. Am J Neuroradiol. 1996;17:129–33.

88. Williamson TH, Smith FW, Forrester JV. Magnetic resonance imaging of intraocular foreign bodies. Br J Ophthalmol. 1989;73:555–8.

89. Nasr AM, Haik BG, Fleming JC, Al-Hussain HM, Karcioglu ZA. Penetrating orbital injury with organic foreign bodies. Ophthalmology. 1999;106:523–32.

90. Gawdat TI, Ahmed RA. Orbital foreign bodies: expect the unexpected. J Pediatr Ophthalmol Strabismus. 2010;47:e1–4.

91. Brock L, Tenenbaum HL. Retention of wooden foreign bodies in the orbit. Can J Ophthalmol. 1980;15:70–2.

92. Macrae JA. Diagnosis and management of a wooden orbital foreign body: case report. Br J Ophthalmol. 1979;63:848–51.

93. Simonton JT, Arthurs BP. Penetrating injuries to the orbit. Adv Ophthalmic Plast Reconstr Surg. 1987;7:217–27.

94. Tate E, Cupples H. Detection of orbital foreign bodies with computed tomography: current limits. Am J Roentgenol. 1981;137:493–5.

95. Adesanya OO, Dawkins DM. Intraorbital wooden foreign body (IOFB): mimicking air on CT. Emerg Radiol. 2007;14(1):45–9.

96. Hansen JE, Gudeman SK, Holgate RC, Saunders RA. Penetrating intracranial wood wounds: clinical limitations of computerized tomography. J Neurosurg. 1988;68(5):752–6.

97. Shelsta HN, Bilyk JR, Rubin PA, Penne RB, Carrasco JR. Wooden intraorbital foreign body injuries: clinical characteristics and outcomes of 23 patients. Ophthal Plast Reconstr Surg. 2010;26(4):238–44.

98. Dalley RW. Intraorbital wood foreign bodies on CT: use of wide bone window settings to distinguish wood from air. AJR Am J Roentgenol. 1995;164(2):434–5.

99. Panda BB, Kim UR. Complications of retained intraorbital wooden foreign body. Oman J Ophthalmol. 2014;7:38–9.

Eyelid Trauma

Adam R. Sweeney and Richard C. Allen

Contents

© Springer Nature Switzerland AG 2021
R. Shinder (ed.), *Pediatric Ophthalmology in the Emergency Room*,
https://doi.org/10.1007/978-3-030-49950-1_5

5.1 Introduction

The eyelid is the periocular component most exposed to superficial trauma. Numerous attachments of the lid provide for the appropriate tension and contour of the eyelid to provide its function and maintain cosmesis. Attention to the delicate anatomy of this structure is imperative for recognition of structures involved, the associated injuries, and possible sequelae of injury.

5.2 Anatomy

The upper eyelid extends from the inferior brow to the superior lid margin, separated from the lower eyelid by the palpebral fissure, which measures approximately 30 mm in horizontal length. The lower eyelid extends from the palpebral fissure to the superior maxilla. The lateral canthus is positioned approximately 1–2 mm superior to the medial canthus creating a gentle slope for tears to drain to the lacrimal drainage apparatus, which originates at the punctum. The tarsus provides the structural backbone for the eyelid and measures approximately 10–12 mm in height in the upper lid and 4 mm in the lower lid. The layers of the eyelid are of particular relevance in the setting of trauma and eyelid reconstruction. From anterior to posterior at the level of the tarsus lie skin, orbicularis oculi muscle, tarsus, and conjunctiva. Superior to the superior tarsus, the layers of the eyelid from anterior to posterior are skin, orbicularis, orbital septum, preaponeurotic fat, levator aponeurosis, Muller muscle, and conjunctiva. The layers of the eyelid inferior to the inferior tarsus are analogous to the upper lid with the capsulopalpebral fascia replacing the levator aponeurosis as the main eyelid retractor. The eyelid margin structures include the lash line anteriorly, the gray line centrally, and the Meibomian glands and mucocutaneous junction posteriorly. Reapproximation of all these layers during eyelid laceration repair is imperative to retain the function of the eyelid.

The medial and lateral canthal angle attachments intricately provide for the struc-tural framework of the eyelids. The medial and lateral canthal tendons are an extension of the superior and inferior tarsal plates. The medial canthal tendon bifurcates just lateral to the lacrimal sac with an anterior limb attaching to the anterior lacrimal crest and a posterior limb attaching to the posterior lacrimal crest. The lateral canthal tendon does not bifurcate but attaches to the lateral orbital tubercle (◻ Fig. 5.1).

The orbicularis oculi circumnavigates the orbital rim and is the eyelid protractor allowing for voluntary and involuntary closure. The orbicularis is divided into pretarsal, preseptal, and orbital portions. The medial orbicularis attachments are particularly important in the setting of medial canthal trauma or avulsion, which is a commonly injured area. The pretarsal orbicularis inserts posteriorly at the posterior lacrimal crest and anteriorly on the medial aspect of the medial canthal tendon. The lateral pretarsal orbicularis fuses to make up the lateral canthal tendon. Medially, the preseptal orbicularis inserts into the common medial canthal tendon and laterally fuses to make up the lateral palpebral raphe. The orbital orbicularis inserts at the anterior canthal tendon medially with various bony attachments around the orbital rim.

The internal and external carotids provide arterial branches to the eyelid to provide an extensive network of collaterals and anasto-

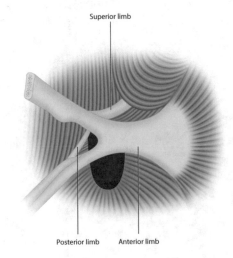

Superior limb

Posterior limb   Anterior limb

◻ **Fig. 5.1** Detailed view of the medial canthal tendon of the right orbit

Table 5.1 Periorbital nerves

Periorbital nerves	Innervated structures
Supraorbital	Eyebrow and forehead
Supratrochlear	Medial canthus, upper eyelid, lacrimal region
Infraorbital	Lower eyelid, upper lip, molars, and part of the nose
Infratrochlear	Medial eyelids, bridge of the nose, conjunctiva, lacrimal sac, and caruncle
Zygomaticofacial	Cheek
Zygomaticotemporal	Lateral canthus and temporalis region

out. It is critical to minimally manipulate the globe and eyelids prior to ruling out globe injury. Thoroughly rinsing and cleaning the eyelids with sterile fluids is helpful to obtain an accurate exam with optimal visualization. Blunt exploration with cotton tip applicators will help reveal the extent and depth of injury. It is imperative to identify any exposed fat in the eyelid as this suggests violation of the septum with orbital penetration, which should raise suspicion for damage to the eyelid retractors or deeper injury to the extraocular muscles or neurovascular structures. Often the lids may be very swollen, and a Desmarres retractor may be used to assist in visualization of the posterior surface of the eyelids to rule out foreign bodies and to obtain a clear view of the medial and lateral canthal angles. Rounding of the canthal angles suggests canthal avulsion.

moses for a robust vascular supply that aids in rapid eyelid healing after trauma or repair. The main arteries of interest in the setting of trauma include the superior and inferior marginal arcades, located approx. 2–4 mm from the margin, and the superior peripheral arcade, located between the retractors of the upper lid. The venous drainage for the eyelid is divided by the septum. Anterior to the septum, the angular vein and superficial temporal vein drain medially and laterally, respectively. Posterior to the septum, the anterior facial vein, pterygoid plexus, and cavernous sinus provide drainage from the eyelid (◘ Table 5.1).

5.3 Eyelid Trauma

5.3.1 Evaluation

When available, a detailed history of the injury is helpful prior to exam. History intake should include the timing and mechanism of injury, blunt vs penetrating nature, surface material of contact with the eyelid, and history of prior trauma or eyelid surgery. Examination of the eyelids should be performed after globe injury has been ruled

5.3.2 Imaging

Imaging for isolated eyelid trauma is not routinely necessary. However, based on the history and exam, a maxillofacial CT scan without contrast is indicated if there is any suspicion of foreign bodies, orbital fractures, or postseptal infection [1]. In the setting of medial canthal rounding, close inspection of CT images for a naso-orbital-ethmoidal fracture is suggested [2]. While providing better soft tissue identification, MRI is typically not indicated in eyelid trauma unless CT is contraindicated or unavailable. MRI may be helpful in instances of suspected organic foreign body. Ultrasound has limited applications in the setting of eyelid trauma.

5.4 Different Presentations of Eyelid Trauma

5.4.1 Eyelid Laceration

Eyelid and eyebrow lacerations account for 40% of facial lacerations presenting to the emergency department [3]. Such lacerations most commonly affect males in their early teenage years [3]. Common presenting signs of eyelid laceration include periocular edema, ecchymosis, tearing, and often bleeding at the site of the laceration. Lacerations should be carefully examined with a cotton tip applicator to identify the length and depth of the laceration and whether it involves the eyelid margin or canaliculus. In the setting of blunt trauma with laceration, orbital CT may be utilized to rule out orbital wall fracture if the mechanism of action is a high-velocity injury [3].

5.4.2 Margin Involving Laceration

Full thickness or partial thickness lacerations involving the eyelid margin raise an added layer of complexity in repair as the smooth border of the eyelid has been compromised. After the lid margin has been lacerated, tension spread across the lid may pull the wound apart, showing a gap, which classically may be mistaken for tissue loss. Patients with margin involving lacerations are at risk of corneal exposure, irregular tear film distribution, and corneal abrasion. Lacerations involving the margin may be vertical, oblique, or compound. Proper attention to closure should provide an equally good outcome despite the orientation of the laceration.

Lacerations involving the medial eyelid margin may involve the canalicular system. Such lacerations, if not repaired with canalicular anastomoses and stenting may result in chronic epiphora, difficult if not impossible for secondary repair through canalicular probing and stenting [4]. In the event of a canalicular involving eyelid laceration, an oculoplastic specialist or a surgeon with experience in canalicular repairs should be consulted.

5.4.3 Extramarginal Eyelid Laceration

Eyelid lacerations not involving the margin may be superficial or deep. Deep extramarginal lacerations may demonstrate violation of the septum, typically seen as exposed orbital fat, which should raise suspicion for retractor muscle injury or deeper injury. Principles of closure in extramarginal lacerations include avoidance of suturing septum and avoidance of vertical traction on the lid with closure. Traction with closure may risk lid retraction and exposure keratopathy. A thorough examination in nonmarginal lacerations should include identification of possible orbital fractures, exploring for foreign bodies, and assessment for lacrimal gland or canalicular involvement.

5.5 Management of Eyelid Lacerations

5.5.1 Medical Management

After the scope of the trauma to the eyelid has been assessed, the examiner must make a determination of the need for surgical intervention. Eyelid injuries that do not require surgical intervention include ecchymosis, eyelid swelling, or eyelid abrasion. These injuries do not require further medical attention, with the exception of a deep or large abrasion, which may be treated with 1 week of antibiotic ointment applied three times per day. If the eyelid does require surgery and the repair is delayed by over 6 hours, application of a topical antibiotic ointment should be considered to provide appropriate antimicrobial coverage and to keep the wound lubricated. Choice of antibiotic should include coverage of gram-positive bacteria as these are the most common offending agents. In margin involving lacerations where there may be exposure of the globe, topical lubricating ointment of the globe should be prescribed with or without an antibiotic component. Steroid and analgesic medications are not necessary for most isolated eyelid traumas.

5.5.2 Surgical Management

The patient's systemic injuries should be considered prior to any surgical repair of eyelid injuries. Evaluation or repair of eyelid injuries should not delay or complicate any vital care provided. The timing of repair may be postponed several days for a patient to become medically stable in almost all circumstances. If such monitoring strategy is implemented, the surgeon should be prepared to freshen up the borders of the wound with a blade to remove unwanted granulation or necrotic tissue to aid in successful repair.

Margin involving lacerations can be performed at bedside or in the operating room. The surgeon should seek a setting with the best lighting possible. Consideration should be made to determine the patient's tolerance of bedside repair. The authors prefer to avoid bedside repair of any margin involving laceration in young children, psychiatrically unstable patients, patients with severe anxiety or fear of needles, or patients with very complex repairs.

Repair of any eyelid or eyebrow laceration should be performed with injection of local anesthetic containing lidocaine with epinephrine for hemostasis and intraoperative pain. The patient should be prepped and draped in the usual sterile ophthalmic fashion. Topical anesthetic may be given in the eyes prior to repair to diminish any irritation caused by betadine, blood, or manipulation during the repair.

5.5.3 Margin Involving Laceration Repair

Repair of a margin involving laceration should start by aligning the lacerated edges of the eyelid with two toothed forceps. This should demonstrate that all eyelid tissue is indeed present in the vast majority of cases. There are multiple ways to repair a margin

involving eyelid laceration. The authors prefer to approximate the tarsus distal to the eyelid margin as this releases tension from the margin and also provides excellent exposure of the vertical length of the tarsus throughout repair. A 5-0 or 6-0 polyglactin suture is placed partial thickness through the anterior surface of the tarsus ensuring that the suture is not passed through the conjunctiva as this may cause postoperative corneal abrasion or irritation. Additional tarsal sutures may need to be similarly passed depending on the vertical length of the laceration (◘ Fig. 5.2a). Up to five deep interrupted passes may be needed for the upper lid and two for the lower lid. Attention is then turned to the margin where a 7-0 polyglactin (or 6-0 silk for older children who would better tolerate suture removal) suture is placed at the level of the Meibomian gland orifice in a vertical mattress fashion (far – far, near – near) to evert the lid margin. A second suture is then placed along the lash line, also in vertical mattress fashion. A third suture is finally placed at the gray line of the eyelid in vertical mattress fashion. In some instances, two marginal sutures will suffice for marginal approximation. It is critical that all sutures placed match each other on each side in terms of depth, length, and height of each pass. Tails of each pass along the eyelid margin are left long in order to incorporate them in subsequent superficial skin closure to keep the tails away to avoid the potential of corneal irritation (◘ Fig. 5.2b). Superficial skin is then closed with interrupted 6-0 plain (or 6-0 silk) gut suture (◘ Fig. 5.2c). A representative case of a margin involving full thickness eyelid laceration repair is shown in ◘ Fig. 5.3.

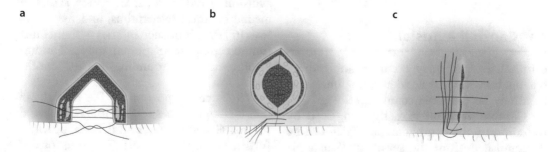

◘ **Fig. 5.2** Margin involving eyelid laceration repair. **a** Tarsal alignment sutures. **b** Margin alignment sutures. **c** Closure of skin. (Photo courtesy of Roman Shinder MD)

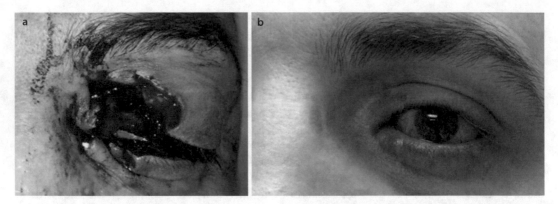

■ **Fig. 5.3** Left upper eyelid margin involving laceration: **a** Preoperative. **b** Postoperative appearance 3 months after repair

5.5.4 Non-margin Eyelid Laceration Repair

Lacerations that do not involve the lid margin are typically more easily repaired. Pillars of repair include avoidance of vertical tension and avoidance of incorporating the septum in the closure as these may cause eyelid retraction. Whenever possible, attempting to use horizontal passes rather than vertical passes may be implemented to avoid vertical tension on the lid. In general, laceration repair should focus on approximating tissues rather than tightly closing the wound. In most cases of isolated eyelid laceration not involving the margin, interrupted, superficial (skin) 6-0 plain gut sutures are sufficient to obtain adequate closure (■ Fig. 5.4). Deep sutures are not necessary and should not be placed. Significantly large lacerations involving other facial structures should be managed in coordination with a facial plastic or general plastic surgeon.

5.6 Canthal Avulsion

Canthal avulsion may occur in any trauma setting; however, car accidents, dog bites, and falls may be the most common etiologies [5, 6]. Canthal avulsion is easily recognized by rounding of the canthal angle, which can be distinguished from the sharp canthal angle borders of the uninvolved eyelid. Routinely, with avulsion of the medial canthus, canalicu-

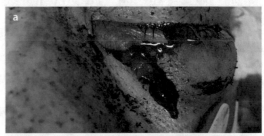

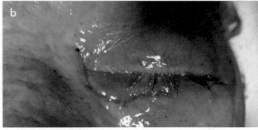

■ **Fig. 5.4** Non-margin involving eyelid laceration repair: **a** Preoperative defect. **b** Postoperative appearance demonstrating tension-free closure

lar laceration can be found (■ Fig. 5.5). Additional findings commonly seen in canthal avulsion include vertical laceration across the medial canthus, telecanthus, and blepharoptosis [6]. Repair of such injuries without attention to canthal repositioning may not address displacement or rounding of the canthal angle.

The superior portion of the medial canthal tendon attaches to the frontal process of the maxilla and the frontal bone providing further structural support. The anterior limb of the medial canthal tendon provides little support to the structure of the lower eyelid

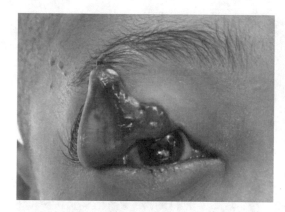

Fig. 5.5 Right upper eyelid full thickness laceration including medial canthal avulsion. (Photo courtesy of Roman Shinder MD)

but is firmly attached to the anterior lacrimal crest. The posterior limb of the medial canthal tendon is weakly attached to the posterior lacrimal crest yet provides the majority of the lower eyelid tension and position. The posterior limb of the medial canthal tendon is thus most likely to detach during trauma and the most important limb to repair.

Following direct closure of any margin involving lacerations and stenting of associated canalicular lacerations, attention is directed at refixation of the medial canthus. If the posterior portion of the tendon remains attached, the avulsed anterior limb may be sutured to the anterior lacrimal crest or to the proximal lacerated stump with a single interrupted 4-0 polyglactin suture. If the posterior tendon is avulsed, significant horizontal laxity may be demonstrated. When posterior tendon avulsion is found, referral to an experienced oculoplastic surgeon is indicated for consideration of microplate fixation, transnasal wiring, or suture refixation to the thin periosteum around the posterior lacrimal crest [7].

5.6.1 Human and Animal Bites

Trauma to the eyelid resulting from human or animal bites is a common presentation to the emergency department, dominated by dog bites in the pediatric setting. Eyelid lacerations from dog bites are four times more likely to occur in children compared to adults [8], demonstrating

the proclivity of dogs to attack the center of the face. Between 20% and 40% of eyelid lacerations from dog bites in children are associated with canalicular laceration [8, 9]. The physician must discuss removal of the animal from the home to ensure the safety of the child.

Large animal attacks may lead to significant morbidity; thus, attention should first be directed to ensuring the patient is primarily stable prior to embarking on a detailed ophthalmic exam. Evaluation of these lacerations should be performed in a similar manner to eyelid trauma from any type described above; however, special attention should be addressed to evaluate for canthal avulsion, infection, penetration into deep structures, globe injury, and canalicular injury. In large animal attacks, CT should be considered to investigate the possibility of facial fractures [9].

Dog and cat bites may be associated with atypical microbial species, including *Pasteurella*, streptococci, staphylococci, *Moraxella*, and *Neisseria* species [10, 11]. The authors routinely prescribe a 7-day course of oral amoxicillin/clavulanate or clindamycin at time of evaluation in bite injuries. Additionally, if the eyelid trauma is from an animal without known rabies immunization, discussion with infectious disease regarding treating the patient prophylactically with a rabies immunization is warranted [12].

The surgical protocol for repair of eyelid lacerations from bites should follow the above guidelines for repair of margin involving and extramarginal eyelid lacerations. Attention should be made to identify and remove any foreign bodies at the time of repair.

5.6.2 Eyebrow Trauma

Defects of the eyebrow resulting from trauma may include laceration, burn, or blunt trauma. Following high-velocity blunt trauma to the brow, CT with thin cuts of the orbits should be performed [13]. Fractures associated with blunt trauma to the brow are more common in children due to incomplete pneumatization of the frontal sinus, which distributes force of impact in adults [14]. Other, more rare complications of blunt force to the brow include

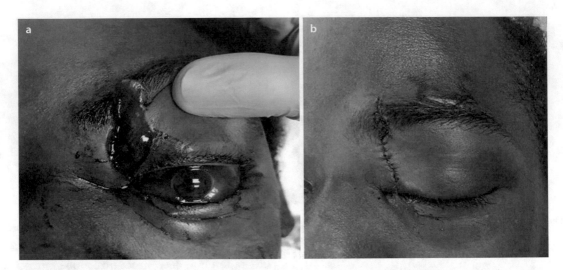

Fig. 5.6 Brow laceration repair. **a** Left medial brow and upper eyelid laceration. **b** Postoperative appearance demonstrating alignment of the brow

intracranial injuries, subperiosteal hematoma, cerebrospinal fluid leak, and retrobulbar hematoma.

Laceration of the brow may be a simple laceration or associated with soft tissue or follicle loss. Simple lacerations may be repaired with careful alignment of the superficial muscle layer with interrupted 4-0 polyglactin sutures followed by closure of the skin with interrupted passes of 5-0 plain gut. Attention should be directed at brow alignment so that there is continuity of the hair follicles after closure. Additionally, vertical tension must be avoided when closing the brow as this may cause upper eyelid retraction and corneal exposure (■ Fig. 5.6).

Lacerations of the brow involving soft tissue or a moderate amount of follicle loss may require local transfer using the remainder of the affected eyebrow to achieve good cosmetic outcomes. Such cases should be referred to a facial surgeon with experience in flap construction.

Large lacerations, degloving injuries, or deep abrasions involving significant brow loss may be best repaired via a free scalp flap, temporal fascia island flap, or V-Y advancement pedicle flap [15]. As grafts involving hair-bearing regions post a challenge to most surgeons, preoperative flap mapping and collaboration with facial plastic surgery colleagues should be considered.

5.6.3 Eyelid Burns

Eyelid burn is seldomly an isolated finding. Typically, eyelid burns present in the setting of other associated facial or full body burns in the setting of flame injury; however, chemical, iatrogenic, or even warm compress-related burns may present with a burn confined to the eyelid region [16]. The eyelids, however, are unique to many other possibly affected burn sites in the associated conditions that may arise from temporarily compromised function [17]. Eyelid burns are associated with corneal injury, ectropion, and severe retraction [18]. Copious lubrication of the eye with lubricating ointments is important in all facial burn settings, often requiring at least three times daily use of a lubricating ointment. Similarly, eyelid burns require aggressive lubrication to limit systemic evaporative fluid loss [19]. If anterior lamellar contracture occurs, skin grafting may be necessary to protect the ocular surface.

In the setting of systemic burns with significant intravenous fluid resuscitation, preseptal eyelid swelling and chemosis may be severe, occasionally creating a compartment syndrome with elevated intraocular pressure, regardless of eyelid burn injury [20]. In this circumstance, diligent monitoring of intraocular pressure is warranted with prompt canthotomy and cantholysis when indicated by an ophthalmologist.

A 16-year-old girl presented to the emergency department following a dog bite to the right periocular region. On examination, there was a full thickness laceration of the central right lower eyelid (■ Fig. 5.7a). The patient was taken to the operating room where the eyelid margin involving laceration was repaired (■ Fig. 5.7b). Postoperatively, the patient had a good cosmetic outcome with excellent eyelid contour.

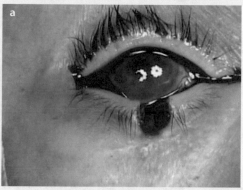
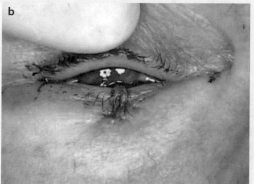

■ **Fig. 5.7** Repair of a full thickness eyelid laceration. **a** Central lower eyelid laceration. **b** Postoperative appearance demonstrating good approximation of the eyelid margin with ideal amount of eversion at the margin

Key Points

- Examination of the eyelids should be performed after ensuring patient is systemically stable and after globe injury has been ruled out.
- Rounding of the canthal angle suggests canthal avulsion.
- High suspicion for canalicular lacerations should be maintained in medial eyelid lacerations – failure to repair canalicular lacerations may result in chronic epiphora.
- Exposed orbital fat should raise suspicion for retractor injury including levator muscle/aponeurosis injury.
- Avoidance of vertical tension and avoidance of incorporation of septum in eyelid laceration closures will assist in minimizing posttraumatic ectropion or retraction.
- Dog and cat bites may be associated with atypical microbial species, and rabies status/vaccination must be considered.

- Evaluation of eyelid or eyebrow lacerations occurring from high-velocity traumas should include CT to rule out fracture.

❓ Review Questions

1. A dog bite to a child results in medial eyelid laceration, rounding of the medial canthus and tearing. What structure is less likely to require repair in this scenario?
   - (a) Canaliculus
   - (b) Lateral canthal tendon
   - (c) Eyelid margin
   - (d) Medial canthal tendon

2. Which of the following signs accompanying presentation with an eyelid laceration indicate CT imaging?
   - (a) Full thickness margin involving laceration
   - (b) Eyelid burn
   - (c) Periorbital hypesthesia
   - (d) Canalicular involving laceration

3. Fat prolapse through a superior eyelid laceration should raise concern for?
   (a) Canthal avulsion
   (b) Levator palpebrae superioris aponeurosis injury
   (c) Fracture
   (d) Foreign body

✔ **Answer**
   1. (b)
   2. (c)
   3. (b)

References

1. Hink EM, Wei LA, Durairaj VD. Clinical features and treatment of pediatric orbit fractures. Ophthalmic Plast Reconstr Surg. 2014;30(2):124–31.
2. Sargent LA, Rogers GF. Nasoethmoid orbital fractures: diagnosis and management. J Craniomaxillofac Trauma. 1999;5(1):19–27.
3. Hwang K, Huan F, Hwang PJ, Sohn IA. Facial lacerations in children. J Craniofac Surg. 2013;24(2):671–5.
4. Murchison AP, Bilyk JR. Pediatric canalicular lacerations: epidemiology and variables affecting repair success. J Pediatr Ophthalmol Strabismus. 2014;51(4):242–8.
5. Priel A, Leelapatranurak K, Oh SR, Korn BS, Kikkawa DO. Medial canthal degloving injuries: the triad of telecanthus, ptosis, and lacrimal trauma. Plast Reconstr Surg. 2011;128(4):300e 5e.
6. Tint NL, Alexander P, Cook AE, Leatherbarrow B. Eyelid avulsion repair with bi-canalicular silicone stenting without medial canthal tendon reconstruction. Br J Ophthalmol. 2011;95(10):1389–92.
7. Howard GR, Nerad JA, Kersten RC. Medial canthoplasty with microplate fixation. Arch Ophthalmol. 1992;110(12):1793–7.
8. Prendes MA, Jian-Amadi A, Chang SH, Shaftel SS. Ocular trauma from dog bites: characterization, associations, and treatment patterns at a regional level I trauma Center over 11 years. Ophthalmic Plast Reconstr Surg. 2016;32(4):279–83.
9. Wei LA, Chen HH, Hink EM, Durairaj VD. Pediatric facial fractures from dog bites. Ophthalmic Plast Reconstr Surg. 2013;29(3):179–82.
10. Talan DA, Citron DM, Abrahamian FM, Moran GJ, Goldstein EJ. Bacteriologic analysis of infected dog and cat bites. Emergency Medicine Animal Bite Infection Study Group. N Engl J Med. 1999;340(2):85–92.
11. Morera Montes J, Lucena Martín MJ, Morera Navarro V, Gómez GM. Pasteurella multocida cellulitis after cat bite and subsequent erythema nodosum. SEMERGEN. 2017;43(4):340–2.
12. Foster MD, Hudson JW. Contemporary update on the treatment of dog bite: injuries to the oral and maxillofacial region. J Oral Maxillofac Surg. 2015;73(5):935–42.
13. Holmgren EP, Dierks EJ, Assael LA, Bell RB, Potter BE. Facial soft tissue injuries as an aid to ordering a combination head and facial computed tomography in trauma patients. J Oral Maxillofac Surg. 2005;63(5):651–4.
14. Oleck NC, Dobitsch AA, Liu FC, et al. Traumatic falls in the pediatric population: facial fracture patterns observed in a leading cause of childhood injury. Ann Plast Surg. 2019;82:S195.
15. Liu HP, Shao Y, Yu XJ, Zhang D. A simplified surgical algorithm for flap reconstruction of eyebrow defects. J Plast Reconstr Aesthet Surg. 2017;70(4):450–8.
16. Jones YJ, Georgesuc D, McCann JD, Anderson RL. Microwave warm compress burns. Ophthalmic Plast Reconstr Surg. 2010;26(3):219.
17. Jovanovic N, Dizdarevic A, Dizdarevic N, Haracic A, Gafurovic L. Case report of Wolfe grafting for the management of bilateral cicatricial eyelid ectropion following severe burn injuries. Ann Med Surg (Lond). 2018;34:58–61.
18. Cabalag MS, Wasiak J, Syed Q, Paul E, Hall AJ, Cleland H. Risk factors for ocular burn injuries requiring surgery. J Burn Care Res. 2017;38(2):71–7.
19. Choi SO, Chung TY, Shin YJ. Impairment of tear film and the ocular surface in patients with facial burns. Burns. 2017;43(8):1748–56.
20. Cabalag MS, Wasiak J, Syed Q, Paul E, Hall AJ, Cleland H. Early and late complications of ocular burn injuries. J Plast Reconstr Aesthet Surg. 2015;68(3):356–61.

The Nasolacrimal System

Nora Siegal and Christopher B. Chambers

Contents

© Springer Nature Switzerland AG 2021
R. Shinder (ed.), *Pediatric Ophthalmology in the Emergency Room*,
https://doi.org/10.1007/978-3-030-49950-1_6

6.1 Introduction

6.1.1 Development of the Nasolacrimal System

The nasolacrimal system begins to develop in utero at approximately 6 weeks. At this time, an epithelial layer of ectodermal tissue is entrapped as a core between the (medial) maxillary process and (lateral) frontonasal process. Fusion of the lateral nasal prominence with the maxillary prominence entraps a double layer of epithelial cells which later canalizes to form the lacrimal outflow system. Over the next several months, this horizontally oriented cord of cells assumes its final, mature vertical position (□ Fig. 6.1). Improper or incomplete development of this system can be associated with epiphora, discharge, dacryocystitis, or cellulitis.

The upper portions of the nasolacrimal system include the puncta, canaliculi, and common canaliculus [1]. Atresia or agenesis of the puncta is not uncommon. Typically, there is a veil or membrane consisting of the conjunctiva that occludes the punctal orifice. Although this may present as a small dimple in the eyelid margin, it is often difficult to appreciate. Gentle pressure along the mucocutaneous junction of

the medial eyelid may aid in the discovery of a hidden punctum. A cutdown of this region can also be performed but is not recommended in the hands of an inexperienced lacrimal surgeon. Congenital absence of the punctum is rare and usually seen in syndromes such as ectrodactyly-ectodermal dysplasia-clefting (EEC) syndrome and lacrimo-dento-digital syndrome (Levy Hollister) [2, 3] (□ Fig. 6.2). Gross examination of the puncta through gentle eversion of the eyelids will reveal whether punctal atresia is present.

Abnormalities of the lower portions of the nasolacrimal system (the lacrimal sac and nasolacrimal duct) typically result from abnormal canalization of the epithelial core. Canalization begins at approximately 16 weeks, and abnormal separation of epithelial cells can result in fistulae between the lacrimal sac and either the nasal cavity (internally) or the skin (externally). External fistulae can often manifest in a pediatric patient as a secondary punctum located inferior and medial to the normal punctum (□ Fig. 6.3). If an internal fistula is present, fluid can get trapped in the nasolacrimal system. The entrapped fluid (which can be mucous, causing a mucocele, or amniotic fluid causing an amniotocele) may present in a neonate as a cystic distention

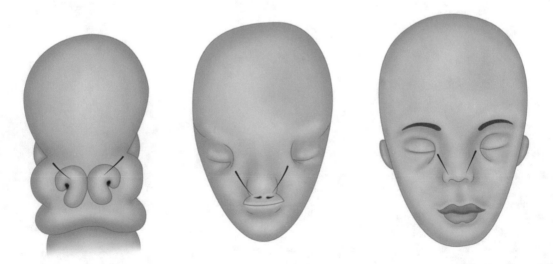

□ **Fig. 6.1** Nasolacrimal duct formation. Fusion of the lateral nasal prominence with the maxillary prominence entraps a double layer of epithelial cells which later canalizes to form the lacrimal outflow system. As

the face develops, this cord of cells (red) shifts from a horizontal orientation to vertical position. (Illustration credit: Christopher B Chambers)

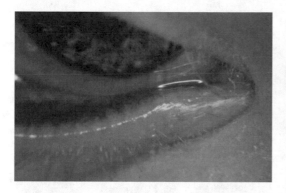

Fig. 6.2 Congenital absence of the punctum of the lower eyelid. (Courtesy of William Katowitz, MD)

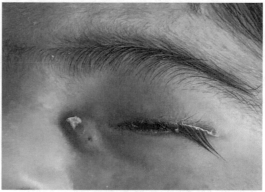

Fig. 6.4 Acute dacryocystitis revealing erythema and induration of the lacrimal sac with early abscess formation. Note mattering of the lashes with mucous discharge lining the eyelid margins

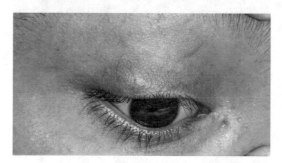

Fig. 6.3 External nasolacrimal fistula can manifest as a secondary punctum located inferior and medial to the normal punctum (arrow)

below the medial canthus. These entities can be evaluated in the emergency room through the use of ultrasonography or simple nasal endoscopy. Importantly, dacryocystoceles have been reported to extend into the nasal cavity and may cause respiratory distress [4].

Infection or inflammation of the nasolacrimal system can occur in the setting of nonpatency. The most common etiology is the presence of a membrane covering the distal nasolacrimal ostium at the valve of Hasner. On exam, this manifests as a resistance to probing in the lower portion of the system. Pediatric patients typically present with tearing and mucopurulent discharge, which is followed by the appearance of an inflamed mass below the medial canthus (**Fig. 6.4**). Stagnant tears within a non-patent system allow bacteria, which typically get drained through the lacrimal system into the nose, to proliferate within the lacrimal system and cause infection. The most common organisms are Gram-positive cocci such as *Streptococcus*

Pneumoniae, *Staphylococcus*, and Gram-negative *Enterobacteriaceae* [5]. Nasolacrimal probing should not be performed in the setting of active infection or inflammation due to the friability of the tissues and the risk of creating a false passage within the system and thus the spread of the infection. Children presenting with evidence of dacryocystitis should receive broad-spectrum antibiotics and should undergo thorough imaging of the orbits if orbital cellulitis is suspected.

Congenital nasolacrimal duct obstructions must be distinguished from other, nonobstructive functional abnormalities in the evaluation of a pediatric patient with tearing. Eyelid malpositions that can also result in tearing include entropion/ectropion, colobomas, masses, or telecanthus/hypertelorism can result in poor punctum-to-globe apposition. Eyelash abnormalities such as trichiasis (inversion of normally located lashes) and distichiasis (accessory row of lashes) can irritate the cornea and conjunctiva resulting in discomfort, redness, and tearing. These conditions are best evaluated with the use of a slit lamp microscope.

The mechanism of tear drainage is facilitated by a combination of positive pressure created by blinking and negative pressure induced by both capillary action and suction within the drainage apparatus. The secretory portion of the lacrimal system is composed of the main and accessory lacrimal glands, located superotemporally to the globe within the lacrimal fossa of the frontal bone and within the palpebral conjunctival stroma, respectively. These glands provide lubrication for the cornea by secreting tears which ultimately accumulate as a tear lake along the margin of each eyelid [6]. The excretory portion of the lacrimal system, which includes the puncta, canaliculi, lacrimal sac, and nasolacrimal duct, allows for drainage of excess tears (◘ Fig. 16.1). The puncta are 0.3 mm concavities located at the medial aspect of both the superior and inferior lid margins. They are continuous with the superior and inferior ampullae, respectively, which are 2 mm in length and oriented perpendicular to the eyelid margin. These ampullae drain tears into the superior and inferior canaliculi (8 mm in length) which usually come together as a common canaliculus. The common canaliculus opens into the lacrimal sac (10–12 mm in length) which is located in the lacrimal sac fossa, comprised anteriorly by the frontal process of the maxillary bone and posteriorly by the lacrimal bone. The sac is continuous with the nasolacrimal duct (12–18 mm) and empties below the inferior turbinate at the inferior meatus within the nasal cavity (◘ Fig. 6.5) (◘ Table 6.1).

◘ **Table 6.1**   Nasolacrimal Anatomy

Lacrimal outflow pathway	Length (mm)	Anatomical pathway
Superior and inferior ampullae	2	Continuous with the puncta and drain tears into the superior and inferior canaliculi
Superior and inferior canaliculi	8	Usually come together as the common canaliculus which opens into the lacrimal sac
Lacrimal sac	10–12	Located in the lacrimal sac fossa (maxillary and lacrimal bones) and is continuous with the nasolacrimal duct
Nasolacrimal duct	12–18	Empties below the inferior turbinate at the inferior meatus within the nasal cavity

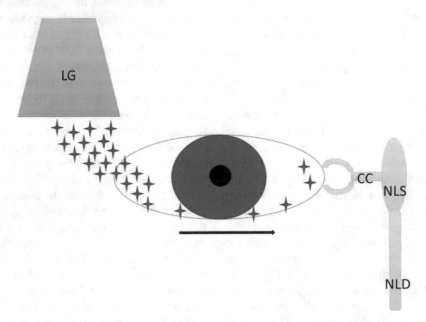

◘ **Fig. 6.5** Schematic representation of the lacrimal apparatus of the right eye. Tears produced in the lacrimal gland (LG) are released onto the surface of the globe and accumulate as a tear lake along the eyelid margin. These tears are drawn into the superior and inferior canaliculi through negative pressure and then travel through the common canaliculus (CC). Tears collect in the lacrimal sac (NLS) where they remain in between each blink. Tears are then forced down the nasolacrimal duct (NLD) and empty into the nose

Normal tear drainage requires proper functioning of the entire nasolacrimal system. At the beginning of a blink, the tear drainage system contains tears that have been provided by the lacrimal gland and accessory glands. Eyelid closure, achieved by contraction of the pretarsal orbicularis oculi muscle, moves the puncta medially and posteriorly and compresses the canaliculi. This action forces tears within the system to move down the nasolacrimal duct into the nasal cavity [6]. After orbicularis relaxation, the components of the lacrimal pump reopen to create a negative pressure in the lacrimal sac which draws tears down into the drainage system (◻ Fig. 16.2). Obstruction at any level can result in epiphora, with proximal obstruction leading to clear tear discharge and distal obstruction leading to mucoid discharge.

6.2 Canalicular Trauma

Eyelid lacerations are very common in both blunt and penetrating trauma to the face due to the delicate nature of eyelid tissues. Penetrating injuries due to sharp objects such as knives, broken glass, or metallic tools require a careful evaluation of both the globe and soft tissues. The presence of foreign bodies and the extent of orbital injury must be evaluated through the use of CT imaging. Dog bites, a common cause of eyelid lacerations in children, are reported to involve canalicular damage in 66% of cases [7]. In a study by Savar et al. [7], the majority of these injuries involved damage to the inferior canaliculus [7]. Canalicular lacerations are common with medial canthal tendon avulsion, which is often the result of shearing forces [8]. If the medial canthal tendon is disinserted, it should be reattached to the posterior lacrimal crest if possible. Normally, the medial canthal tendon has two limbs that surround the lacrimal sac within the lacrimal sac fossa (◻ Fig. 16.2). The anterior limb attaches to the frontal process of the maxilla (anterior lacrimal crest), while the posterior limb attaches to the lacrimal bone (posterior lacrimal crest). Appropriate repositioning of the medial canthal tendon establishes normal, anatomic tone of the lower lid

around the globe and decreases the likelihood of post-traumatic epiphora.

In the emergency department, physicians should determine the tetanus status of the patient and administer broad-spectrum antibiotics and pain control prior to wound exploration [9]. Soft tissue lacerations can be irrigated with saline via a high-pressure syringe and cleaned with hydrogen peroxide to ensure that all foreign bodies and dried blood are removed. Canalicular injuries can be missed upon gross inspection, and it should be presumed that the canaliculus has been violated if an eyelid margin laceration is full thickness and medial to the punctum [8, 10]. Magnification using a slit lamp or surgical loupes can aid in the assessment of canalicular trauma. Damage to the canalicular system is diagnosed through punctal probing. A topical anesthetic is instilled into the fornix, and a punctal dilator can be used to dilate the punctum. A series of lacrimal probes are then introduced into the nasolacrimal system in the following fashion: perpendicular to the eyelid margin for 2 mm and then turned at a sharp 90° angle to be parallel to the lid margin toward the medial canthus. Providing slight lateral tension on the eyelid facilitates the easier movement of the probe through the canaliculus. If the end of the lacrimal probe can be visualized during this procedure, a canalicular laceration is confirmed. Another method of evaluating canalicular trauma is through the use of lacrimal irrigation. A 1 or 3 mL syringe filled with normal saline can be attached to a blunt irrigation cannula. This can be inserted into the punctum and proximal canaliculus so that saline is instilled slowly. If the canalicular system is lacerated, the saline will efflux out of the system instead of traveling down into the nasopharynx. Simple probing is the preferred method as it may be difficult to differentiate reflux from true efflux in a lacerated canalicular system.

6.3 Canalicular Laceration Repair

Many studies have revealed that canalicular injuries are more common in young, male patients. Reports cite between 54% and 83% of canalicular lacerations being in this patient population [11–13]. Common mechanisms of injury include physical altercations, accidents in high-speed vehicles, dog bites, and sport-related injuries. Most oculoplastic surgeons agree that canalicular repair should occur within 72 hours of trauma to prevent granulation tissue from obscuring anatomy and leading to stenosis of the nasolacrimal system and possible fistula formation [14, 15]. There are several factors that determine whether repair at the bedside or in the operating room is undertaken, including the patient's age, health status, level of comfort, other associated injuries, and the experience and preference of the surgeon. Studies have suggested that the success of canalicular repair is highly dependent upon the surgeon's training level, and when possible, oculoplastic surgeons should be consulted for such repairs [13].

The debate regarding mono- vs bicanalicular stenting for canalicular repair is ongoing with no clear difference in outcome. Repair using a monocanalicular stent (Mini Monoka stent, FCI Ophthalmics Inc., Pembroke, MA) involves only the injured canaliculus. Bicanalicular stenting through the use of a Crawford tube (FCI Ophthalmics Inc., Pembroke, MA) requires that the stent be passed through the uninjured canaliculus and thus puts it at risk for injury [15]. When a Mini Monoka stent is used, it gets seated in place at the level of the punctum. Although monocanalicular stents have the advantage of easy removal with only forceps in the office, their placement at the level of the punctum prevents tear drainage while they are in place. Patients who receive a monocanalicular stent should be counseled that tearing will likely occur while the tube is in place and the tissues are healing. Bicanalicular stents are typically secured endonasally during canalicular repair, and removal in the office can be more complex, sometimes requiring the use of an endoscope and/or endonasal anesthesia. In young children, there may be a need to return to the operat-

ing room for sedation in order to safely remove a bicanalicular stent.

Canalicular repair can be performed under local anesthesia at the bedside or on under general anesthesia in the operating room. The ideal setting is determined by the patient's age, level of cooperation, and the surgeon's comfort level. All young children must be taken to the operating room for optimal repair. Once the eyelids have been cleaned and infiltrated with a local anesthetic, the distal end of the canalicular laceration must be found. This step is best achieved in good lighting with the use of a headlight and an assistant who can help with retraction and hemostasis. The lacerated ends of the canaliculus look like blood vessels cut in the coronal plane or small holes lined by mucosa [16]. If the distal cut end cannot be found by examination with surgical loupes or a microscope, injection of saline or fluorescein solution can be performed into the uninjured canaliculus. Efflux of fluid can be seen coming from the distal cut end. Another technique is to instill a few drops of 2.5% phenylephrine into the laceration, which may cause the pouting of the cut canaliculus [15–17]. After the distal end is found, a lacrimal probe should be passed through the cut end to ensure a hard-stop on the lacrimal bone. The monocanalicular stent can then be cut to size and threaded through the proximal end of the laceration and through the distal end. Trimming of the stent should be minimal to allow proper bridging of the distance between the cut ends. The trimmed edge of the stent is then threaded into the nasolacrimal system using either non-toothed forceps to prevent stent trauma or a needle driver in a hand-over-hand technique. This step can be challenging and requires patience as the stent has a tendency to prolapse back especially if the stent is left overly long. Once the stent is partially threaded into the nasolacrimal system, the pericanalicular soft tissues can be reapproximated. This step is best achieved through the use of an assistant who can help realign the tissues and prevent stent prolapse. A 5-0 polyglactin suture on a small, half-circle needle can help facilitate suture passes in the pericanalicular tissue and also in the medial canthal region in the setting of an avulsed medial canthus. Proper alignment of the two ends of the laceration reestablishes the eyelid anatomy and increases the likelihood of nasolacrimal system patency after healing has taken place. Once the repair is complete, the lower eyelid should be well approximated to the globe. Antibiotic ointment is applied to the wounds for 1–2 weeks. The monocanalicular stent can be removed in the office 3 months following repair (◻ Figs. 6.6 and 6.7).

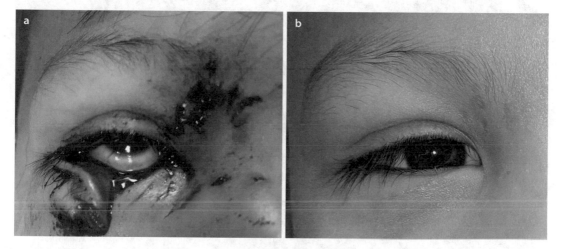

◻ **Fig. 6.6** Five-year-old boy who suffered a dog bite with resultant right lower eyelid canaliculus-involving laceration and medial canthal avulsion **a**. Postoperative month 3 status post-repair of the lower eyelid **b**

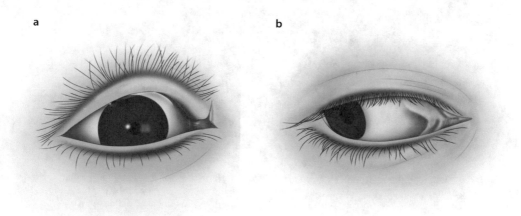

◻ **Fig. 6.7** A 17-year-old male who suffered a basketball injury resulting in a laceration of the upper canaliculus and medial conjunctiva **a**. Postoperative week 1.5 status post-repair of upper eyelid laceration and conjunctiva **b**

6

A 4-year-old boy presented to the emergency room after running into a wire fence during recess at school. Exam was notable for a left lower eyelid laceration involving the inferior canaliculus (◘ Fig. 6.8a). Lacrimal probing revealed the distal cut end of the canalicular laceration (◘ Fig. 6.8b). CT of the orbits did not reveal any fractures. The patient underwent immediate surgical repair with placement of a Mini Monoka stent. At postoperative month 3, the monocanalicular stent was removed. The lower lid was nicely apposed to the globe, and there was a normal tear lake, suggesting proper alignment of the nasolacrimal system (◘ Fig. 6.8c).

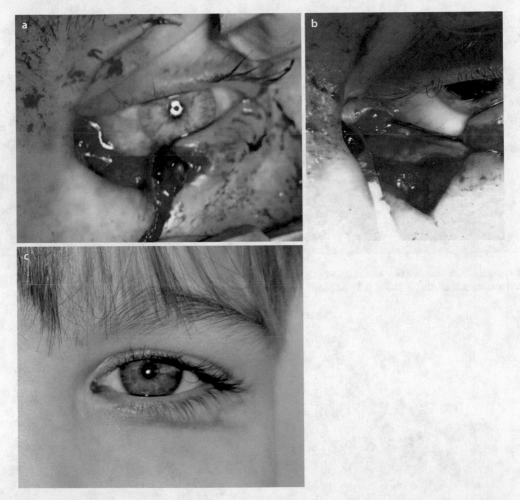

◘ **Fig. 6.8** Clinical photograph showing full-thickness medial left lower eyelid laceration including canalicular laceration **a**. Intraoperative photograph showing a lacrimal probe placed within the distal cut end of the canaliculus **b**. Postoperative photograph showing good lid position **c**

Key Points

- The nasolacrimal system begins to develop in utero at 6 weeks. Improper or incomplete development of this system can be associated with epiphora, discharge, dacryocystitis, or cellulitis.
- The secretory portion of the lacrimal system is composed of the main and accessory lacrimal glands, located superotemporally to the globe within the lacrimal fossa of the frontal bone and within the palpebral conjunctival stroma, respectively. These glands provide lubrication for the cornea by secreting tears which ultimately accumulate as a tear lake along the margin of each eyelid.
- The excretory portion of the lacrimal system, which includes the puncta, canaliculi, lacrimal sac, and nasolacrimal duct, allows for drainage of excess tears.
- Canalicular trauma is common in children and can be the result of either blunt or penetrating injury.
- Evaluation of canalicular trauma should be performed urgently and referral to an oculoplastic surgeon for repair should be made.
- Canalicular repair can be performed under local anesthesia at the bedside or on under general anesthesia in the operating room within 72 hours of trauma.

❓ Review Questions

1. The anatomic pathway of the nasolacrimal system is punctum → canaliculus → common canaliculus, then?
   (a) Semilunar fold → lacrimal sac → nasolacrimal duct → valve of Hasner
   (b) Valve of Rosenmüller → lacrimal sac → nasolacrimal duct → valve of Hasner
   (c) Valve of Hasner → lacrimal sac → nasolacrimal duct → valve of Rosenmüller
   (d) Semilunar fold → lacrimal sac → nasolacrimal duct → valve of Hasner

2. The nasolacrimal duct opens below the:
   (a) Inferior turbinate
   (b) Superior turbinate
   (c) Middle turbinate
   (d) Middle meatus

3. Which bones comprise the lacrimal sac fossa?
   (a) Maxillary and lacrimal
   (b) Maxillary and ethmoid
   (c) Ethmoid and lacrimal
   (d) Maxillary and zygoma

✅ Answer

1. (b)
2. (a)
3. (a)

References

1. Herzum H, Holle P, Hintschich C. Eyelid injuries: epidemiological aspects. Ophthalmologe. 2001;98:1079–82.
2. Low JE, Johnson MA, Katowitz JA. Management of pediatric upper system problems: punctal and canalicular surgery. In: Katowitz JA, editor. Pediatric oculoplastic surgery. New York: Springer-Verlag; 2002. p. 337–46.
3. Hurwitz JJ. Embryology of the lacrimal drainage system. In: Hurwitz JJ, editor. The lacrimal system. Philadelphia: Lippincott-Raven; 1996. p. 9–13.
4. Grin TR, Mertz JS, Stass-Isern M. Congenital nasolacrimal duct cysts in dacryocystocele. Ophthalmology. 1991;98(8):1238–42.
5. Huber-Spitzy V, Steinkogler FJ, Haselberger C. The pathogen spectrum in noenatal dacryocystitis. Klin Monatsbl Augenheilkd. 1987;190(5):445–6.
6. Records RE. The conjunctiva and lacrimal system. In: Tasman W, Jaeger EA, editors. Duane's clinical ophthalmology (2005 Ed [CD ROM]). Philadelphia: Lippincott, Williams & Wilkins; 2010.
7. Savar A, Kirszrot J, Rubin PA. Canalicular involvement in dog bite related eyelid lacerations. Ophthal Plast Reconstr Surg. 2008;24(4):296–8.

8. Nerad JA. Eyelid and orbital trauma. In: Nerad JA, editor. Techniques in ophthalmic plastic surgery. New York: Saunders Elsevier; 2010. p. 356–67.

9. Katowitz JA. Pediatric orbital trauma. In: Katowitz JA, editor. Pediatric oculoplastic surgery. 2nd ed. New York: Springer; 2002. p. 648.

10. Rattan GH, Kulwin DR, Levine M, et al. Management of ocular adnexal trauma. In: Black EH, Nesi FA, Calvano CJ, Gladstone GJ, Levine MR, editors. Smith and Nesi's ophthalmic plastic and reconstructive surgery. 3rd ed. New York: Springer; 2012. p. 207–29.

11. Kennedy RH, May J, Dailey J, Flanagan JC. Canalicular laceration: an 11-year epidemiologic and clinical study. Ophthal Plast Reconstr Surg. 1990;6(1):46–53.

12. Naik M, Kelapure A, Rath S, Honavar SG. Management of canalicular lacerations: epidemiological aspects and experience with mini-monoka monocanalicular stent. Am J Ophthalmol. 2008;145(2): 375–80.

13. Murchison A, Bilyk J. Canalicular laceration repair: an analysis of variables affecting success. Ophthal Plast Reconstr Surg. 2014;30(5):410–4.

14. Jordan DR. To reconstruct or not. Ophthalmology. 2000;107(6):1022–3.

15. Kalin-Hajdu E, Cadet N, Boulos P. Controversies of the lacrimal system. Surv Ophthalmol. 2015;61:309.

16. Eo S, Park J, Cho S, Azari KK. Microsugrical reconstruction for canalicular laceration using monostent and mini-monoka. Ann Plast Surg. 2010;64(4): 421–7.

17. Cho SH, Hyun DW, Kang HJ, Ha MS. A simple new method for identifying the proximal cut end in lower canalicular laceration. Korean J Ophthalmol. 2008;22(2):73–6.

Pediatric Corneal Emergencies

Douglas R. Lazzaro and Jennifer Barger

Contents

© Springer Nature Switzerland AG 2021
R. Shinder (ed.), *Pediatric Ophthalmology in the Emergency Room*,
https://doi.org/10.1007/978-3-030-49950-1_7

7.1 **Introduction**

The cornea is contiguous with the sclera and helps form the outer tunic of the eye. The cornea is a five-layered structure that protects the inner structures of the eye but also serves as a refractive surface (● Fig. 7.1). The cornea must remain clear in order for the eye to see well.

The tear film sits on the corneal epithelium, the outermost part of the cornea. This multilayered nonkeratinized epithelium regenerates itself normally and in disease. It is firmly anchored to its underlying basement membrane by hemi-desmosomes [1]. Bowman's layer sits between the epithelium and the stromal layer. At the posterior stroma resides Descemet's membrane, a true basement membrane. Internal to Descemet's membrane is a single layer of hexagonal cells comprising the corneal endothelium.

Many disorders affect various parts of the cornea. The cornea can be examined grossly in the emergency room with a penlight. For further magnification, a penlight can be used in conjunction with a 20-diopter lens. The slit lamp microscope is the ideal exam tool which offers great illumination, optical viewing, and much higher magnification. After concluding whether the cornea is clear or hazy, one can use topical anesthesia with fluorescein strips to determine corneal epithelial integrity. Using fluorescein and a cobalt blue light, one can detect a violation of the epithelium (● Fig. 7.2). One can also look for a positive Seidel test where aqueous humor is streaming out of the eye in anterior ruptured globes, thereby diluting the fluorescein [2].

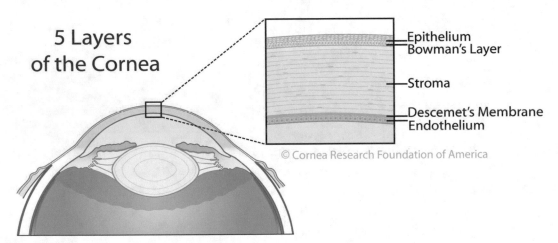

● **Fig. 7.1** Schematic diagram showing the layers of the cornea. (Used with permission from the Cornea Research Foundation of America)

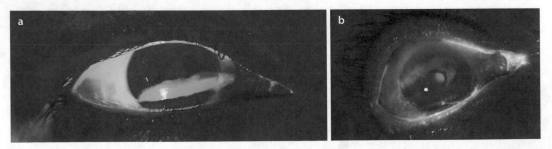

● **Fig. 7.2** Slit lamp and external photographs displaying fluorescein staining where the corneal epithelium is violated in corneal abrasions. One classic pattern is an abrasion within the interpalpebral fissure **a**. There may be more focal loss resulting in punctate staining defects **b**

7.2 Emergency Diseases Affecting the Cornea

7.2.1 Corneal Abrasion

The cornea can be abraded from innumerable sources. These abrasions can vary from very small to very large and even affect the entire corneal epithelium. The history often aids in making the diagnosis, indicating the cause and nature of the abrasion. Fingernails, paper, leaves and branches, hairbrushes, eyeliner wands, toys, and pet claws are among the common etiologies.

After ascertaining the nature of the injury, ask about any treatment prior to presentation. The use of contact lenses should be specifically asked about. The patient with corneal abrasion presents with pain, tearing, light sensitivity, and decreased vision.

Visual changes should be assessed with a near card, and pupils also should be examined thoroughly. There have been cases of ruptured globes being misdiagnosed as a corneal abrasion, and sometimes, the shape of the pupil can help in proper diagnosis. In cases of suspected foreign bodies (cutting wood or metal on a machine), it is important to not only inspect the cornea but also evert the lids and examine the fornices to identify additional foreign bodies. Fluorescein staining is very helpful in detecting a corneal abrasion (◘ Fig. 7.2). Measure the abrasion size if possible at the slit lamp. Anterior chamber inflammation is sometimes present on slit lamp exam as well.

The treatment of corneal abrasion includes topical prophylactic antibiotics (generally fluoroquinolones or aminoglycosides) and sometimes cycloplegic agents (such as cyclopentolate1% twice daily) for comfort. The use of a patch depends on the size and type of abrasion. If a contact-lens-related infection or contact with wood matter are possible causes of the abrasion, patching should be avoided. A bandage contact lens can be used in small or large abrasions, but we prefer to patch large abrasions. Similar time to healing [3] and similar percent of healing [4] were observed with both patching and topical therapy. However, patching does temporarily limit depth perception by preventing binocular vision [3, 4]. Patching may represent a good strategy in young children, as the need for topical medication applied several times daily is obviated. Additionally, keeping the eye closed under a patch will keep the child more comfortable rather than feel the discomfort that comes with each blink over an abraded cornea. Pain will likely persist until the epithelium regenerates.

Case Presentation

A child experienced a scratch by a fingernail. Note the epithelial defect with fluorescein uptake (◘ Fig. 7.3). The fluorescein is also taken up by tear film at the lid margins.

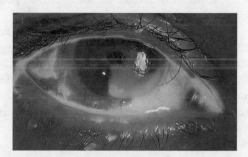

◘ **Fig. 7.3** Clinical photograph of an inferomedial corneal abrasion with fluorescein staining

7.2.2 Chemical Burn

The cornea is very susceptible to both acid and alkali burns (the latter tend to be more severe). Take a careful history, and determine what the toxic substance is. Try to figure out the pH and obtain the data sheet on the chemical with the help of poison control. In children, battery acid and laundry detergent pods have been noted to cause ocular injury. These eyes need to be irrigated extensively and have antibiotics applied promptly.

The time of injury and any treatment prior to the emergency department visit should be ascertained. Chemical burn patients require a complete eye exam. Most of these patients have severe pain, tearing, and decreased vision. In the cases of severe burns, a "white" eye can be indicative of an ischemic process which carries a poor prognosis.

The mainstay of treatment is determining the pH and trying to normalize it through copious irrigation with sterile water or a balanced saline solution [5]. A Morgan lens used with topical anesthesia can be very helpful to administer the irrigation. It's important to sweep the fornices with a cotton tip applicator to remove any toxin or toxin-containing particulates from the ocular adnexa. Restoring the pH of tears to the physiologic range (7.3–7.7) may require prolonged irrigation and repeated forniceal sweeping. The corneal exam will reveal superficial punctate keratitis or frank abrasion upon the application of fluorescein. If a very large abrasion or ischemia is noted, a Seidel test may be appropriate to ensure the burn has not penetrated the full thickness of the cornea.

The treatment of chemical burns includes antibiotic drops, copious use of preservative-free artificial tears, and very close follow-up. Surgical management may take place at a later time if the burn is severe and may involve amniotic membrane graft, keratoprosthesis, or limbal cell transplant.

> Patients who present with a suspected ocular chemical burn should be examined immediately. Irrigation must be initiated emergently after checking a visual acuity and initial pH of the tear film if equipment is available. Use urine pH paper or a wider-range pH paper. Check pH prior to the instillation of topical anesthesia and irrigation if possible; however, do not delay initiation of irrigation if these tools are not immediately available. Pause irrigation for 10 minutes to allow tear film pH to reflect its true pH and not that of the irrigation fluid once appropriate pH paper is available.

7.2.3 Corneal Foreign Body

When a corneal foreign body is suspected, the examiner should take a thorough history, and determine the nature of the injury. Was it while walking outside or while cutting something? Did something enter the eye and remain there, or was it removed by the patient or someone else? When did the injury occur? Patients sometimes present immediately after suspected foreign body injury but also sometimes present days later due to persistent ocular irritation.

Inspect the everted lid and fornices as more than one foreign body can be present. It is important to assess the size and depth of the corneal foreign body. If very deep or partially in the anterior chamber, it may be best to remove under microscopic control in the operating room. For very superficial corneal foreign bodies, a cotton tip applicator may suffice for removal, but in the vast majority, it is necessary to use a bent needle carefully at the slit lamp as the foreign body is generally embedded partially in the corneal stroma. An epithelial defect will remain after the removal of the foreign body. If perforation is suspected, Seidel testing should also be performed before the foreign body removal and again afterward if removal at the slit lamp occurs.

> – Superficial corneal foreign bodies not associated with full-thickness corneal injury typically can be safely removed at the slit lamp with sufficient patient cooperation.
> – Very superficial foreign bodies may be removed with the use of a cotton tip applicator by gently brushing the foreign body in parallel with the corneal surface.
> – If this is not sufficient, use a very fine-gauge needle (the authors recommend a 30 gauge; however, 27 and 29 gauges such as sometimes found on a tuberculin syringe can be used). Bend the needle 30 degrees toward the examiner with the bevel also facing the examiner. Hold the eyelids open, and using the edge of the bevel gently, scrape the base of the foreign body in parallel with the corneal surface.

- After removing as much of the lodged material as possible, instill topical antibiotic drops and repeat Seidel testing to ensure that the corneal damage has not violated deeper layers or become full thickness.
- Sweep the everted eyelids with a cotton-tip applicator again to remove any loosened foreign material to prevent repeated injury.

An additional examination should also occur for concurrent injury to other ocular structures, including conjunctival or scleral lacerations, anterior chamber inflammation or hemorrhage, iris injury, or pupil peaking. There is a low likelihood of a concurrent intraocular foreign body [6].

The treatment of corneal foreign bodies is the prompt removal and use of topical antibiotics. In the case of wood matter, the possibility of fungus has to be considered if an infection develops. Corneal foreign bodies incurred while gardening can also carry a number of organisms including bacteria and fungi. Counsel patients to use protective eyewear as a preventative measure against recurrent injury [7].

Case Presentation

A child complained of pain after cutting metal during shop class due to a corneal foreign body (■ Fig. 7.4).

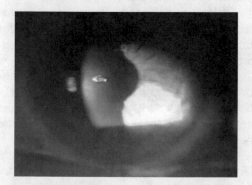

■ **Fig. 7.4** Slit lamp photograph displaying a superficial metallic corneal foreign body in the center of the visual axis

7.2.4 Corneal Laceration and Ruptured Globe

Open globe injuries in childhood are uncommon. The source of injury can be determined in most cases by a careful history. The object can be blunt or sharp, penetrating or perforating, and single or multiple. Examples of offending agents include pencils, pens, toys, balls, knives, and fences [8, 9].

The examination should start by assessing visual acuity and pupils. In the appropriate age group, visual acuity at presentation is the most important factor in visual and ocular prognosis; however, ensure the patient can tolerate examination without squeezing the eye which causes undue pressure on the globe [9]. It is important not to press on the eye (such as with an ultrasound probe) and provide adequate systemic analgesia in suspected cases of globe rupture, as the pressure can lead to intraocular content protrusion [10].

Look at the lids carefully—in the case of full-thickness lid lacerations, a cut into the sclera may sometimes be visible. The diagnosis of a corneal laceration can be made easily in some cases such as when uvea (iris) is protruding through the cornea (■ Figs. 7.5 and 7.6). In cases where the pupil is normal and there is no iris protrusion, a careful slit lamp exam is necessary. The depth of the anterior chamber and the integrity of the cornea can be helpful in making the diagnosis. A positive

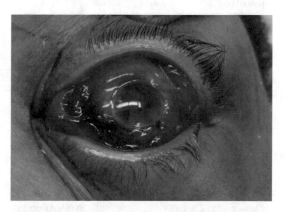

■ **Fig. 7.5** Clinical photograph of a full-thickness scleral laceration ruptured globe of the left eye showing uveal prolapse through the wound and a traumatic pupil. (Photo courtesy of Roman Shinder, MD)

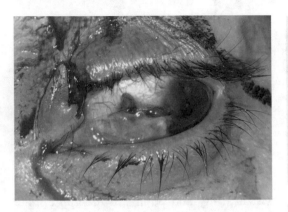

Place a clear rigid shield over an affected eye once a corneal laceration or any type of ruptured globe is identified. This provides protection from external pressure including the patient's hands. The clear material allows the patient to still appreciate the vision they have in the affected eye and notice any visual decline. Patients should be counseled to alert their provider if they notice any visual decline.

● **Fig. 7.6** Clinical photograph of a full-thickness corneoscleral laceration ruptured globe showing uveal prolapse through the wound and a traumatic pupil. (Photo courtesy of Solly Elman, MD)

CT is the preferred imaging modality if a ruptured globe is suspected. If there is any concern for a retained intraocular foreign body that is metallic, MRI is contraindicated. Ultrasound often requires applying pressure to the eye which could cause further ocular damage in addition to intraocular tissue expulsion from a wound. Wood material is difficult to visualize on many imaging modalities and a greater index of suspicion should be employed.

Seidel test is indicative of a leak and an open globe. CT can be helpful in posterior ruptures. Imaging can also be obtained if an intraocular foreign body is suspected but not visualized though MRI is contraindicated in this context given the possibility of a metallic foreign body [10]. In cases where the diagnosis is still in doubt but suspected, an exam under anesthesia may be warranted.

When the diagnosis of a ruptured globe is made, the evaluation can be stopped, and a clear rigid shield should be placed over the eye. Do not patch the eye as this may put additional pressure on the globe and also prevent the patient from appreciating visual changes. In the vast majority of cases, the lacerations do not self-seal, thus requiring repair in the operating room under general anesthesia.

The treatment of a ruptured cornea or globe is surgical in almost all cases. In the sterile environment of the operating room, the wound is carefully inspected and closed appropriately. Antibiotics are used intraoperatively and postoperatively to prevent endophthalmitis and direct extension of infection into surrounding tissues. The surgery should be performed within 24 hours of presentation, and prognosis depends on the extent of the injury and amount of damage to vital structures [8]. Further steps include patching and glasses use to prevent deprivation amblyopia in the operative eye, as well as a consistent follow-up to identify and manage further ocular morbidity [8].

7.2.5 Contact Lens Related Infection

Children are prescribed contact lenses typically around age 12. Although most contact lens wearers do not incur serious injuries, there are a number of problems that can arise from contact lens use. We will touch on some of the more common issues that can bring the patient to the emergency department.

Patients can overwear lenses, which causes redness and discomfort. The treatment for this is to stop the use of lenses and take a contact lens "holiday."

Giant papillary conjunctivitis is a condition seen in chronic lens users. The conjunctiva develops giant papillae on the undersurface of the upper lid, and the eye can become red with discharge. The treatment is usually a change in the lens (in addition to a lens holiday) and topical anti-inflammatory drops to reduce inflammation. We prefer topical antihistamines and low-dose steroids.

Contact-lens-related infections will be covered in ► Chap. 11.

Many contact-lens-related issues can be alleviated with a contact lens "holiday." Additional therapeutic strategies are targeted at the specific secondary infected or inflamed tissue.

Contact-lens-associated conditions: This patient is a 16-year-old contact lens wearer with a corneal infection (keratitis) as evidenced by round whitish stromal infiltrates with hazy margins inferiorly (□ Fig. 7.6).

Key Points

1. Corneal abrasions are extremely common and often easy to diagnose. Patients present with pain and tearing and a variable change in vision. Use fluorescein staining to determine size and location, and treatment should start soon after diagnosis. The goal of treatment is corneal re-epithelialization, pain control, and prevention of infection through antibiotic use.

2. Chemical injury can cause serious ocular morbidity. The patients look clinically much like the corneal abrasion patient: history distinguishes the two pathologies. The goal of treatment is the normalization of the surface pH through copious irrigation which in some severe cases may take 24–48 hours. Upon discharge, the patient should be using frequent artificial tears and topical antibiotics.

3. A corneal foreign body can be diagnosed in the emergency department by use of the slit lamp after taking a careful history. Removal of the foreign body is done at the slit lamp under high magnification and using topical anesthesia. Topical antibiotics and close follow-up should be arranged.

4. A pediatric ruptured globe is a true ophthalmic emergency requiring emergency intervention. Once the diagnosis

is made, a clear rigid shield (not a patch) is placed over the eye without placing any pressure on the globe. Topical and systemic antibiotics should be promptly begun and preparation for the operating room made for repair under general anesthesia.

5. Contact lens wearers presenting to the emergency room with a red eye need a careful eye exam to the emergency room must have infection ruled out by slit lamp examination. The patient may have just an epithelial defect on presentation and some inflammatory cells in the corneal stroma (not yet a well-defined corneal infectious infiltrate), and it is important to recognize the infection early. Treatment with a broad spectrum combination of antibacterial antibiotics should be initiated once the diagnosis is made to distinguish the possible entities including infection, overwear, and corneal abrasion, among others.

❓ Review Questions

1. A 6-year-old boy presents for evaluation after hitting his eye on the corner of a wooden table at home and is found to have a corneal foreign body. Which of the following would be included in the examination?
   (a) Fluorescein exam
   (b) Visual acuity
   (c) CT orbits
   (d) A and B
   (e) B and C
   (f) A, B, and C

(D: no CT typically indicated given the very low likelihood of concurrent intraocular foreign body if a corneal foreign body is identified)

2. Which imaging modality is most appropriate when there is concern for a full-thickness corneal laceration?
   (a) MRI
   (b) Ultrasound
   (c) CT
   (d) X-ray

3. Which finding present on the exam would **NOT** be expected secondary to contact-lens-related issues alone?
   (a) Papillary conjunctivitis
   (b) Punctate corneal abrasions
   (c) Follicular conjunctivitis
   (d) Bulbar conjunctival injection

4. True or false: A negative Seidel test indicates that a full-thickness corneal injury is present.

✅ Answers

1. (d)
2. (c)
3. (c)
4. False

References

1. DelMonte DW, Kim T. Anatomy and physiology of the cornea. J Cataract Refract Surg. 2011;37(3):588–98. https://doi.org/10.1016/j.jcrs.2010.12.037.

2. Seidel E. WeitereexperimentelleUnter-suchungen uber die Quelle und den Verlauf der intraokularenSafstromung: XII. Ueber den manometrischenNachweis des physiologischenDruckgefalleszwichenVoderkammer und SchlemmschemKanal. Arch Ophthalmol. 1921;107:101–4.

3. Lim CHL, Turner A, Lim BX. Patching for corneal abrasion.*Cochrane Database of Systematic Reviews* [Internet] 2016 [cited 2019Aug 6]. Available from:https://www.cochranelibrary.com/cdsr/doi/10.1002/14651858.CD004764.pub3/full.

4. Michael JG, Hug D, Dowd MD. Management of corneal abrasion in children: a randomized clinical trial. Ann Emerg Med. 2002;40:67–72. https://doi.org/10.1067/mem.2002.124757.

5. Herr RD, White GL Jr, Bernhisel K, Mamalis N, Swanson E. Clinical comparison of ocular irrigation fluids following chemical injury. Am J Emerg Med. 1991;9(3):228–31.

6. Luo Z, Gardiner M. The incidence of intraocular foreign bodies and other intraocular findings in patients with corneal metal foreign bodies. Ophthalmol. 2010;117(11):2218–21. https://doi.org/10.1016/j.ophtha.2010.02.034.

7. Kehat R, Bonsall DJ. Recurrent corneal metallic foreign bodies in children with autism spectrum disorders. J AAPOS. 2009;13(6):621–2. https://doi.org/10.1016/j.jaapos.2009.10.005.

8. Li X, Zarbin MA, Bhagat N. Pediatric open globe injury: a review of the literature. J Emerg Trauma Shock. 2015;8(4):216–23. https://doi.org/10.4103/0974-2700.166663.

9. Segev F, El A, Harizman N, Barequet I, Almer Z, Raz J, Moisseiev J. Corneal laceration by sharp objects in children ages seven years of age and younger. Cornea. 2007;26(3):319–23.

10. Kubal WS. Imaging of orbital trauma. Radiographics. 2008;28(6):1729–39. https://doi.org/10.1148/rg.286085523.

7

Anterior Chamber and Lens

Laura Palazzolo, Nicole Lanza, and Allison E. Rizzuti

Contents

© Springer Nature Switzerland AG 2021
R. Shinder (ed.), *Pediatric Ophthalmology in the Emergency Room*,
https://doi.org/10.1007/978-3-030-49950-1_8

8.1 Introduction

The anterior chamber of the eye is the aqueous humor-filled space bordered by the cornea anteriorly and the iris and lens posteriorly. The *iridocorneal angle* created by the intersection of the iris root and the peripheral cornea is an important anatomical landmark which houses the ciliary body, scleral spur, Schlemm's canal, and the trabecular meshwork. These structures are responsible for the production and drainage of aqueous humor and for controlling the size of the pupillary aperture.

The crystalline lens lies directly posterior to the pupillary diaphragm. It is held in place by suspensory ligaments called *zonules of Zinn*, which extend from the ciliary body to the lens. The normal lens is a transparent structure responsible for maintaining its own clarity, refracting light, and providing accommodation.

Slit lamp biomicroscopy is used to directly visualize the anterior chamber, while a mirrored lens called a gonioscope must be placed directly on the cornea to view the internal angle structures. Gonioscopy may be difficult to perform on a child, as the examination can be uncomfortable and requires stable positioning at the slit lamp. Other imaging modalities such as ultrasound biomicroscopy (UBM) and anterior segment ocular coherence tomography (AS-OCT) are non-contact methods of visualizing the anterior chamber and angle and may be better tolerated in children.

While trauma to the anterior chamber can occur in isolation after blunt trauma to the eye, it often occurs in conjunction with injury to adjacent ocular tissues such as the cornea or retina. A complete ophthalmologic examination of the anterior and posterior segment is essential for all children presenting with eye trauma. B-scan ultrasonography is often necessary as the view to the fundus may be obscured by blood, inflammation, or another anterior segment pathology. MRI or CT should be obtained if there is a concern for open globe or orbital injury. Examination under anesthesia may be required if a complete ophthalmologic exam is unable to be performed in an uncooperative child.

8.1.1 Subconjunctival Hemorrhage

▪▪ Introduction

Subconjunctival hemorrhage (SCH) is an accumulation of blood in the subconjunctival space due to bleeding from a conjunctival or episcleral blood vessel. In young patients, trauma followed by contact lens wear is the most common causes of SCH [1]. The differential diagnosis for SCH in a child without a history of trauma is extensive and is outlined in ◘ Table 8.1. Non-accidental trauma is a rare but important cause of SCH that should be considered in the absence of other etiologies.

▪▪ Clinical Presentation and Diagnosis

Children with SCH typically present to the emergency room after trauma to the eye or, in cases of spontaneous subconjunctival hemorrhage, are brought in by their parents who notice the striking red spot of blood. Because SCH often accompanies trauma to other ocular structures, presenting symptoms can be

◘ **Table 8.1**   Differential diagnosis of subconjunctival hemorrhages

Causes	Examples
Traumatic	Blunt or penetrating trauma Birth trauma Surgical traumaContact lens associated Acute thoracic compression syndrome Non-accidental trauma
Acute hemorrhagic conjunctivitis	Enterovirus, Coxsackievirus, Kawasaki disease, Adenovirus
Valsalva maneuvers	Coughing, vomiting, straining
Oncologic	Neuroblastoma, leukemia, rhabdomyosarcoma
Hematologic	Hemophilia, thrombocytopenia
Vascular	Hypertension, diabetes, atherosclerosis
Drugs	Anticoagulants

variable; however, when SCH occurs in isolation, it is asymptomatic.

The diagnosis of SCH is made on physical examination alone, which reveals a flat, sharply circumscribed, localized collection of blood in the subconjunctival space (■ Fig. 8.1). It is typically described as involving a certain number of degrees of the conjunctiva (0–360). A complete anterior and posterior segment examination is important to rule out any coexisting injury. Three hundred sixty degrees of SCH is suspicious for globe rupture and may warrant surgical exploration.

■■ Management
Though the appearance of SCH may be alarming, patients must be reassured that SCH alone will resolve spontaneously and does not require treatment. Blood degradation and absorption will cause the red color of SCH to evolve into orange or yellow before complete absorption usually occurring between 1 and 2 weeks from onset [2].

8.1.2 Hyphema

■■ Introduction
A hyphema is the presence of blood within the anterior chamber of the eye. It most commonly occurs after blunt or penetrating trauma, with the presumed source of bleeding from tears in the anterior ciliary body and iris blood vessels [3]. Traumatic hyphema occurs at a rate of 17 per 100,000 per year with 70–75% of patients being children [4]. The majority of cases occur during sports, but other important causes include airbag, paintball, and nerf gun injuries [5–7].

Non-traumatic causes of hyphema are uncommon in children but include intraocular surgery, iris neovascularization, anterior chamber tumors, myotonic dystrophy, keratouveitis, leukemia, and bleeding disorders [8, 9]. A spontaneous hyphema from vascularized iris nodules is the most common presenting symptom of juvenile xanthogranuloma (JXG), a benign dermatologic disorder affecting infants and young children. Patients also present with a single (or rarely multiple) asymptomatic yellow and brown skin nodule. The nodules in JXG are benign and are the result of histiocyte proliferation [10].

As in the case of subconjunctival hemorrhage, a hyphema in the absence of known trauma or predisposing ocular or systemic disease should raise suspicion for non-accidental injury.

■■ Clinical Presentation and Diagnosis
Children with hyphema typically present after eye trauma with pain, photophobia, and decreased vision. The hyphema may be visualized via penlight or slit lamp examination as a layering of blood within the anterior chamber (■ Fig. 8.2) and can be graded as the percent of space it occupies (■ Table 8.2). A *microhyphema* refers to the presence of red blood cells suspended in the anterior chamber, and an *8-ball hyphema* describes an anterior chamber

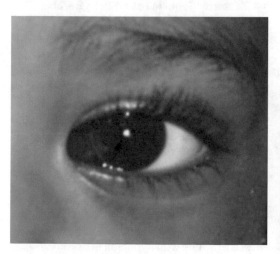

■ **Fig. 8.1** Clinical photograph of nasal subconjunctival hemorrhage

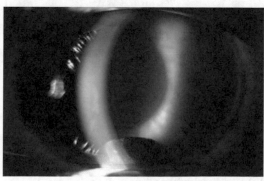

■ **Fig. 8.2** Clinical photograph showing hyphema

◾ **Table 8.2** Hyphema grading

Microhyphema	Circulating red blood cells
Grade I	≤ 1/3 anterior chamber volume
Grade II	1/3 to 1/2 anterior chamber volume
Grade III	> 1/2 anterior chamber volume
Grade IV	Total anterior chamber volume

that is completely filled with dark-clotted blood.

A complete ophthalmologic examination must be performed, as hyphema can signify severe ocular injury and damage to adjacent tissues. Dilated fundus exam should be attempted to evaluate concomitant posterior segment trauma, but B-scan ultrasound may be necessary as blood may obscure the view to the fundus. CT scan or MRI of the orbits may also be indicated if there is suspicion for globe rupture. Sickle cell prep and, if indicated, hemoglobin electrophoresis should be ordered, as the presence of sickle cell hemoglobinopathy will change management and prognosis. Laboratory workup including complete blood count, prothrombin time, partial thromboplastin time, liver function tests, and bleeding time should be considered in patients with bleeding disorders.

▪ Complications of Hyphema

Because of the complications that can be associated with hyphema, close follow-up is recommended until resolution of the layered clot. A secondary hemorrhage, or rebleed, can occur between 2 and 5 days of the initial trauma, and so daily follow-up is often recommended during this time. A rebleed carries a poor prognosis as it has been associated with increased intraocular pressure, corneal bloodstaining, and amblyopia. Rebleeds are more common in African American patients and patients with sickle cell disease [11].

▪ Elevated Intraocular Pressure and Optic Atrophy

Elevations in intraocular pressure (IOP) can occur from hyphemas of any size, and so IOP should be checked and closely monitored. The iCare tonometer (Tiolat Oy, Helsinki, Finland) is a newer, non-contact method of measuring intraocular pressure which is useful in the pediatric population. Elevated intraocular pressure (>22 mm hg) can lead to glaucoma or optic atrophy resulting in permanent vision loss. Particular attention must be given to the sickle cell patient with hyphema as sickled red blood cells can clog the trabecular meshwork leading to persistently elevated intraocular pressure in eyes that are more prone to optic atrophy. Lower thresholds for surgical intervention exist for these patients.

▪ Corneal Bloodstaining

Corneal bloodstaining occurs when hemoglobin and hemosiderin deposit into the corneal stroma typically due to severe and prolonged hyphema. The incidence is 5% of patients with hyphema, with risk factors including compromised corneal endothelium, large hyphemas, elevated intraocular pressure, and rebleed [4]. The pigment deposition results in a straw-yellow opacification of the cornea and subsequent vision loss. Corneal bloodstaining may take several months to 2 years to clear, which in children is problematic due to the risk of amblyopia. A corneal transplant may be indicated depending on the severity and duration of vision loss and the age of the child.

▪ Posterior Synechiae and Peripheral Anterior Synechiae

Prolonged inflammation and clot organization may produce both posterior synechiae (adhesions between the iris and lens) and peripheral anterior synechiae (adhesions between the iris and the trabecular meshwork). Both conditions can result in angle-closure glaucoma and vision loss if left untreated.

▪ Amblyopia

Visual deprivation due to the hyphema itself or from corneal bloodstaining obstructing the visual axis may lead to amblyopia. Though eye shields in adults with hyphema are often utilized to prevent additional trauma leading to rebleed, eye shields are avoided in children in order to reduce the risk of amblyopia [8]. The risk of traumatic hyphema-induced amblyopia may be overstated, however. In a study of 316 children with traumatic hyphema, only two patients developed amblyopia, and those two patients had concurrent traumatic cataracts [12].

■ ■ Management

All patients with hyphema are instructed to refrain from physical activity to prevent secondary hemorrhage and to elevate the head to promote gravitational layering and clot formation. Admission to the hospital should be considered if it seems unlikely that the child and/or caregivers will be able to follow the recommendations.

Most cases of traumatic hyphema respond well to medical management. Topical cycloplegics are prescribed for symptom relief and for the prevention of posterior synechiae. Topical steroids are routinely used to decrease inflammation and prevent subsequent peripheral anterior synechiae formation. Topical steroids carry their own risks however, namely, glaucoma and cataract formation, and so should be used cautiously in children. In a Cochrane meta-analysis comparing topical steroid use to controls, no significant difference was seen in time to resolution of primary hemorrhage, risk of secondary hemorrhage, or risk of elevated intraocular pressure; however they are used routinely in cases of hyphema to control inflammation and prevent synechiae [13]. Antifibrinolytics have been shown to decrease the rate of secondary rebleed, but they may delay clot resorption [8].

Aggressive treatment of elevated IOP is necessary to prevent corneal bloodstaining, optic atrophy, and glaucoma. Topical beta blockers are the first-line treatment of elevated IOP in children. An alternative or adjunctive option is a topical carbonic anhydrase inhibitor. Adrenergic agonists such as brimonidine are contraindicated in children due to the risk of central nervous system depression [14]. Systemic carbonic anhydrase inhibitors are used when topical medications fail to control the intraocular pressure.

Surgical evacuation of the hyphema or *anterior chamber washout* should be considered in the setting of non-resolving hyphema, persistently elevated IOP unresponsive to medical therapy, or visual deprivation in children who are at risk for amblyopia. In patients with sickle cell disease or trait, there should be a low threshold for surgical evacuation because of the increased risk of optic atrophy.

8.1.3 Traumatic Iritis

■ ■ Introduction

Traumatic iritis, or traumatic acute anterior uveitis, refers to inflammation of the iris and/or ciliary body following ocular trauma. It is the most common cause of uveitis in children accounting for up to 25% of childhood uveitis diagnoses [15]. Traumatic iritis is thought to be caused by the inflammatory response to cell injury and necrosis following trauma. Inflammatory mediators are released after injury, resulting in vasodilation, increased vascular permeability, and chemotaxis of inflammatory cells.

■ ■ Clinical Presentation and Diagnosis

Patients with traumatic iritis typically present 24–48 hours after traumatic eye injury complaining of photophobia, tearing, and blurry vision. Inflammatory cells and aqueous flare in the anterior chamber are visible on slit lamp examination. Irritation of the iris and ciliary body can cause spasm of accommodation and often results in a poorly dilating pupil. Intraocular pressure may initially be low due to transient shutdown of the ciliary body but may later rise secondary to trabecular meshwork swelling and obstruction by inflammatory debris [16].

■ ■ Management

Traumatic iritis is a self-limited process and will resolve on its own in 7–14 days; however, most patients are treated with topical cycloplegics and topical steroids for patient comfort and to prevent the formation of posterior synechiae and peripheral anterior synechiae. With the resolution of iritis, cycloplegics can be discontinued and steroids tapered to prevent rebound inflammation.

8.1.4 Iris Trauma: Sphincter Tear

Introduction Blunt trauma to the eye can cause tears in the iris sphincter muscle, resulting in pupillary abnormalities. Compressive forces generate horizontal stretching within the pupillary aperture in opposition to the resistance provided by the lens, resulting in disruption of the marginal sphincter fibers [17].

■■ **Clinical Presentation and Diagnosis**

Patients with iris sphincter tears commonly present after blunt trauma to the eye. Symptoms are dependent on the extent and severity of associated injuries but can include pain, photophobia, and blurry vision. Iris sphincter tears can be seen on slit lamp examination as scalloped notches in the iris sphincter at the pupillary margin. Depending on the extent of tearing, the pupil may appear irregular or dilated and may be minimally reactive to light. Evaluation requires careful slit lamp examination as hyphema and traumatic iritis often occur in conjunction with iris sphincter tears. In cases where the pupil appears dilated, it is important to rule out a third nerve palsy, which can present with mydriasis, ptosis, and extraocular muscle abnormalities on the affected side. Neuroimaging is indicated if third nerve palsy is suspected.

■■ **Management**

Topical corticosteroids and cycloplegics are used to treat accompanying iritis and/or hyphema. If pupillary function does not return after a period of observation, patients may report persistent debilitating glare, photophobia, and monocular diplopia. Prosthetic contact lenses employ the pinhole effect to alleviate these symptoms [18]. Surgical pupilloplasty may be considered in cases of multiple or large tears [19].

8.1.5 Iris Trauma: Iridodialysis

■■ **Introduction**

Iridodialysis is the separation of the iris root from the ciliary body. The iris root is the thinnest portion of the iris stroma, leaving it particularly vulnerable to damage [20]. Blunt or

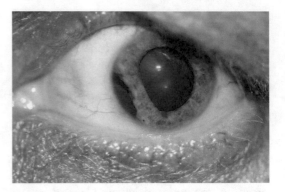

☐ **Fig. 8.3** Clinical photograph showing irregular D-shaped pupil, clinically significant for iridodialysis. (Reprinted with permission from the American Academy of Ophthalmology. © 2019 American Academy of Ophthalmology)

penetrating trauma is the most common cause of iridodialysis in all age groups. Airsoft toy guns, bottle rockets, and water balloon slingshots are important causes of iridodialysis in the pediatric population [5, 21, 22].

■■ **Clinical Presentation and Diagnosis**

Symptoms of iridodialysis depend on its size and associated inflammatory response. Small dialyses may be asymptomatic, while larger dialyses may cause monocular diplopia, glare, and photophobia. The disinserted iris root appears on slit lamp examination as *polycoria*, or the presence of an additional "D-shaped" pupil (☐ Fig. 8.3). Accompanying hyphema and/or traumatic iritis are common findings.

■■ **Management**

Topical corticosteroids and cycloplegics may be given to treat the accompanying traumatic iritis and/or hyphema. Small asymptomatic iridodialyses require no further intervention, but a larger or symptomatic iridodialysis presents both functional and cosmetic concerns. Treatment is either a prosthetic contact lens or surgical repair of the iridodialysis [23, 24].

8.1.6 Iris Trauma: Cyclodialysis

■■ **Introduction**

Cyclodialysis describes a separation of the longitudinal fibers of the ciliary muscle from the scleral spur. This separation, or cleft, provides a pathway for aqueous humor to drain into the suprachoroidal space and results in ocular hypotony (IOP lower than or equal to 5 mmHg). The primary cause of cyclodialysis in all age groups is blunt trauma [25]. Less frequently, cyclodialysis may be iatrogenic from surgical iris manipulation. Aminlari described a 4.5-month-old girl who had cyclodialysis following trabeculotomy for congenital glaucoma [26].

▪▪ Clinical Presentation and Diagnosis

All patients with cyclodialysis will present with a very low IOP often less than 5 mmHg. In a case review of 32 eyes with cyclodialysis, mean presenting IOP was 3.2 mm Hg [27]. Clinical studies repeatedly demonstrate that the size of the cyclodialysis cleft does not correlate with the degree of hypotony [26, 27]. Patient's history should correlate with clinical findings, for example, report of recent blunt injury or ocular surgery. Concurrent clinical evidence of severe ocular trauma, such as iris sphincter tears or hyphema, can also aid in the diagnosis. Complications of severe ocular hypotony may be observed on initial clinical presentation, including shallow anterior chamber, cataract, optic disc edema, macular edema, choroidal effusion, and retinal or choroidal folds [25, 26, 28].

Gonioscopy is the primary method to confirm the diagnosis of cyclodialysis, but it has several limitations. Gonioscopy is difficult to perform on a child, and it is especially difficult on a hypotonous eye with a shallow anterior chamber. Ultrasound biomicroscopy and anterior segment OCT are noninvasive imaging modalities that minimize patient discomfort because they do not require direct contact with the eye. Both AS-OCT and UBM are easy to repeat in order to monitor response to treatment [27, 29].

▪▪ Management

The size of the cyclodialysis guides treatment. For small clefts (<4 clock hours), treatment should begin conservatively with medical management consisting of 1% atropine, one to two times daily for a period of 6 to 8 weeks. It is hypothesized that by relaxing the ciliary muscle with atropine, the detached muscle

fibers are brought closer to the sclera to permit cleft closure [30]. Topical corticosteroids should be limited because they can delay healing of the cleft.

Noninvasive methods of closure such as laser photocoagulation [31], transscleral diathermy [32], or transconjunctival cryotherapy [33] can be considered for moderate sized clefts. Surgical approaches are reserved for larger clefts, or if noninvasive methods have failed [34, 35]. Overall, the prognosis of cyclodialysis is favorable. Good visual outcomes have been reported following cyclodialysis closure regardless of cleft size or time until receiving treatment [26, 36].

8.1.7 Traumatic Cataract

▪▪ Introduction

Cataract, or opacification of the crystalline lens, is a major preventable cause of blindness in children worldwide. While a cataract in an adult can be successfully managed at any point after its development, delayed treatment of a cataract in a child can lead to deprivation amblyopia, in which improper development of the visual pathways leads to permanent vision loss. In developed countries, 0.1 to 0.4 per 10,000 children are blind from childhood cataracts, and the number increases tenfold in developing countries with limited access to healthcare [37]. Trauma to the globe can induce monocular cataract formation, which carries the highest risk of amblyopia in children. The percentage of childhood cataracts from a traumatic etiology has been reported from 11.6% to 57% [38–40]. Cataract in a child can also be congenital, which may be genetic (autosomal dominant), associated with a systemic disease, or idiopathic [41].

Traumatic cataract is precipitated by blunt injury to the eye or direct penetrating injury to the crystalline lens and can occur acutely or years after the inciting injury. Blunt trauma causes a "shock wave" to advance through the eye, which stimulates cataract formation. Penetrating injury leads to opacification at the site of penetrating trauma and can rapidly progress to complete lens opacification. The mechanism of traumatic cataract in children varies based on geographic location. The majority of injuries are accidental while children are playing or involved in sports [42, 43]. In a review of patients in Colorado, United States, the most common cause of monocular cataract was from metallic objects including knives or BB guns, while bilateral cataracts were often associated with chronic self-injurious hitting or firework injuries [44].

■■ Clinical Presentation and Diagnosis
The clinical presentation of cataract is variable in a child. Patients typically have a recent, or sometimes remote, history of ocular trauma and may or may not complain of decreased visual acuity. Other presenting signs and symptoms include photophobia, strabismus, or the parents noting an abnormal opacification or discoloration of the child's eye. Leukocoria or "white pupil" is the loss of the pupillary red reflex and may be present. Small cataracts may not cause any symptoms and may be found incidentally during a routine eye exam. The diagnosis of cataract is made by slit lamp examination which demonstrates focal or complete opacification of the crystalline lens. Contusion-related traumatic cataracts classically form a rosette or stellate opacification (□ Fig. 8.4). Total white lens opacification may also be seen.

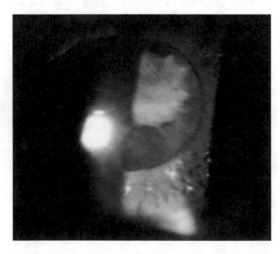

□ **Fig. 8.4** Slit lamp photograph showing stellate traumatic cataract following blunt trauma

■■ Management
Visually significant traumatic cataracts should be removed surgically within weeks of the injury, especially for children less than 6 years of age who are at greatest risk of developing deprivation amblyopia [45]. Surgical planning can be complex for these patients and varies depending on the age of the child and the extent of ocular injury. Postoperatively, pediatric patients have a higher tendency for inflammation, intraocular pressure increases, hyphema, posterior capsular opacification, lens-iris capture with intraocular lens decentration, and long-term increased risk of glaucoma [46–48]. However the prognosis is overall favorable. Patients with traumatic cataract often have good visual outcomes [49, 50].

8.1.8 Ectopia Lentis and Lens Subluxation

■■ Introduction
Ectopia lentis describes displacement or malposition of the crystalline lens. The lens may be *subluxed*, partially displaced while remaining in the pupillary space, or it may be *luxed*, completely dislocated and found free floating in the vitreous, anterior chamber or laying directly on the retina. Ectopia lentis is most commonly the result of blunt trauma to the globe, in which shearing forces stretch and break the lens zonules resulting in zonular dehiscence and subsequent dislocation. Other causes of ectopia lentis include congenital conditions that predispose to zonular weakness such as Marfan syndrome, homocystinuria, or Ehlers-Danlos syndrome. These conditions should be considered in non-traumatic cases, or when lens dislocation occurs after a minor injury.

■■ Clinical Presentation and Diagnosis
Symptoms of ectopia lentis depend on the degree of lens dislocation. In cases of mild subluxation, vision may be minimally affected due to refractive changes or not affected at all. Complete dislocation will cause severe vision loss. Slit lamp examination is necessary to evaluate the position of the lens, and the edge

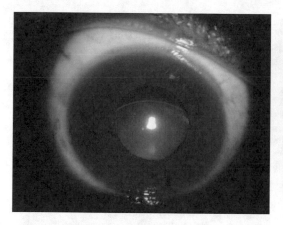

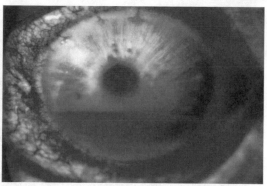

Fig. 8.5 Clinical photograph showing lens subluxation (ectopia lentis) inferiorly

Fig. 8.6 Clinical photograph showing layered hyphema. (Reprinted with permission from the American Academy of Ophthalmology. © 2019 American Academy of Ophthalmology)

of a subluxed lens may be visible through a dilated pupil (■ Fig. 8.5). Iridodonesis (quivering of the iris) or phacodonesis (quivering of the lens) may be present. A posteriorly luxed lens may be visualized on dilated funduscopic exam, B-scan ultrasonography, UBM, or CT scan. An anteriorly luxed lens will be visualized in the anterior chamber and can cause pain and a rise in intraocular pressure due to pupillary block.

■■ Management
Management of ectopia lentis in children initially involves optimization of optical refraction in order to prevent amblyopia. Cataract extraction with intraocular lens implantation may be considered when functional visual acuity cannot be achieved with refraction, the refraction is unstable due to lens mobility, or when displacement of the lens causes secondary ocular hypertension [51]. Following surgical correction, patients should be monitored for late intraocular lens (IOL) decentration or subluxation, especially if there is a sutured IOL which has long-term risks of suture breakage 5 or more years following insertion [52–54]. Overall, prognosis is good for these patients with the majority experiencing an improvement in visual acuity after surgery [55]. Despite the risks of long-term suture breakage, overall good outcomes have been reported with both iris-fixated [56] and

scleral-fixated [57, 58] intraocular lenses in children. Long-term follow-up shows stability of corrected vision [59].

8.1.9 Case Study

A 7-year-old boy presented to the emergency department after being hit in the left eye with a soccer ball. He complained of ocular pain and blurry vision. Visual acuity was 20/20 in the right eye and 20/100 in the left eye. A 3 mm layered hyphema was visible inferiorly in the anterior chamber (■ Fig. 8.6). Initial intraocular pressure (IOP) measurements were within normal limits. A B-scan was performed because of the poor view to the fundus and was within normal limits. A sickle cell screen was negative. The patient was started on prednisolone acetate 1% eye drops four times a day to the left eye and cyclopentolate hydrochloride eye drops three times a day to his left eye. The patient was advised to maintain strict bed rest and was given daily follow-up. On day 1, intraocular pressure was found to be elevated to 35 mm hg. The patient was started on timolol eye drops twice a day with improvement in intraocular pressure. After 10 days, the clot resorbed and intraocular pressure remained stable after cessation of timolol. His visual acuity returned to 20/20.

Key Points
- For all childhood ocular trauma, early intervention is critical to decrease the risk of amblyopia, in which improper development of the visual pathways leads to permanent vision loss.
- Subconjunctival hemorrhage resolves spontaneously and does not require treatment.
- Patients with hyphema must be closely monitored for complications, which include rebleed, elevations in intraocular pressure, optic atrophy, corneal bloodstaining, synechiae formation, and amblyopia.
- Traumatic hyphemas are typically managed with topical cycloplegics, steroids, and, if necessary, intraocular pressure lowering medications.
- Traumatic iritis presents 24–48 hours after traumatic eye injury, and patients present with photophobia, tearing, and blurry vision.
- Iris sphincter tears appear as scalloped notches in the iris sphincter at the pupillary margin and may coincide with the presence of hyphema and traumatic iritis.
- Cyclodialysis is a separation of the longitudinal fibers of the ciliary muscle from the scleral spur. Patients will have low intraocular pressure, and early management is medical with topical cycloplegics.
- Traumatic cataract may form after blunt or penetrating injury to the eye, and patients will have decreased visual acuity in the affected eye. Early surgical management is indicated in children.
- Ectopia lentis describes displacement or malposition of the crystalline lens, and usually occurs following blunt ocular trauma.

❓ Review Questions

1. Subconjunctival hemorrhages are best managed by
   (a) Observation
   (b) Topical cycloplegics
   (c) Topical steroids
   (d) Stopping use of blood thinners

2. An 8-year-old boy presents to the emergency room after being hit in the right eye with a basketball. He reports blurry vision, eye pain, headache, and sensitivity to light. The intraocular pressure of the right eye is 34 mm Hg, and a 2 mm layered hyphema is found in the anterior chamber. Sickle cell prep is negative. The best next step is
   (a) Surgical evacuation of the anterior chamber
   (b) Placement of an eye shield, bed rest, and observation
   (c) Topical cycloplegics, steroids, and intraocular pressure lowering drops
   (d) Topical and oral NSAIDs

3. Traumatic iritis typically presents __ after a traumatic eye injury
   (a) Immediately
   (b) Several hours
   (c) 24–48 hours
   (d) 1 week

4. Iridodialysis is
   (a) The separation of the longitudinal fibers of the ciliary muscle from the scleral spur
   (b) The separation of the iris root from the ciliary body
   (c) The separation of the anterior layer of iris stroma is separated from the posterior iris stroma
   (d) The disruption of the marginal sphincter fibers of the iris

5. What is the typical clinical presentation of traumatic cyclodialysis?
   (a) Elevated intraocular pressure > 35 mmHg
   (b) Very low intraocular pressure < 5 mmHg
   (c) Irregularly shaped pupillary margins
   (d) Blood in the anterior chamber (hyphema)

6. A 2-year-old girl with no past medical history and normal development to date was a passenger in a motor vehicle accident and on examination is noted

to have a "white pupil" with loss of the pupillary light reflex. What is the likely diagnosis?

(a) Traumatic cataract

(b) Hyphema

(c) Ptosis

(d) Strabismus

✅ **Answer**

1. (a)
2. (c)
3. (c)
4. (b)
5. (b)
6. (a)

References

Subconjunctival Hemorrhage

1. Mimura T, Usui T, Yamagami S, Funatsu H, Noma H, Honda N, Amano S. Recent causes of subconjunctival hemorrhage. Ophthalmologica. 2010;224(3):133–7.
2. Hu DN, Mou CH, Chao SC, Lin CY, NIen CW, Kuan PT, Jonas JB, Sung FC. Incidence of Non-Traumatic Subconjunctival Hemorrhage in a Nationwide Study in Taiwan from 2000 to 2011. PLoS One. 2015;10(6):e0132762.

Hyphema

3. Turkcu FM, Yuksei H, Sahin A, Cingu K, Ari S, Cinar Y, Sahin M, Yildirim A, Caca I. Demographic and etiologic characteristics of children with traumatic serious hyphema. Ulus Travma Acil Cerrahi Derg. 2013;19(4):357–62.
4. Trief D, Adebona OT, Turaiba AV, Shah AS. The pediatric traumatic hyphema. Int Ophthalmol Clin. 2013;53(4):43–57.
5. Shazly TA, Al Hussaini AK. Pediatric ocular injuries from airsoft toy guns. J Pediatr Ophthalmol Strabismus. 2012;49(1):54–7.
6. Motley WW 3rd, Kaufman AH, West CE. Pediatric airbag-associated ocular trauma and endothelial cell loss. J AAPOS. 2003;7(6):380–3.
7. Leuder GT. Air bag-associated ocular trauma in children. Ophthalmology. 2000;107(8):1472–5.
8. Bansal S, Gunasekeran DV, Ang B, Lee J, Khandelwal R, Sullivan P, Agrawal R. Controversies in the pathophysiology and management of hyphema. Surv Ophthalmol. 2016;61(3):297–308.
9. Shields JA, Shields CL, Materin M. Diffuse infiltrating retinoblastoma presenting as a spontaneous hyphema. J Pediatr Ophthalmol Strabismus. 2000;37(5):311–2.
10. Karcioglu ZA, Mullaney PB. Diagnosis and management of iris juvenile xanthogranuloma. J Pediatr Ophthalmol Strabismus. 1997;34(1):44–51.
11. Lai JC, Fekrat S, Barron Y, Golberg MF. Traumatic hyphema in children: risk factors for complications. Arch Ophthalmol. 2001;119(1):64–70.
12. Agapitos PJ, Noel LP, Clarke WN. Traumatic hyphema in children. Ophthalmology. 1987;94(10):1238–41.
13. Gharaibeh A, Savage HI, Scherer RW, Goldberg MF, Lindsley K. Medical interventions for traumatic hyphema. Cochrane Database Syst Rev. 2019;1:CD005431.
14. Oh DJ, Chen JL, Vajaranant TS, Dikopf MS. Brimonidine tartrate for the treatment of glaucoma. Expert Opin Pharmacother. 2018;8:1–8.

Traumatic Iritis

15. Engelhard SB, Bajwa A, Reddy AK. Causes of uveitis in children without juvenile idiopathic arthritis. Clin Ophthalmol. 2015;9:1121–8.
16. Kaur S, Kaushik S, Singh PS. Traumatic Glaucoma in children. J Curr Glaucoma Pract. 2014;8(2):58–62.

Iris Trauma: Sphincter Tear

17. Pujari A, Agarwal D, Kumar Behera A, Bhaskaran K, Sharma N. Pathomechanism of iris sphincter tear. Med Hypotheses. 2019;122:147–9.
18. Weissbart SB, Ayres BD. Management of aniridia and iris defects: an update on iris prosthesis options. Curr Opin Ophthalmol. 2016;27(3):244–9.
19. Younif M. Single suture customized loop for large iridodialysis repair. Clin Ophthalmol. 2016;10:1883–90.

Iris Trauma: Iridodialysis

20. Kumar S, Miller D, Atebara N, Blance E. A quantitative animal model of traumatic iridodialysis. Acta Ophthalmol. 1990;68(5):591–6.
21. Khan M, Reichstein DM, Recchia F. Ocular consequences of bottle rocket injuries in children and adolescents. Arch Ophthalmol. 2011;129(5):639–42.
22. Bullock JD, Ballal DR, Johnson DA, Bullock RJ. Ocular and orbital traumat from water balloon slingshots. A clinical, epidemiological, and experimental study. Ophthalmology. 1997;104(5):878–87.
23. Pandav SS, Gupta PC, Singh RR, Das K, Kaushik S, Raj S, Ram J. Cobbler's technique for iridodialysis repair. Middle East Afr J Ophthalmol. 2016;23(1):142–4.
24. Okamoto Y, Yamada S, Akimoto M. Suturing repair of subtotal iridodialysis. Int Ophthalmol. 2018;38(1):395–8.

Iris Trauma: Cyclodialysis

25. González-Martín-Moro J, Contreras-Martín I, Muñoz-Negrete FJ, Gómez-sanz F, Zarallo-Gallardo J. Cyclodialysis: an update. Int Ophthalmol. 2017;37(2):441–57.
26. Aminlari A, Callahan CE. Medical, laser, and surgical management of inadvertent cyclodialysis cleft with hypotony. Arch Ophthalmol. 2004;122(3):399–404.

27. Hwang JM, Ahn K, Kim C, Park KA, Kee C. Ultrasonic biomicroscopic evaluation of cyclodialysis before and after direct cyclopexy. Arch Ophthalmol. 2008;126(9):1222–5.

28. Ioannidis AS, Barton K. Cyclodialysis cleft: causes and repair. Curr Opin Ophthalmol. 2010;21(2):150–4.

29. Mateo-Montoya A, Dreifuss S. Anterior segment optical coherence tomography as a diagnostic tool for cyclodialysis clefts. Arch Ophthalmol. 2009;127(1):109–10.

30. Prata TS, Palmiero PM, De Moraes CG, et al. Imaging of a traumatic cyclodialysis cleft in a child using slit-lamp-adapted optical coherence tomography. Eye (Lond). 2009;23(7):1618–9.

31. Han JC, Kwun YK, Cho SH, Kee C. Long-term outcomes of argon laser photocoagulation in small size cyclodialysis cleft. BMC Ophthalmol. 2015; 15:123.

32. Ormerod LD, Baerveldt G, Sunalp MA, Riekhof FT. Management of the hypotonous cyclodialysis cleft. Ophthalmology. 1991;98(9):1384–93.

33. Ceruti P, Tosi R, Marchini G. Gas tamponade and cyclocryotherapy of a chronic cyclodialysis cleft. Br J Ophthalmol. 2009;93(3):414–6.

34. Agrawal P, Shah P. Long-term outcomes following the surgical repair of traumatic cyclodialysis clefts. Eye (Lond). 2013;27(12):1347–52.

35. Ioannidis AS, Bunce C, Barton K. The evaluation and surgical management of cyclodialysis clefts that have failed to respond to conservative management. Br J Ophthalmol. 2014;98(4):544–9.

36. Delgado MF, Daniels S, Pascal S, Dickens CJ. Hypotony maculopathy: improvement of visual acuity after 7 years. Am J Ophthalmol. 2001; 132(6):931–3.

Traumatic Cataract

37. Lim Z, Rubab S, Chan YH, Levin AV. Pediatric cataract: the Toronto experience-etiology. Am J Ophthalmol. 2010;149(6):887–92.

38. Khokhar S, Agarwal T, Kumar G, Kushmesh R, Tejwani LK. Lenticular abnormalities in children. J Pediatr Ophthalmol Strabismus. 2012;49(1):32–7.

39. Johar SR, Savalia NK, Vasavada AR, Gupta PD. Epidemiology based etiological study of pediatric cataract in western India. Indian J Med Sci. 2004;58(3):115–21.

40. Xu YN, Huang YS, Xie LX. Pediatric traumatic cataract and surgery outcomes in eastern China: a hospital-based study. Int J Ophthalmol. 2013;6(2):160–4.

41. Deng H, Yuan L. Molecular genetics of congenital nuclear cataract. Eur J Med Genet. 2014;57(2–3):113–22.

42. Pandey SK, Ram J, Werner L, et al. Visual results and postoperative complications of capsular bag and ciliary sulcus fixation of posterior chamber intraocular lenses in children with traumatic cataracts. J Cataract Refract Surg. 1999;25(12):1576–84.

43. Sen P, Shah C, Sen A, Jain E, Mohan A. Primary versus secondary intraocular lens implantation in traumatic cataract after open-globe injury in pediatric patients. J Cataract Refract Surg. 2018;44(12):1446–53.

44. Qiu H, Fischer NA, Patnaik JL, Jung JL, Singh JK, Mccourt EA. Frequency of pediatric traumatic cataract and simultaneous retinal detachment. J AAPOS. 2018;22(6):429–32.

45. Shah M, Shah S, Upadhyay P, Agrawal R. Controversies in traumatic cataract classification and management: a review. Can J Ophthalmol. 2013;48(4):251–8.

46. Lacmanović Loncar V, Petric I. Surgical treatment, clinical outcomes, and complications of traumatic cataract: retrospective study. Croat Med J. 2004;45(3):310–3.

47. Trivedi RH, Wilson ME. Posterior capsule opacification in pediatric eyes with and without traumatic cataract. J Cataract Refract Surg. 2015;41(7): 1461–4.

48. Haargaard B, Ritz C, Oudin A, et al. Risk of glaucoma after pediatric cataract surgery. Invest Ophthalmol Vis Sci. 2008;49(5):1791–6.

49. Birch EE, Cheng C, Stager DR, Felius J. Visual acuity development after the implantation of unilateral intraocular lenses in infants and young children. J AAPOS. 2005;9(6):527–32.

50. Lambert SR, Lynn MJ, Hartmann EE, et al. Comparison of contact lens and intraocular lens correction of monocular aphakia during infancy: a randomized clinical trial of HOTV optotype acuity at age 4.5 years and clinical findings at age 5 years. JAMA Ophthalmol. 2014;132(6):676–82.

Ectopia Lentis and Lens Subluxation

51. Neely DE, Plager DA. Management of ectopia lentis in children. Ophthalmol Clin N Am. 2001;14(3):493–9.

52. Buckley EG. Pediatric sutured intraocular lenses: trouble waiting to happen. Am J Ophthalmol. 2009;147(1):3–4.

53. Price MO, Price FW, Werner L, Berlie C, Mamalis N. Late dislocation of scleral-sutured posterior chamber intraocular lenses. J Cataract Refract Surg. 2005;31(7):1320–6.

54. Asadi R, Kheirkhah A. Long-term results of scleral fixation of posterior chamber intraocular lenses in children. Ophthalmology. 2008;115(1):67–72.

55. Bardorf CM, Epley KD, Lueder GT, Tychsen L. Pediatric transscleral sutured intraocular lenses: efficacy and safety in 43 eyes followed an average of 3 years. J AAPOS. 2004;8(4):318–24.

8

56. Yen KG, Reddy AK, Weikert MP, Song Y, Hamill MB. Iris-fixated posterior chamber intraocular lenses in children. Am J Ophthalmol. 2009; 147(1):121–6.

57. Konradsen T, Kugelberg M, Zetterström C. Visual outcomes and complications in surgery for ectopia lentis in children. J Cataract Refract Surg. 2007; 33(5):819–24.

58. Hyun DW, Lee TG, Cho SW. Unilateral scleral fixation of posterior chamber intraocular lenses in pediatric complicated traumatic cataracts. Korean J Ophthalmol. 2009;23(3):148–52.

59. Anteby I, Isaac M, Benezra D. Hereditary subluxated lenses: visual performances and long-term follow-up after surgery. Ophthalmology. 2003;110(7): 1344–8.

Retina and the Posterior Segment

Ekjyot S. Gill, Eric M. Shrier, and Ilya Leskov

Contents

© Springer Nature Switzerland AG 2021
R. Shinder (ed.), *Pediatric Ophthalmology in the Emergency Room*,
https://doi.org/10.1007/978-3-030-49950-1_9

9.1 Introduction

Trauma to the posterior segment can drastically impact vision and result in permanent visual loss. This chapter will review posterior segment anatomy and techniques for its examination in the emergency room and will describe the effects of trauma on various structures of the posterior segment with a focus on diagnosis and management. The goal is to help guide patient evaluation and appropriate referral.

9.2 Ocular Anatomy

A basic understanding of eye anatomy is necessary prior to examining the eye. Similar to a camera, the eye consists of structures that gather and focus incoming light and structures that sense the resulting images and transmit them to the brain.

The main light-sensing structure of the eye, the retina, and the tissues that support its function (sclera, vitreous humor, optic nerve, choroid) make up the posterior segment. The sclera is a dense, collagen-rich structure that is between 0.3 and 1 mm thick and forms the outer wall of the posterior four-fifths of the eye and gives it the characteristic globe-like shape [1]. Extraocular muscles attach directly to the sclera. Most of the volume of the posterior segment is occupied by the vitreous humor, a gel-like substance composed of hyaluronic acid and water. The neurosensory retina lines the inner wall of the posterior segment. It is a translucent tissue between 0.1 and 0.5 mm thick, composed of several layers of photoreceptors, neuronal cells, and other cell types, that provides support [2]. Retinal photoreceptors convert light into electrical signals that are then transmitted to the brain via the optic nerve. The posterior-most aspect of the retina is called the macula, an area where photoreceptor density is highest and visual acuity is best [3]. The optic disc, located at the nasal edge of the macula, is the location where retinal nerve fibers collect and exit the eye, forming the optic nerve (cranial nerve II). A central retinal artery and vein

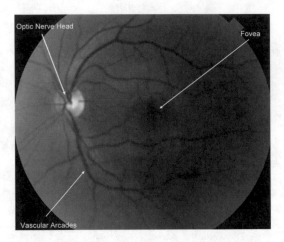

◘ Fig. 9.1   Fundus photo of left eye

run within the optic nerve. These prominent vessels provide blood supply to the superficial 2/3 of the retina (so-called inner retina) via their smaller subdivisions (branch retinal arteries and veins), which can be readily seen on fundus examination. The deeper 1/3 of the retina (so-called outer retina) contains retinal photoreceptor cells and is supported by an adjacent monolayer of pigmented cells called the retinal pigmented epithelium (RPE). [3] Between the RPE and the sclera lies the choroid, a network of small arterioles, capillaries, and venules that provides nutritional support to the RPE and to the outer retina. The choroid extends anteriorly, almost to the anterior segment. At its anterior edge, the choroid abuts the ciliary body, a tissue that produces the aqueous humor and supports the crystalline lens. The iris, choroid, and ciliary body considered together form the uvea (◘ Fig. 9.1).

9.3 Posterior Segment

Common abbreviations in posterior segment examination:
- Vit: vitreous humor
- ON: optic nerve
- Mac: macula
- AV: arteries and veins
- P: peripheral retina

The structures visible on posterior segment examination include the vitreous, optic nerve head, the retina, with its associated arteries and veins. Many of these may be seen, at least partially, using a direct ophthalmoscope via an undilated pupil. A much better view of these structures can be obtained with pharmacologic pupil dilation. Typical dilating drops are 1% tropicamide and 2.5% phenylephrine (with dilation lasting approximately 4 hours) or cyclopentolate (dilation lasting approximately 8 or more hours). Atropine 1% drops can cause dilation for over 1 week and thus should be avoided as a first-line agent.

In the emergency room setting, direct ophthalmoscopy is a useful technique to view some aspects of the posterior segment. The limitations of direct ophthalmoscopy include a very narrow field of view (a typical ophthalmoscope provides only ~5 degrees of view of the retina) and a very short working distance, which may be uncomfortable for some patients and physicians. An alternative to the traditional direct ophthalmoscope is the PanOptic™ Ophthalmoscope (Welch Allyn, New York), which provides an expanded 25-degree field of view and has a longer working distance, which may make its use more comfortable.

Traumatic abnormal findings in the posterior segment include vitreous hemorrhage, intra- and subretinal hemorrhages, retinal tears and/or detachments, macular holes, retinal edema (commotio), choroidal rupture and hemorrhage, optic nerve edema or avulsion, and intraocular foreign bodies.

If media opacity (dense hemorrhage in the anterior chamber or vitreous, dense corneal haze, dense cataract) or poor pupil dilation precludes visualization of the posterior segment, a sonographic examination of the eye is needed to determine if there are any gross retinal or choroidal abnormalities, such as retinal detachment or choroidal hemorrhage, as well as intraocular foreign bodies. Most detailed images are obtained using ultrasound machines specialized for ocular use, but if one is not available, machines specialized for abdominal/obstetric sonography can be used as well.

CT and MRI scans are commonly used to assess intraorbital pathology, such as fractures, infections, inflammation, and tumors. CT may also be used to detect a presence of an otherwise occult intraocular foreign body. Not infrequently, these foreign bodies are ferromagnetic, so care must be taken before ordering MRI for patients with severe eye trauma, as the magnet can cause secondary damage via induced foreign body movement [4].

> "Care must be taken before ordering MRI for patients with severe eye trauma, as the magnet can cause secondary damage via induced foreign body movement."

Ophthalmologists have other imaging modalities that document the status of the eye and its changes over time. Retinal vasculature may be monitored using color fundus photographs and retinal angiography, while retinal layers and structures can be visualized with the aid of optical coherence tomography (OCT). These modalities, however, require non-portable equipment and high degree of patient cooperation, and so are most useful in outpatient, non-urgent settings.

9.4 Vitreous

The posterior segment of the eye is normally filled with the vitreous humor – a thick gel-like fluid, similar in consistency to raw chicken egg white [5]. The vitreous is strongly adherent to the retina in children but liquefies and becomes less adherent with age, often detaching from the posterior retina. In most cases, such posterior vitreous detachments (PVD) are atraumatic, but in some patients, tractional forces from the vitreous may result in nicking of retinal blood vessels, mild bleeding into the vitreous, or even a retinal tear or detachment. Most frequently, tears occur in the peripheral retina, where the vitreous attachment to the retina is strongest [6].

Bleeding into the vitreous cavity is referred to as vitreous hemorrhage. Such vitreous hemorrhage may be due to damaged retinal vessels, ruptured retinal vessel aneurysms, blood seeping from ectopic blood vessels that develop superficial to or deep to the retina (neovascularization) in such common conditions as diabetic retinopathy and age-related macular degeneration, as well as due to eye trauma with resulting choroidal rupture [7].

Vitreous hemorrhage without associated anterior segment injury typically presents with a painless reduction in visual acuity and floaters (some resembling cobwebs or dark swirls). Symptoms can worsen overnight with complaints of severe vision loss in the morning due to blood pooling, while the patient lays supine. Therefore, if the diagnosis of vitreous hemorrhage is made early, it is important to emphasize sleeping with the head of the bed elevated, or even sleeping sitting upright overnight, to promote the hemorrhage settling inferiorly. In a case of vitreous hemorrhage, evaluation of the retina is necessary to detect a tear or detachment, preferably by visualization, or with sonography if the hemorrhage is dense and does not permit a view of the fundus.

Infectious or inflammatory processes in the posterior segment can result in the appearance of white blood cells in the vitreous, called vitritis. Inflammatory material in the vitreous is perceived by the patient as haze or fog in their vision. Examination will often reveal conjunctival redness and refractile cells in the anterior and/or posterior segment. Vitritis and hypopyon after an eye trauma suggest post-traumatic endophthalmitis, and ophthalmology should be urgently consulted [8].

> "Vitritis and hypopyon after an eye trauma suggest post-traumatic endophthalmitis and ophthalmology should be urgently consulted."

9.5   Retina

The retina is a thin, translucent tissue that converts light stimuli into electrical signals, which in turn are carried by the optic nerve to the brain's visual processing centers. Damage to the retina may result in vision loss. Below, we describe traumatic conditions specific to the retina and structures adjacent to it.

9.5.1   Commotio Retinae

Blunt force trauma produces shock waves that are transmitted to the retina through the vitreous. The resultant damage to retinal photoreceptors and underlying retinal pigmented epithelium is called commotio retinae (◘ Fig. 9.2). When the macula is affected, the condition is also referred to as Berlin's edema. Because traumatic shock waves are more readily transmitted through formed vitreous [9], the condition is more common among younger patients [10]. Commotio retinae manifests as patches of retinal whitening in the affected areas, where profound photoreceptor damage may be permanent. Most cases, however, have a good prognosis, with spontaneous resolution and visual recovery. Exceptions have coincident choroidal ruptures, vitreous or subretinal hemorrhage, and retinal tears or detachments.

9.5.2   Retinal Tears and Detachments

Retinal detachment (RD) is a sight-threatening condition in which the neurosensory retina becomes separated from underlying retinal pigment epithelium and the choroid. Patients who had sustained ocular trauma should be asked about symptoms of

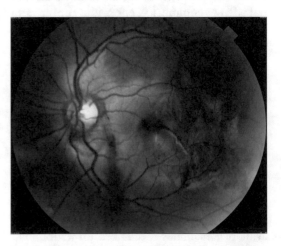

◘ **Fig. 9.2** Fundus photograph of left eye showing retinal whitening indicative of comotio retina (Berlin's edema)

retinal detachment including seeing flashes of light, new floaters, or curtain-like obscurations of vision. Traumatic retinal detachments are often rhegmatogenous – that is, they are caused by retinal tears. Retinal tears, often flap-shaped, occur in areas of the retina (most often in the periphery) that are tightly adherent to the vitreous [11]. Separation of the posterior vitreous from the retina, whether traumatic or spontaneous, exerts traction on the retina and will sometimes cause it to tear (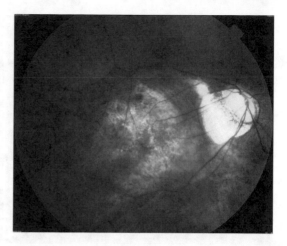 Fig. 9.3). Ongoing vitreous traction on the tear, combined with intraocular fluid currents that occur with eye movements, together promotes entry of liquefied vitreous fluid through the tear into the subretinal space, resulting in retinal detachment. Less commonly, ocular trauma may cause the most peripheral edge of the retina to detach and allow subretinal entry of fluid without any retinal tearing; this is called a retinal dialysis [12].

Two common conditions that make the retina more susceptible to post-traumatic tears and detachment are myopia and lattice degeneration. Myopia, commonly called nearsightedness, is often due to an elongated globe shape that results in increased susceptibility to tears (◼ Fig. 9.4) [13]. Lattice degeneration describes patches of thin peripheral retina that appear to have a lattice-like structure. These may arise spontaneously or may be associated with other ocular or systemic conditions such as myo-

Fig. 9.4 The posterior pole of a highly myopic individual. The optic disc is somewhat tilted. There is broad peri-papillary atrophy and macular pigmentary mottling

pia and Stickler syndrome. Retina within patches of lattice is therefore more likely to tear and detach with traction or after trauma [14].

Retinal detachments are broadly divided into peripheral detachments (macula-on) (◼ Fig. 9.5a, b) and detachments involving the macula (macula-off, ◼ Fig. 9.5c). Retinal detachments are also described in terms of clock hours in which they are present. A consultation with a retinal surgeon should be obtained to localize any retinal tears, to determine whether there is any chronic inflammation in the eye that may result in retinal scarring and foreshortening and to determine the correct treatment of the condition. Reassuringly, single-surgery success rate for retinal detachment is usually greater than 90% [15].

The urgency of retinal detachment repair is primarily determined by the state of the macula. A macula-sparing retinal detachment (macula-on RD) requires surgical repair within 24 hours in order to prevent spread of the detachment and to protect central visual acuity. A macula-involving retinal detachment (macula-off RD) has poor prognosis for visual recovery, and urgent repair is thus less critical. In these cases, studies show that repair should be performed within 7–10 days for the best visual outcome [16].

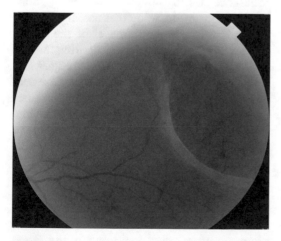

Fig. 9.3 Fundus photograph showing a giant retinal tear

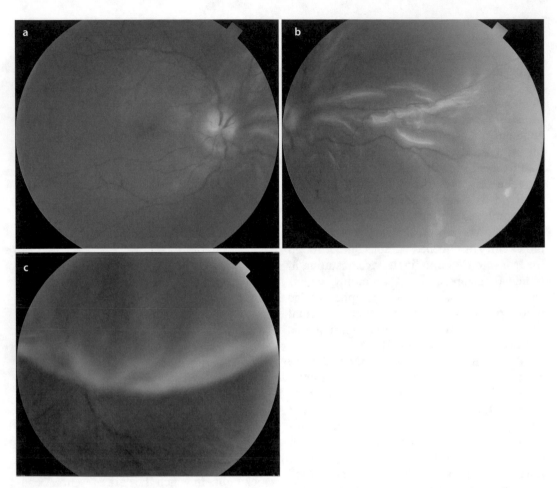

Fig. 9.5 **a, b** Fundus photos of a macula-sparing retinal detachment in the left eye with subretinal fluid noted nasal to the optic nerve. **c** Fundus photo of a macula-involving retinal detachment

9.5.3 **Macular Hole**

A macular hole is a break in the central macula that may develop spontaneously or secondary to vitreous traction from a variety of etiologies, including trauma. Patients with small macular holes often report metamorphopsia, a visual distortion wherein images appear to be wavy or warped [17]. An Amsler grid may be used to test for metamorphopsia – patients with this condition are often able to localize the area on the grid (in their visual field) where the straight lines of the grid appear wavy or curved. Patients with larger macular holes present with reduced central visual acuity, a non-specific complaint. Ophthalmologists are often able to discern a macular hole by its appearance, but most also obtain additional imaging of the macula to

supplement their clinical assessment. Optical coherence tomography (OCT) is a non-invasive form of imaging that uses light waves to create cross-sectional images of the retina. OCT is an excellent tool for evaluating the size and thickness of a macular hole (Fig. 9.6a). Macular holes, especially ones that arise secondary to ocular trauma, may close spontaneously, with some improvement in visual acuity. Persistent macular holes require surgical intervention (Fig. 9.6b).

9.5.4 **Solar and Laser Injuries**

Solar retinopathy is damage to the retinal photoreceptors, most commonly in the fovea, due to the toxic effects of UV radiation. Patients with solar retinopathy tend to be

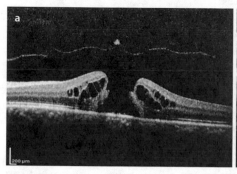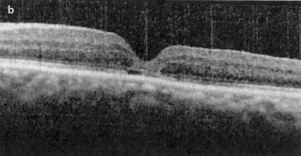

☐ **Fig. 9.6** **a** OCT of full-thickness macular hole. **b** OCT of the same eye following surgical repair

younger and usually report looking directly into sunlight, such as gazing at a solar eclipse [18]. The associated vision loss is transient and often improves over months, although there may be permanent visual sequelae.

Laser light propagates at shorter wavelengths than solar UV radiation, thereby transmitting more energy. Similar to UV radiation, laser light can cause phototoxic reactions in the eye but can also transfer direct thermal energy into the sensitive structures in the retina and the underlying retinal pigment epithelium. Symptoms are dependent on the severity of the retinal damage and the location of the injury and may range from minor visual changes to permanent vision loss. Direct laser damage to the fovea is much more likely to result in significant vision changes than damage to the peripheral retina. Laser retinopathy is typically due to accidental trauma from laser pointers or workplace injuries [19]. The rate of accidental eye trauma has increased as the unregulated market for higher power lasers has grown [20]. If laser retinopathy is suspected, the patient should be given an outpatient appointment with an ophthalmologist for evaluation of damage and for further management.

9.5.5 Terson's Syndrome

Terson's syndrome is vitreous and retinal hemorrhaging associated with intracranial hemorrhages, including subarachnoid hemorrhage and traumatic brain injury [21]. It is a condition that usually occurs in adults, but it has been reported in children as young as 7 months

old [22]. A commonly accepted mechanism of Terson's syndrome is that a sudden rise in intracranial pressure results in dilatation of retinal venules, some of which break open and bleed in all parts of the retina and into the vitreous [23]. Given the association of Terson's syndrome with potentially life-threatening intracranial pathology, pharmacologic pupil dilation should be deferred until monitoring for possible brain herniation via pupillary reactivity is no longer required. Treatment of the inciting intracranial pathology takes precedence to treatment of intraocular hemorrhage. The ophthalmology service should be consulted once the patient is stabilized.

9.5.6 Purtscher's Retinopathy

Purtscher's retinopathy is a rare condition which develops after trauma, usually associated with head or chest compression or long-bone fractures [24]. Observed retinal abnormalities include foci of nerve fiber layer whitening ("cotton-wool spots"), patches of retinal non-perfusion, macular edema, and intraretinal hemorrhages. Loss of vision in these patients may occur immediately after the injury or may be delayed for up to 48 hours [25]. The mechanism of retinal injury remains unclear and may involve systemic release of platelet or fibrin aggregates, fat or air emboli, as well as complement-mediated intravascular inflammation, which may then result in retinal vascular micro-infarctions. There is no retina-specific treatment. Systemic administration of high-dose IV corticosteroids has not shown success in visual improvement [26].

9.5.7 Non-accidental Pediatric Trauma (Shaken Baby Syndrome)

Shaken baby syndrome, non-accidental trauma due to acceleration-deceleration forces during a shaking episode, affects approximately 1400 children per year [27]. The typical child suffering from such non-accidental trauma presents obtunded, with illness and dehydration as the default diagnosis. However, once non-accidental trauma is suspected, a detailed eye exam is warranted. Bilateral vitreous, intraretinal, and subretinal hemorrhages are the hallmark findings of pediatric non-accidental trauma (◘ Fig. 9.7) [28]. However, care must be taken to distinguish this serious condition from intraretinal hemorrhages that may be the sequelae of normal vaginal birth. Children that present with intraocular bleeding have poor visual and neurologic outcomes; conversely, reassuring initial neurological examination is usually correlated with a good visual prognosis.

9.6 Ciliary Body

The ciliary body, located posterior to the iris plane, consists of secretory cells that generate the aqueous humor filling the anterior chamber. It also includes muscle and fine connec-tive tissue that support the crystalline lens capsule, maintaining its proper positioning along the visual axis and enabling it to change shape during accommodation [29]. Blunt trauma may cause the tearing of the delicate muscles within the ciliary body which is termed angle recession. Subsequent scarring and fibrosis of the damaged structures may lead to elevated intraocular pressures and traumatic glaucoma years later. Trauma may also cause the ciliary body to separate from the underlying sclera entirely, creating a so-called cyclodialysis cleft. Such clefts create a relatively unimpeded pathway for aqueous humor to drain from the eye, resulting in hypotony and consequent chorioretinal folds and decreased vision [30]. Because the signs of ciliary body trauma may be subtle (minimal hemorrhages, a slight distortion in iris or pupil shape), while the effects of such trauma may not manifest for months or even years, it is vital that injured eyes be examined by an ophthalmologist during or soon after the patient's visit to the emergency room [31].

9.7 Choroid

Contiguous with the ciliary body, the choroid is a dense network of arterioles and capillaries located between the sclera and the retinal pigment epithelium (RPE). Choroidal vessels

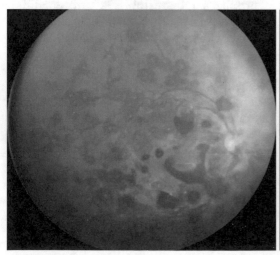 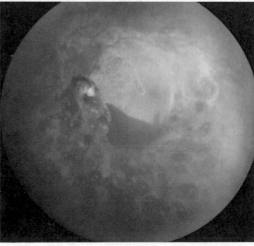

◘ **Fig. 9.7** Fundus photograph of the right and left eye of a child with non-accidental trauma demonstrating diffuse pre-retinal bleeding as well as numerous dot-blot and flame intraretinal hemorrhages extending from the posterior pole to the periphery. (Image courtesy of Neelakshi Bhagat, MD)

provide the RPE and the deeper part of the retina (outer retina) with nutritional and oxygen support [32].

Sudden significant differences between intra-arterial pressure and intraocular pressure (as in penetrating eye trauma or some types of ocular surgery) may result in effusions into the potential space between the choroid and the sclera. These are called choroidal detachments. They may be serous, which tend to be painless and are due to serum transudation, or hemorrhagic, which are characterized by a sudden onset of severe eye pain due to shearing of choroidal vessels [33]. Choroidal detachments may enlarge to the point of blocking some or most of a patient's visual field. Depending on etiology and severity, they may be managed by topical or oral steroids and/or by surgical drainage.

Compressive eye trauma may cause a momentary but significant deformation of the globe and result in linear breaks in the RPE and its underlying basement membrane and choroid.

Such breaks are called choroidal ruptures and may result in subretinal, intraretinal, and vitreous hemorrhage (■ Fig. 9.8). Ruptures in the macula will result in a greater degree of vision loss. Although the hemorrhages typically resolve within weeks, discontinuities of the RPE and its basement membrane persist and may lead to development of ectopic and disorganized blood vessels deep to the retina (choroidal neovascularization). These, in turn, may result

in additional subretinal bleeding, scarring, and further vision loss [34]. An ophthalmologist will usually follow patients with history of choroidal rupture closely, monitoring for development of neovascularization and treating any abnormal vasculature that may arise.

9.8 Sclera

The sclera is the connective tissue outer casing (the "white") of the eye that provides structure and shape to the eye. Although the sclera is resilient, substantial trauma to the eye can result in disruption of the scleral structure, which may present as a scleral laceration/rupture. Typical presenting symptoms are pain, light sensitivity, and conjunctival chemosis.

Suspected scleral laceration should be examined further, with the goal of determining the depth of the injury. A full-thickness scleral laceration may also damage the underlying choroid, resulting in notable subconjunctival hemorrhage in all quadrants. If the scleral laceration does not result in hemorrhage, the Seidel test may nevertheless be useful in determining whether colorless intraocular contents (such as vitreous or subretinal fluid) are being extruded through the wound. A positive Seidel test result warrants an urgent ophthalmology consult for globe rupture. Patients with a suspected scleral laceration should receive an urgent non-contrast CT of the orbits to determine if any intraocular foreign bodies are present. Posterior scleral lacerations are not visible at the slit lamp but may present with low intraocular pressure (hypotony) and with resulting chorioretinal or even corneal folds.

Treatment of partial-thickness scleral lacerations includes broad-spectrum topical antibiotics and possible surgical repair. Full-thickness scleral lacerations represent a globe rupture and as such require emergent evaluation and surgical repair [35].

9.9 Intraocular Foreign Body

Presence of an intraocular foreign body (IOFB) indicates a penetrating ocular injury has occurred, and the case should be treated

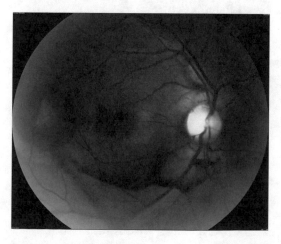

■ **Fig. 9.8** Fundus photograph of the right eye showing a choroidal rupture deep to the macula

as an open globe. The extent of ocular damage caused by foreign body penetration depends on the route of the projectile, structures penetrated, and the size, shape, and composition of the penetrating material. For example, a smaller foreign body entering the vitreous cavity directly through the sclera causes less damage to fewer structures than a larger one passing through the cornea, iris, and the crystalline lens.

IOFB composition imparts different post-injury risks. Metallic IOFBs, particularly ones made of iron or copper, will result in long-term retinal toxicity if left embedded in the eye, unlike IOFBs made of inert substances like glass, stone, or plastic (◻ Fig. 9.9). Conversely, metallic IOFBs may be relatively hot when entering the eye (as in the case of shrapnel) and, as such, be relatively sterile and less likely to cause a post-injury endophthalmitis than IOFBs that contain or carry vegetable matter or other organic materials [36].

The overall risk of post-traumatic endophthalmitis is approximately 1% [37]. This risk is increased to 6.9–16.5% in cases of retained foreign body material and even higher if the retained material is composed of organic matter [38].

Aspects of the eye examination that suggest the presence of an intraocular foreign body include signs of an open globe (scleral or corneal perforations), as well as signs of intraocular damage, such as focal iris trans-illumination defects, unilateral cataract in the injured eye, or hemorrhage in the anterior chamber or vitreous cavity.

Further evaluation of a possible IOFB should include a CT scan of the orbits and possibly an ocular ultrasound. MRI should be avoided if the foreign body is suspected to be ferromagnetic. If presence of an intraocular foreign body is suspected, the ophthalmology service should be notified in order to assess and provide appropriate treatment.

Key Points
- The macula is responsible for central visual acuity, and damage to the macula may be visually devastating.
- The PanOptic™ has advantages to the traditional direct ophthalmoscope including a wider field of view and a longer working distance.
- Ophthalmic ultrasonography is required to assess the status of the retina when a view of the posterior pole is not attainable.
- Symptoms of a retinal detachment include new onset flashes, shower of floaters, and/or a curtain over the visual field.
- Macula-sparing retinal detachments require more urgent repair than macula-involving retinal detachments in order to protect central visual acuity.
- Cases of suspected non-accidental trauma in infants require a dilated fundus exam.
- MRI must be avoided in cases of suspected metallic intraocular foreign body.

? Review Questions
1. A 56-year-old woman presents to the emergency department with decreased vision in her right eye after a mechanical fall. Her vision is 20/200 in the right eye with a pressure of 16. No afferent pupillary defect is noted on exam. A photo of her fundus is shown (◻ Fig. 9.10). What is the most likely diagnosis?

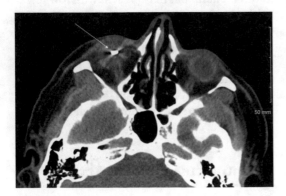

◻ **Fig. 9.9** CT image showing a metallic foreign body within the vitreous cavity of the right eye

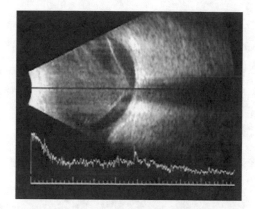

Fig. 9.10 A photo of her fundus is shown. What is the most likely diagnosis?

2. A 48-year-old man presents to the emergency department reporting a 2-day history of worsening floaters in his right eye. The onset of floaters was accompanied by flashes. The patient also states that earlier today, a shadow appeared in the periphery of his vision in his right eye. His visual acuity in his right eye is 20/30, pressure is 14mmHg, and no afferent pupillary defect is noted. A photo of his fundus is shown (Fig. 9.11). What is the most likely diagnosis and what are the next steps?

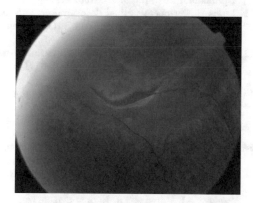

Fig. 9.11 What is the most likely diagnosis and what are the next steps?

3. A 26-year-old man presents to the emergency department after feeling a sharp pain in his left eye, while he was working on a construction project. He was not wearing eye protection at the time. His vision is 20/25 in the left eye,

the intraocular pressure is 12mmHg, and there is no afferent pupillary defect. What is the likely diagnosis in this case? What additional testing would confirm or disprove the likely diagnosis?

✅ **Answer**

1. The fundus photograph shows a round spot in the center of the macula surrounded by a gray halo. The patient likely has a macular hole as evidenced by her history of trauma and sudden decrease in vision to 20/200. Of note, the patient does not have an afferent pupillary defect because the surrounding retina and optic nerve remain unharmed. Based on the photo, the differential diagnosis is full-thickness macular hole, partial-thickness lamellar hole, epiretinal membrane (macular pucker), solar retinopathy, or an intraretinal cyst among others. In the ophthalmologist's office, the patient will undergo testing to determine the diagnosis.

2. Fundus photo of the right eye showing a temporal retinal tear with associated detachment.

    The most likely diagnosis is a rhegmatogenous retinal detachment with macula attached. It is important to ask the patient the duration of symptoms, history of trauma, previous eye surgery/procedures, or myopia. On exam, look for associated vitreous hemorrhage. This condition requires urgent evaluation by an ophthalmologist in order to preserve vision. Correcting a retinal detachment in which the macula is still attached is often done surgically within 24 hours of patient presentation.

3. Slit lamp photograph shows a round irregularity in the lens. After an eye examination including Seidel testing, CT scan is warranted. Image of a CT scan is shown. There is a foreign body noted in the posterior vitreous in the left eye. Due to presence of an intraocular foreign body, this case is considered an open globe and requires urgent ophthalmology evaluation.

Case Presentation

A 16-year-old boy with a recent history of multiple presentations after altercations with peers presents again, this time reporting decreased vision in the left eye. He reports that a dark curtain has descended over his central vision over the last several days and that his vision has continued to worsen. An external exam of the face and left eye shows faint periocular bruising. His vision is hand motion in the left eye, and dilated fundus exam shows retinal dialysis (disinsertion of the peripheral retina at the ora serrata) as well as total retinal detachment. Ophthalmic ultrasound confirms retinal dialysis, and the retina is detached with only a posterior attachment at the optic nerve (◘ Fig. 9.12). This is considered a macula-off retinal detachment in an open-funnel configuration. The patient required repair in the operating room.

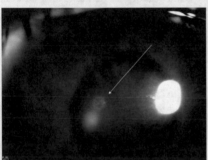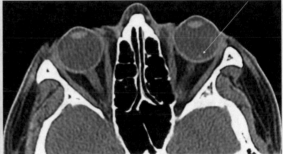

◘ **Fig. 9.12** Ophthalmic ultrasound confirms retinal dialysis and the retina is detached with only a posterior attachment at the optic nerve

References

1. Davson H, Graham L. The eye. New York: Academic Press; 1969. p. 289 92.
2. Krause WJ II. Krause's essential human histology for medical students. Boca Raton: Universal Publishers; 2005.
3. Yanoff M, Sassani J. Ocular pathology. Elsevier Health Sciences. p. 393–6.
4. Kubal WS. Imaging of orbital trauma. Radiographics. 2008;28(6):1729–39. https://doi.org/10.1148/rg.286085523.. Review
5. Standring S. Gray's anatomy: the anatomical basis of clinical practice. London: Elsevier; 2016. p. 2371–8.
6. Kun E. Gross and microscopic pathology in autopsy eyes. Part III. Retinal breaks without detachment. Am J Ophthalmol. 1961;51:369–91.
7. Spraul CW, Grossniklaus HE. Vitreous hemorrhage. Surv Ophthalmol. 1997;42:3–39.
8. Peyman GA, Lee PJ, Seal DV. Endophthalmitis: diagnosis and management. London: Taylor & Francis; 2004. p. 90–1.
9. Liu W, Grzybowski A. Current management of traumatic macular holes. J Ophthalmol. 2017;2017:1–8.
10. Ahn SJ, Woo SJ, Kim KE, Jo DH, Ahn J, Park KH. Optical coherence tomography morphologic grading of macular commotio retinae and its association with anatomic and visual outcomes. Am J Ophthalmol. 2013;156(5):994–1001.e1.
11. Lewis H. Peripheral retinal degenerations and the risk of retinal detachment. Am J Ophthalmol. 2003;136(1):155–60.
12. Vote BJ, Casswell AG. Retinal dialysis: are we missing diagnostic opportunities? Eye (Lond). 2004;18(7):709–13.
13. Smith MJ, Walline JJ. Controlling myopia progression in children and adolescents. Adolesc Health Med Ther. 2015;6:133–40. https://doi.org/10.2147/AHMT.S55834. eCollection 2015. Review.
14. Wilkinson CP. Interventions for asymptomatic retinal breaks and lattice degeneration for preventing retinal detachment. Cochrane Database Syst Rev. 2014;9:CD003170.
15. Brucker AJ, Hopkins TB. Retinal detachment surgery: the latest in current management. Retina. 2006;26:S28–33.
16. Yang CH, Lin HY, Huang JS, Ho TC, Lin CP, Chen MS, Yang CM. Visual outcome in primary macula-off rhegmatogenous retinal detachment treated with scleral buckling. J Formos Med Assoc. 2004;103(3):212–7.
17. Miller JB, Yonekawa Y, Eliott D, Kim IK, Kim LA, Loewenstein JI, Sobrin L, Young LH, Mukai S, Vavvas DG. Long-term follow-up and outcomes

in traumatic macular holes. Am J Ophthalmol. 2015;160(6):1255–1258.e1.

18. Gregory-Roberts E, Chen Y, Harper CA, Ong T, Maclean MA, Fagan XJ, Carden SM. Solar retinopathy in children. J AAPOS. 2015;19(4): 349–51.

19. Turaka K, Bryan JS, Gordon AJ, Reddy R, Kwong HM Jr, Sell CH. Laser pointer induced macular damage: case report and mini review. Int Ophthalmol. 2012;32(3):293–7.

20. Consumer health information: illuminating the hazards of powerful laser products. Silver Spring, MD: Food and Drug Administration, 2009. Available at: http://www.fda.gov/downloads/ForConsumers/ConsumerUpdates/UCM167564.pdf.

21. Czorlich P, Skevas C, Knospe V, et al. Terson syndrome in subarachnoid hemorrhage, intracerebral hemorrhage, and traumatic brain injury. Neurosurg Rev. 38:129–3. Epub 2014 Aug 31.

22. Bhardwaj G, Jacobs MB, Moran KT, Tan K. Terson syndrome with ipsilateral severe hemorrhagic retinopathy in a 7-month-old child. J AAPOS. 2010;14:441–3.

23. Mazurek M, Krzystolik K, Lachowicz E, Kubasik-Kladna K, Czepita D. Terson syndrome--a literature review. Klin Ocz. 2014;116(1):59–63. Review.

24. Agrawal A, McKibbin M. Purtscher's retinopathy: epidemiology, clinical features and outcome. Br J Ophthalmol. 2007;91(11):1456–9.

25. Behrens-Baumann W, Scheurer G, Schroer H. Pathogenesis of Purtscher's retinopathy. Graefes Arch Clin Exp Ophthalmol. 1992;230(3):286–91.

26. Gil P, Pires J, Costa E, Matos R, Cardoso MS, Mariano M. Purtscher retinopathy: to treat or not to treat? Eur J Ophthalmol. 2015;25(6):e112–5.

27. All About SBS/AHT. The National Center on Shaken Baby Syndrome. Available at: http://www.dontshake.org/sbs.php?topnavid=3&subnavid=27.

28. Kivlin JD, Simons KB, Lazoritz S, Ruttum MS. Shaken baby syndrome. Ophthalmology. 2000;107(7):1246–54.

29. Standring S. Gray's anatomy: the anatomical basis of clinical practice. London: Elsevier; 2016. p. 1825–61.

30. Wang M, Hu S, Zhao Z, Xiao T. A novel method for the localization and management of traumatic cyclodialysis cleft. J Ophthalmol. 2014;2014:761851.

31. Gentile R, Pavlin C, Liebmann J, Easterbrook M, Tello C, Foster F, et al. Diagnosis of traumatic cyclodialysis by ultrasound biomicroscopy. Ophthalmic Surg Lasers. 1996;27(2):97.

32. Vuong VS, Moisseiev E, Cunefare D, Farsiu S, Moshiri A, Yiu G. Repeatability of choroidal thickness measurements on enhanced depth imaging optical coherence tomography using different posterior boundaries. Am J Ophthalmol. 2016;169:104–12.

33. Robert B, Leo C, Thomas HB. Choroidal detachment: clinical manifestation. Ther Mech Form Ophthalmol. 1981;88(11):1107–15.

34. Aguilar J, Green W. Choroidal rupture. Retina. 1984;4(4):269–75.

35. George CW, Slack WJ. Corneal and scleral lacerations. A five-year review. Am J Ophthalmol. 1962;54:119.

36. Justin G, Baker K, Brooks D, Ryan D, Weichel E, Colyer M. Intraocular foreign body trauma in operation iraqi freedom and operation enduring freedom. Ophthalmology. 125(11):1675–82.

37. Andreoli CM, Andreoli MT, Kloek CE, Ahuero AE, Vawas D, Durand ML. Low rate of endophthalmitis in a large series of open globe injuries. Am J Ophthalmol. 2009;147(4):601–8. (reference for 1% endophthalmitis) Ophthalmology 2018;125(11):1675–1682.

38. Essex RW, Yi Q, Charles PG, Allen PJ. Post-traumatic endophthalmitis. Ophthalmology. 2004;111:2015–22.

Neuro-Ophthalmic Trauma

Laura Palazzolo, Daniel Wang, and Valerie I. Elmalem

Contents

© Springer Nature Switzerland AG 2021
R. Shinder (ed.), *Pediatric Ophthalmology in the Emergency Room*,
https://doi.org/10.1007/978-3-030-49950-1_10

10.1 Introduction

10.1.1 Optic Nerve Anatomy

Cranial nerve II, the optic nerve, is composed of 1.1 million retinal ganglion cell (RGC) axons that transmit afferent visual input from the retina. The optic nerve has four anatomical subdivisions: intraocular (1 mm), intraorbital (24 mm), intracanalicular (9 mm), and intracranial (16 mm). As the RGC axons exit the globe to form the optic nerve, they are supported by the lamina cribrosa, a system of 10 connective tissue plates. The optic nerve fibers are myelinated by oligodendrocytes posterior to the lamina cribrosa and surrounded by a meningeal sheath (pia mater, arachnoid mater, and dura mater). The intracanalicular segment travels through the optic canal within the lesser wing of the sphenoid bone, and at this segment the dural sheath surrounding the optic nerve fuses with the periosteum and immobilizes the nerve. The optic nerves converge at the optic chiasm and the neural fibers continue posteriorly as the optic tracts.

The short posterior ciliary arteries, branches from the ophthalmic artery, provide vascular supply to the optic nerve head. These arteries have few anastomoses and are susceptible to ischemia. The remainder of the optic nerve obtains its primary blood supply from pial branches of the surrounding meninges.

10.1.2 Traumatic Optic Neuropathy

10.1.2.1 Definition

In traumatic optic neuropathy (TON), damage of optic nerve fibers leads to complete or partial impairment of visual function [1]. TON may be caused by direct or indirect injury. In direct TON, penetrating trauma with optic nerve transection, optic nerve avulsion, hemorrhage, or hematoma leads to direct optic nerve damage [2]. Indirect TON is the more common mechanism of TON and involves severe closed head trauma with coup and contrecoup shearing forces disrupting optic nerve fibers [3]. The damage is most often at fixed segments of the optic nerve, with highest frequency at the intracanalicular segment where the nerve is adherent to the periosteum in the optic canal [4].

10.1.2.2 Epidemiology

TON is most frequently diagnosed in younger patients and has a male predilection [5]. The estimated annual incidence for pediatric traumatic optic neuropathy is 0.99 cases per million [6]. In a case review of pediatric patients with visual pathway injuries following ocular trauma, TON made up the majority (86.1%) of injury types [7]. The most common mechanisms for TON in pediatric populations are falls from a height, motor vehicle accidents, and sports-related injuries [8–10].

10.1.2.3 Clinical Presentation

The diagnosis of TON is primarily clinical, and early diagnosis is often delayed due to impaired consciousness or unstable condition with multisystem trauma. If able, patients may describe a subjective decrease in visual acuity. Non-accidental forms of trauma should be ruled out for all pediatric patients.

10.1.2.4 Diagnosis

On clinical examination, patients will have severely reduced visual acuity reported as 20/400 or worse in the affected eye [11]. A relative afferent pupillary defect in the affected eye is an early sign of optic nerve dysfunction and can be easily tested regardless of a patient's level of consciousness. In addition, patients may have visual field limitations and impaired color vision. A direct ophthalmoscope can be used to visualize the optic nerve. In the case of posterior optic nerve injury the nerve can appear normal. For acute anterior optic nerve injury, there may be optic disc swelling, dilated retinal veins, and retinal hemorrhage.

Patients should have a complete examination by an ophthalmologist including fundus examination to directly visualize the optic nerve and rule out other ocular injury. Other serious injuries often coexist, including ante-

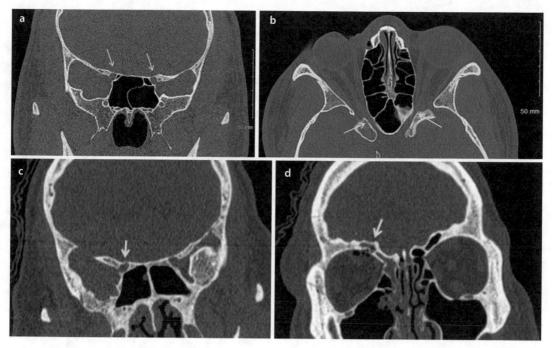

☐ **Fig. 10.1** **a** Coronal CT with normal optic canal (arrow), **b** Axial CT with normal optic canal (arrow), **c** Coronal CT with optic canal fracture (arrow) and traumatic optic neuropathy, **d** Coronal CT showing associated orbital roof fracture (arrow)

rior or posterior segment ocular injury, orbital wall fractures, skull fractures, or intracranial bleeding [7, 12].

Imaging studies are advised in the setting of head trauma, although it has uncertain clinical value for the diagnosis of TON [4]. CT scan is preferable for examining bony structures and can evaluate for causes of direct TON such as optic canal fracture. If a patient has an orbital roof fracture there is also a high likelihood of optic canal fracture, and careful clinical and radiologic examination should be made to rule out direct TON (☐ Fig. 10.1). In one case series of pediatric traumatic optic neuropathy, 14% were associated with optic canal fracture [8]. To limit radiation exposure, MRI evaluation of the optic nerve may be preferable in the pediatric population. However, MRI should not be used if there is a possibility of a metallic foreign body. In addition, B-scan ultrasonography is a noninvasive and inexpensive option that has shown utility for diagnosing optic nerve avulsion anteriorly [13].

10.1.2.5 Management

Primary nerve injury is irreversible, and TON treatment focuses on limiting further secondary injury. The main approach for TON is conservative, with patients observed for visual recovery [14]. Reports of spontaneous visual improvement following indirect TON are encouraging for conservative management, with a recovery rate of 30–60% [15]. The prognosis for spontaneous recovery is positively related to the patient's presenting visual acuity [16].

Based on research with spinal cord injury and corticosteroid use, it is hypothesized that high-dose corticosteroids administered soon after trauma may relieve optic nerve edema within the optic canal and decrease risk of damage to retinal ganglion cells [17]. Research has been undertaken regarding the use of high-dose IV steroids for treatment in TON with mixed results [18–21]. As per the most recent Cochrane Eyes and Vision Group review in 2013, there is not enough evidence to support the use of steroids over observation alone [16]. In addition, the Corticosteroid

Randomization After Significant Head Injury (CRASH) trial demonstrated higher mortality rates for patients receiving high-dose steroids after head injury, and high-dose steroids should not be given to the large subgroup of patients with both TON and head injury [22].

Surgical decompression may be indicated and should be evaluated on a case-by-case basis [23]. With retrobulbar hematoma or optic nerve sheath hematoma, urgent surgical decompression and evacuation of the hematoma are imperative to relieve optic nerve compression and improve potential for visual recovery [24]. The use of optic canal decompression for other forms of TON such as optic canal fracture is currently debated. Optic canal fracture has been identified as a poor prognostic factor, regardless of surgical intervention, and further research is being conducted in this area [16].

10.1.2.6 Prognosis

For indirect TON, potential for visual recovery is related to visual acuity on initial presentation. Patients who have no light perception vision on presentation have poor visual prognosis regardless of treatment [9, 21]. If there is no visual improvement within 48 hours after injury, there is also a poor prognosis [25]. Direct TON has a poor prognosis in all cases [26].

10.1.3 Pupil Abnormalities: Acquired Horner Syndrome

10.1.3.1 Anatomy

Problems with pupillary response may be related to either interruption of sympathetic activity, responsible for pupillary dilation (mydriasis), or parasympathetic activity, responsible for pupillary constriction (miosis).

Pupillary Light Reflex   The pupillary light reflex pathway is responsible for equal and simultaneous pupillary constriction in response to light. Afferent fibers first travel along the optic nerve to synapse in the pretectal nucleus, located in the midbrain at the level of the superior colliculus. Then, efferent fibers travel to both the ipsilateral

and contralateral Edinger-Westphal nuclei. The Edinger-Westphal nucleus gives rise to preganglionic parasympathetic fibers that exit with cranial nerve III. The fibers synapse in the ciliary ganglion and give rise to postganglionic myelinated short ciliary nerves, which innervate the iris sphincter muscle for pupillary constriction.

Sympathetic Pathway to Head and Neck   The sympathetic pathway leading to pupillary dilation involves three neuron synapses (◘ Fig. 10.2). The first-order neuron originates in the ipsilateral hypothalamus and descends the spinal cord to synapse in the inferomediolateral gray matter at C8, T1, and T2, also called the ciliospinal center of Budge-Waller. The second-order preganglionic neuron exits the spinal cord, passes over the pulmonary apex, and synapses in the superior cervical ganglion. The third-order postganglionic neuron

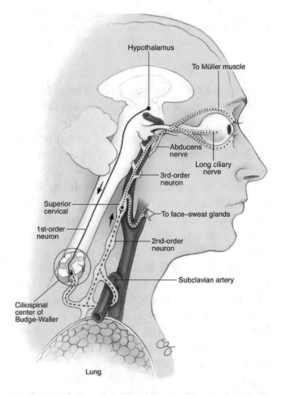

◘ Fig. 10.2   Sympathetic pathway. (Reproduced from BCSC Neuro-ophthalmology, ◘ Figs. 1–41: Anatomy of the Sympathetic Pathway with permission from American Academy of Ophthalmology. Illustration by Christine Gralapp. © 2020 American Academy of Ophthalmology [92])

ascends in the paravertebral chain and along the wall of the carotid artery, entering the cavernous sinus and then traveling with the abducens nerve (cranial nerve VI) to enter the orbit.

10.1.3.2 Definition

Horner syndrome describes an interruption at any point along the three neuron sympathetic pathway supplying the head and neck, with subsequent clinical manifestations including the classic triad of ipsilateral ptosis (related to Müller muscle dysfunction), miosis (pupillary dilator dysfunction), and anhidrosis.

10.1.3.3 Epidemiology

Pediatric Horner syndrome is rare, with a reported incidence of 1.42 per 100,000 patients under 19 years of age [27]. Trauma is the most common cause of acquired Horner syndrome in children, with the most cited mechanisms including birth trauma or iatrogenic injury [27]. Birth trauma is associated with the use of forceps or vacuum extraction, shoulder dystocia, fetal rotation, or post-term delivery, all of which can result in brachial plexus injury or damage to vascular structures [28]. In several case reports, birth trauma was linked to carotid artery dissection and associated Horner syndrome [29, 30]. Iatrogenic trauma leading to pediatric Horner syndrome has been identified in several case reports, including secondary to thyroid surgery and following pulmonary hydatid cyst removal [31, 32]. Nontraumatic causes of Horner syndrome in children include neuroblastoma or other malignancy, and these causes should still be considered even if there is a history of trauma or surgery [33, 34]. See ▶ Chap. 15 for more information on neuroblastoma.

10.1.3.4 Clinical Presentation

Patients will present with ipsilateral ptosis, miosis, and anhidrosis to varying degrees based on the location of sympathetic fiber disruption. Anisocoria is more pronounced in dim lighting.

Patients with first- and second-order neuron Horner syndrome have complete ipsilateral face anhidrosis, while those with third-order neuron lesions will only have anhidrosis involving the ipsilateral forehead. The

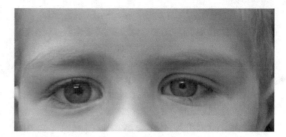

■ **Fig. 10.3** Pediatric Horner syndrome on the left side showing iris heterochromia, anisocoria, ipsilateral miosis, and ptosis. There is usually straighter hair on the ipsilateral side. (Adapted from Smith et al. [93], ■ Fig. 1. Reproduced under a Creative Commons Attribution 4.0 International license [▶ https://creativecommons.org/licenses/by/4.0/])

iris melanocytes are derived from neural crest cells, and when Horner syndrome is acquired prior to 2 years of age, melanocyte innervation needed for early melanin pigmentation of the iris is disrupted. This leads to a difference in eye color with the ipsilateral iris being lighter, termed iris heterochromia [35] (■ Fig. 10.3a).

Signs of Horner syndrome in the pediatric population: ipsilateral
- Ptosis
- Miosis
- Anhidrosis (first- and second-order neuron)
- Iris heterochromia (congenital or onset prior to age 2)
- Straighter hair

Patients with Horner syndrome secondary to carotid artery dissection may also demonstrate focal cerebral deficits and cranial nerve palsies. In one rare clinical case, unilateral straight hair was the first sign of pediatric Horner syndrome [36] (■ Fig. 10.3b).

10.1.3.5 Diagnosis

Diagnosis is largely clinical as above, combined with MRI and MRA studies to identify the cause of Horner syndrome. Imaging workup is especially important to rule out life-threatening causes of Horner syndrome such as carotid dissection or malignancy [29, 37]. Pharmacologic testing can also aid in the diagnosis of Horner syndrome. Topical apraclonidine eye drops (0.5% or 1%) will cause reversal of anisocoria with the Horner pupil becoming larger than the normal pupil, as well as reversal of the ptosis. The Horner pupil will poorly dilate with topical cocaine eye drops 4% or 10%, while the normal pupil dilates, thus increasing the anisocoria. Cocaine testing has been used safely in children with no systemic side effects; however, apraclonidine should be used with caution due to the risk of central nervous system depression in children, especially if less than 2 years old [38].

10.1.3.6 Management

Treatment of Horner syndrome is dependent on the etiology. In the case of carotid dissection, antiplatelets or anticoagulation is imperative to reduce the risk of stroke [34]. Patients who fail medical management of carotid artery dissection may be closely monitored or undergo surgical intervention, such as intravascular stenting. For iatrogenic causes of Horner syndrome or other non-life-threatening mechanisms, observation is preferred. Spontaneous resolution over months has been reported [31].

10.1.4 Head Trauma: Overview

10.1.4.1 Epidemiology

Head trauma is a frequent cause of emergency room visits, with isolated head trauma reported as 30% of all major pediatric trauma in one large case series [39]. Young males are the primary demographic affected, and motor vehicle accidents are the primary reported cause of accidental severe head injury in children [40, 41]. Patients presenting with a Glasgow Coma Scale score less than or equal to 8 have more severe head injuries, and those who lose consciousness following head injury are more likely to have permanent neurologic injury [42].

Patients with head injury and visual complications should be evaluated for skull base fracture, arterial or venous injury, traumatic brain injury, or direct penetrating trauma to visual pathways. These diagnoses will be reviewed in the remainder of the chapter.

10.1.5 Skull Base Fractures

10.1.5.1 Anatomy

A skull base (or basilar skull) fracture extends through any of the cranial floor bone and can damage vascular and nerve structures at foramina as they exit or enter the skull base (◘ Fig. 10.4).

The anterior skull base is composed of the frontal bone. There is risk of injury to CN I as it exits the cribriform plate. The middle skull base is composed of the sphenoid bone. The middle skull base has several important structures at risk for damage, including the optic nerve (CN II) and ophthalmic artery in the optic canal; the superior orbital fissure with CN III, IV, ophthalmic nerve (V1), VI, and superior ophthalmic vein; the foramen rotundum with the maxillary nerve (CN V2), foramen ovale with the mandibular nerve (CN V3); and the carotid canal with the internal carotid artery and sympathetic plexus.

The posterior skull base is composed of the temporal bone and occipital bone. In the posterior skull base, there is the internal acoustic meatus where CN VII and VIII exit; the jugular foramen is passage for the internal jugular vein, CN IX, CN X, CN XI, inferior petrosal sinus, and posterior meningeal artery; the hypoglossal canal with CN XII; and the foramen magnum with CN XI, vertebral artery, spinal vein, and spinal arteries.

10.1.5.2 Epidemiology

Skull base fractures are due to high-impact trauma [43]. The rate of skull base fractures in children with head trauma ranges from 4% to 20% [44]. Blunt head trauma causes over 90% of skull base fractures, and the most common mechanisms in children are motor vehicle accidents or falls from a height [45–47]. Less commonly, skull base fractures are due to iatrogenic injury, including complications of endoscopic sinus surgery, or direct penetrating injury, such as a gunshot wound through the skull base [48, 49].

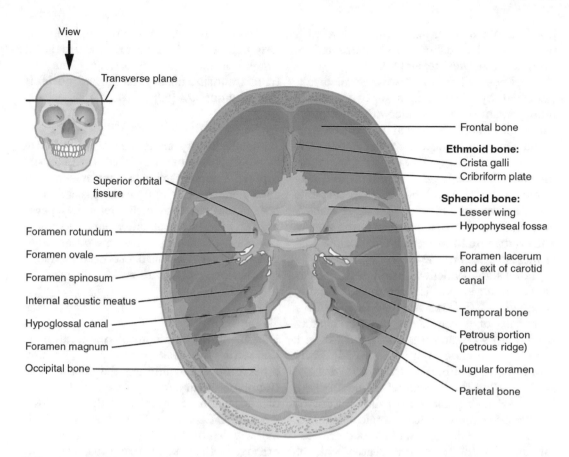

◨ Fig. 10.4 Skull base anatomy. (Adapted from ◨ Fig. 7.8 Skull base anatomy superior view, Betts et al. [100]. ©Jan 16, 2020 OpenStax ▶ https://openstax.org/books/anatomy-and-physiology/pages/7-2-the-skull)

10.1.5.3 Clinical Presentation

The clinical presentation can vary greatly based on the location and severity of the fracture. Physical examination may be limited due to the state of the patient following high-impact trauma. If able, physical examination should look for evidence of skull base injury, such as cranial nerve deficits, periorbital ecchymosis, and hemotympanum. Clinically, cerebrospinal fluid (CSF) leak may present as otorrhea or rhinorrhea, with increase on Valsalva or other high-pressure maneuvers. CSF leak is a critical finding that provides evidence of dural break with associated risk for meningitis.

10.1.5.4 Diagnosis

If there is suspected CSF otorrhea or rhinorrhea, the fluid can be sent for β-2 transferrin or β-trace protein laboratory testing. Clinical examination should be paired with imaging studies to aid with identifying the site of skull base fracture and CSF leak. For immediate diagnosis, plain x-ray of the head and cervical spine and a standard non-contrast head CT can rule out associated intracranial hemorrhage or other acute life-threatening conditions. CT scan can be paired with more detailed imaging to aid with localization of CSF leak and possible surgical planning, including high-resolution CT, angiographic studies including CT or MR angiography, and venography. CT scan is the preferred modality for early investigations of head injury, and MRI is used as a secondary evaluation of soft tissue, because MRI has been shown to have a high false positive rate for localizing fractures and CSF fistulas [50].

10.1.5.5 Management

Management is individualized based on the patient's clinical presentation, severity of skull base fracture, and other comorbid injuries

[51, 52]. A closed basilar skull fracture with no associated vascular or nerve damage does not require surgical repair [47].

Basilar skull fractures with dural break, indicated by CSF leak, have two primary management options: conservative and surgical management. The goal of conservative management is to decrease intracranial pressure and rate of CSF leak, with measures including bed rest, head elevation, and carbonic anhydrase inhibitors [53]. Patients should avoid nose blowing and other maneuvers that may increase pressure in the sinuses and contribute to worsening CSF leak as well as increased risk of meningitis.

For a stable patient with CSF leak, conservative management is encouraged because traumatic CSF leaks are associated with a high rate of spontaneous closure, ranging from 50 to 90%, and often observed within 1 week of traumatic injury [45, 53, 54]. Early prophylactic antibiotics have not demonstrated utility for preventing meningitis [44]. If a CSF leak persists following 1 week of conservative management, surgical management is favored due to low likelihood of spontaneous resolution and increased risk of meningitis [50, 55].

10.1.6 Traumatic Aneurysm

Traumatic aneurysms are "false" aneurysms. Trauma induces complete disruption of the arterial wall, and a false lumen is formed by a surrounding hematoma. These are unstable, with a poorly defined shape and irregular neck. The majority (90%) of traumatic aneurysms occur in the anterior fossa at the skull base or on distal, small cerebral branches [56].

10.1.6.1 Epidemiology
Traumatic intracranial aneurysms are rare, representing less than 1% of all intracranial aneurysms [56]. They are more prevalent in children than adults, and it is estimated that 30% of traumatic aneurysms occur in patients less than 20 years of age [57, 58]. The primary mechanism is penetrating trauma, particularly stab wounds [59]. There is a severe risk of delayed intracranial hemorrhage, and ruptured traumatic aneurysms have a mortality rate of about 50% [60].

10.1.6.2 Clinical Presentation
Traumatic aneurysm may be asymptomatic or have symptoms of mass effect or aneurysm rupture. Symptoms may become evident only a few minutes after injury if there is early rupture, or may develop slowly over time depending on the size, stability, and location. Common presenting symptoms of aneurysmal rupture include headache, decreased level of consciousness, seizure, and focal neurological deficits [60].

10.1.6.3 Diagnosis
Due to nonspecific clinical presentation in the setting of head trauma with possible other intracranial injuries, the diagnosis of traumatic aneurysm requires a high degree of suspicion combined with radiologic workup. CT scan can be performed quickly and will demonstrate acute intracranial hemorrhage in the case of a ruptured traumatic aneurysm. CT scan should be followed with angiography if CT scan identifies intracranial hemorrhage, skull fracture, or if there is continued clinical suspicion for an aneurysm [61]. CT angiography (CTA) is preferred as the first line study in emergencies; however, digital subtraction angiography (DSA) is the gold standard for diagnosing aneurysm. DSA should be used to confirm and document the location of an aneurysm initially identified with CTA [57]. Traumatic aneurysms may take some time to develop, and repeat imaging is recommended 2–4 weeks after the injury.

10.1.6.4 Management
Early neurosurgical or endovascular management of traumatic aneurysm is imperative due to the high risk of aneurysmal rupture and associated mortality rate [56, 58]. The appropriate treatment option is based on the location of aneurysm and its structure.

10.1.7 Traumatic Intracranial Hemorrhage

Intracranial hemorrhage (ICH) is defined as bleeding within the intracranial vault and is defined by its anatomic site: subarachnoid, intraparenchymal, epidural, or subdural (◘ Fig. 10.5).

10.1.7.1 Subarachnoid Hemorrhage

Subarachnoid hemorrhage (SAH) is bleeding within the subarachnoid space. Overall, traumatic SAH is reported to occur at a rate of 28–61% following moderate to severe head injury with an average age of 40 years old [62–64]. Children are at decreased risk of developing traumatic SAH compared to adults. The

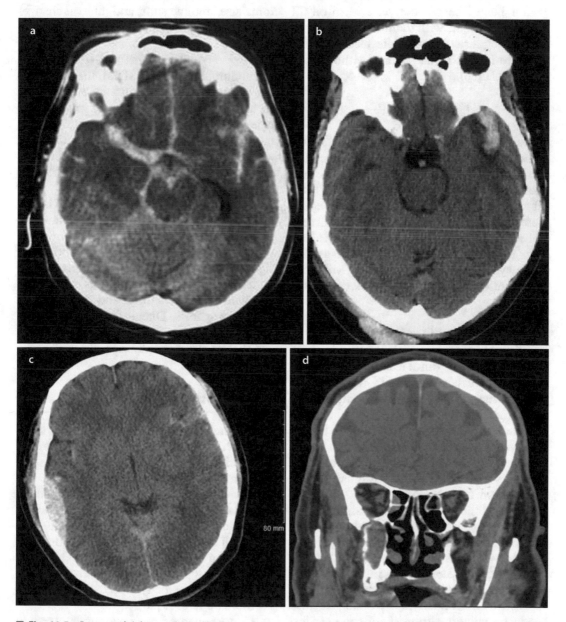

◘ **Fig. 10.5** Intracranial hemorrhage on CT. **a** Subarachnoid hemorrhage (Reproduced Wilson et al. [101] with permission from John Wiley and Sons. ©2005 John Wiley & Sons, Inc.). **b** Intraparenchymal hemorrhage (Adapted from Chang et al. [102] with permission from Oxford University Press. © 2006 Oxford University Press). **c** Epidural hematoma (arrow). **d** Subdural hematoma (arrow)

clinical presentation includes severe headache, vomiting, altered mental status, and possible loss of consciousness. CT scan has high sensitivity and specificity for diagnosis [65]. Lumbar puncture is the gold standard for diagnosis and should be performed if CT scan is negative but high clinical suspicion remains. Macroscopic blood in the CSF, termed xanthochromia, identifies the presence of SAH even if hemorrhage is not yet evident on CT scan [65]. Patients with traumatic SAH have a worse prognosis for complete recovery compared to head trauma patients without traumatic SAH [66].

10.1.7.2 Intraparenchymal Hemorrhage

Intraparenchymal hemorrhage (IPH) describes hemorrhage into the brain parenchyma. The hemorrhage can possibly extend into the ventricles and the subarachnoid space. The earliest symptom is headache from rapidly increased intracranial pressure, and focal deficits evolve over a period of minutes to half an hour based on location of hemorrhage [67]. Other symptoms include stiff neck, vomiting, and seizures. IPH is best diagnosed with CT scan.

10.1.7.3 Epidural Hematoma

In epidural hematoma (EDH), there is bleeding external to the dural membrane following rupture of vessels that run in the periosteal layer of the dura. It may be associated with skull fracture [68]. The incidence of EDH is reported between 1 and 6% in children following severe head trauma and most often associated with falls from a height [69]. Reported mortality in children with traumatic EDH ranges from 1 to 12% [55].

The classic clinical presentation of an EDH describes a "lucid interval" during which the patient appears awake and alert, followed by a loss of consciousness and rapid neurological decline secondary to mass effect [70]. Other clinical signs include scalp hematoma suggestive of underlying cranial fracture, headache, vomiting, transient or complete loss of consciousness, amnesia, and epistaxis [40]. There is risk of cerebral herniation with increasing size of EDH. Diagnosis is made

with CT scan, which will demonstrate a biconvex hyperdensity that can cross the midline.

In pediatric patients, conservative management with close observation is advocated for asymptomatic patients, or those with no mass effect and EDH volume less than 15 mL on initial CT scan [71–73]. Surgical management is indicated with poor neurological status or dependent on characteristics such as hematoma size, midline shift, and interval changes on repeat imaging [74].

10.1.7.4 Subdural Hematoma

In subdural hematoma (SDH), there is bleeding under the dural membrane, often caused by tears of the cerebral bridging veins as they enter the dural sinus [68]. Traumatic SDH is more common in adults than children, although it has been reported as a frequent finding in children who were victims of abusive head trauma [75].

Compared to EDH, SDH has a higher association of intraparenchymal brain damage and worse prognosis [76]. Patients may present with headache, seizures, and other signs of raised intracranial pressure. If the patient has unreactive pupils, this may signify transtentorial herniation and worsens the overall prognosis. Diagnosis is made by CT scan and seen as a crescent-shaped hyperdensity that does not usually cross the midline.

10.1.8 Traumatic Brain Injury

The definition of TBI is not standardized, although it typically describes external mechanical injury to the brain resulting in primary and secondary outcomes [77].

Primary TBI describes the immediate impact of trauma with possible damage to the skull and brain parenchyma and includes basilar skull fractures, intracranial hemorrhage, penetrating injury, contusions, and diffuse axonal injury. Contusions are very common following high-velocity closed head trauma, reported up to 89% [78].

Contusions are caused by coup-contrecoup forces causing brain parenchyma to hit against the cranial fossa, falx cerebri, or tentorium cerebelli with subsequent tissue damage.

Diffuse axonal injury (DAI) is a severe form of TBI. It describes widespread axonal damage from shearing forces during rapid rotational movement, especially fast acceleration or deceleration, which stretch and deform brain parenchyma and vasculature [79]. DAI most greatly affects interfaces of different tissue density, including the corpus callosum, gray-white matter junctions, deep white matter, periventricular regions, hippocampal regions, and the brainstem [80].

Secondary TBI describes the long-term neuropsychiatric and functional impairment that follows primary TBI, a spectrum that is closely linked to the severity of initial injury.

10.1.8.1 Epidemiology

TBI is the leading cause of disability and death in children [81, 82]. According to surveillance data from the CDC's National Center for Injury Prevention and Control, approximately 1.7 million people in the United States suffer traumatic brain injuries each year [83]. The rate of TBI is higher in younger age groups and males, with about 30% in children aged less than 14 years old [84]. The primary mechanism is high velocity falls [83].

> Traumatic brain injury is the leading cause of disability and death in children and is most frequent in males less than 14 years old.

10.1.8.2 Clinical Presentation

Patients with DAI may present with loss of consciousness or persistent vegetative state following head trauma [85]. Secondary TBI has been reported months to years following the inciting event [86]. Frequently reported sequelae of secondary TBI include headache, dizziness, irritability, impaired concentration, memory deficits, fatigue, depression, anxiety, judgment problems, noise sensitivity, photophobia, oculomotor deficits with resultant diplopia, and visual field loss [87]. Post-traumatic seizures are common, with increased frequency for children who were injured at a younger age, trauma by abuse or

assault, and in those who had associated subdural hemorrhage [88].

10.1.8.3 Diagnosis

CT scan may identify areas of contusion. MRI is the best imaging modality for DAI [89].

10.1.8.4 Management

Early neuropsychological rehabilitation may decrease the long-term morbidity of TBI [90]. The main focus of early management of severe TBI is to prevent secondary injury by avoiding hypotension and hypoxia with close ICU monitoring and treatment [84, 91]. For patients with secondary TBI, rehabilitation, including referral to a low vision specialist, may help with the adaptation to long-term visual and neurological sequelae.

10.1.9 Oculomotor System

The oculomotor system is a complex set of interconnected regions throughout the central nervous system that controls various eye movements. Furthermore, the oculomotor system maintains the stability of eye position and directs eye movements in a coordinated fashion. Dysfunction of the system may lead to ocular misalignment and associated symptoms of blurry vision and/or diplopia. A child with extraocular nerve palsies may present differently than adults due to their inability to properly verbalize/describe their complaints such as diplopia. A high level of suspicion is required to properly diagnose and subsequently treat a child with an oculomotor deficit secondary to trauma.

10.1.10 Overview of Anatomy

10.1.10.1 The Orbit

There are seven bones that form the orbit: frontal, zygomatic, maxillary, ethmoid, sphenoid, lacrimal, and palatine bone (◘ Fig. 10.6). The orbital roof is comprised of two bones including the frontal bone and the lesser wing of the sphenoid; together the two bones separate the orbit from the above frontal sinus and intracranial cavity. The lateral wall is formed by the

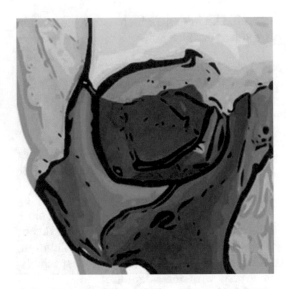

◘ Fig. 10.6 Depiction of the seven orbital bones. Yellow = frontal bone; red = sphenoid bone; green = lacrimal bone; brown = ethmoid bone; blue = Zygomatic bone; purple = maxillary bone; turquoise = palatine bone (Reproduction of a lithograph plate from Gray's Anatomy ◘ Fig. 190, a two-dimensional work of art. Permission permitted under the Creative Commons Attribution License 2.5. Created on 12.15.2006, no further changes were made to the figure. ▶ https://commons.wikimedia.org/wiki/File:Orbital_bones.png)

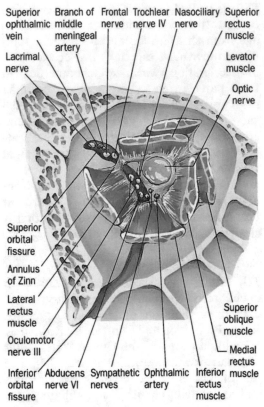

◘ Fig. 10.7 Extraocular muscles of the right eye, with the five muscles that form the annulus of Zinn. (Reproduced with permission from ▶ https://www.aao.org/image/fibrous-annulus-of-zinn © 2020 American Academy of Ophthalmology)

zygomatic bone and the greater wing of the sphenoid. The maxilla along with the palatine bone and orbital plate of the zygomatic bone make up the orbital floor. Lastly, the medial wall is comprised of the lesser wing of the sphenoid along with the lacrimal bone, the orbital plate of the ethmoid, and the frontal process of the maxilla. Important neurovascular structures pass through the orbital apex via the optic canal, and the superior and inferior orbital fissures.

The Extraocular Muscles

There are seven extraocular muscles of the eye consisting of four rectus muscles, two oblique muscles, and one palpebral muscle. The four rectus muscles include the superior, inferior, medial, and lateral. The rectus muscles as well as the levator palpebrae superioris (levator muscle) originate from the annulus of Zinn, which is a tendinous ring at the orbital apex (◘ Fig. 10.7). The superior oblique originates from the periosteum of the body of the sphenoid bone and inserts onto the eye beneath the insertion of the superior rectus. The infe-

rior oblique has an origin from the periosteum of the maxillary bone and inserts on the posterior inferior temporal surface of the eye. Lastly, the levator muscle originates from the lesser wing of the sphenoid bone and eventually travels anteriorly to become the levator aponeurosis with insertion into the eyelid.

The Ocular Motor Cranial Nerves, in Brief

There are three ocular motor cranial nerves that control eye movements: the third nerve (oculomotor), the fourth nerve (trochlear), and the sixth nerve (abducens). These nerves arise from their nuclei located in the midbrain and pons, then course through the subarachnoid cistern and the cavernous sinus before entering the orbit via the superior orbital fissure to innervate their respective extraocular muscles (◘ Fig. 10.8).

10.1.10.2 Cranial Nerve III: The Oculomotor Nerve

Anatomy

The oculomotor nerve (third nerve) originates in the midbrain and travels through the subarachnoid space, and eventually into the lateral wall of the cavernous sinus. The nerve then divides into superior and inferior branches before terminating at the extraocular muscles, levator muscle in the eyelid, and pupillary sphincter muscle. The superior division of the third nerve innervates the levator muscle and superior rectus, while the inferior division innervates the medial rectus, lateral rectus, inferior rectus, and inferior oblique muscles (◘ Fig. 10.9).

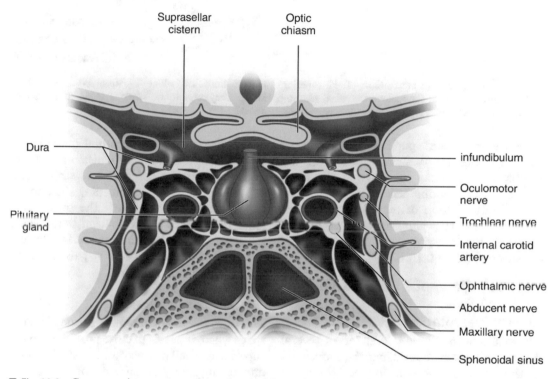

◘ **Fig. 10.8** Cavernous sinus anatomy. (Reproduced with permission from Chowdhury et al. [103])

◘ **Fig. 10.9** Superior and inferior divisions of the oculomotor nerve. (Adapted from Eye nerve pathways diagram. Patrick J. Lynch, medical illustrator; C. Carl Jaffe, MD, cardiologist. Creative commons attribution 2.5 license 2006)

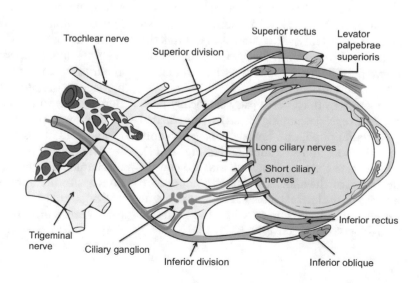

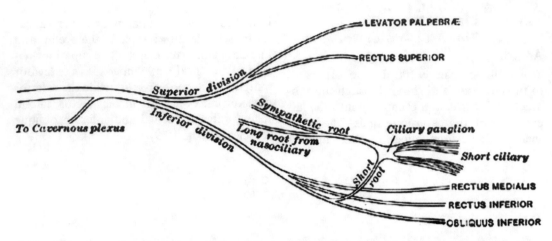

Fig. 10.10 Respective innervations of the superior and inferior divisions of the oculomotor nerve. (Reproduced from Henry Gray, Warren Lewis, Anatomy of the Human Body, 1918. Plate 775 from Wikimedia Commons: Grey's Anatomy. Work is listed in the public domain)

Parasympathetic pupillary fibers travel from the Edinger-Westphal nucleus in the midbrain and follow the path of the third nerve. The parasympathetic fibers then follow the inferior division of the third nerve, synapse in the ciliary ganglion, and eventually innervate the iris sphincter muscle (pupillary constrictor) (■ Fig. 10.10).

10.1.10.3 Traumatic Third Nerve Palsy

Clinical Presentation

The oculomotor nerve (CN3) serves several functions, namely, controlling the movement of the medial rectus, superior rectus, inferior rectus, inferior oblique, and levator muscles. Functionally, this translates into inward, upward, and downward movement and torsion of the eye. Levator control maintains the upper eyelid position. Lastly, the oculomotor nerve permits the pupil to constrict and facilitates accommodation.

Complete third nerve palsy classically presents with eyelid drooping (ptosis), a fixed dilated (mydriatic) pupil, and limitation of adduction, infraduction, and supraduction (■ Fig. 10.11). There is usually an outward and downward deviation of the affected eye due to unopposed activity of the lateral rectus and superior oblique muscles, which are innervated by the sixth and fourth nerves, respectively.

Trauma to the third cranial nerve is the second most common mechanism of dysfunction, occurring by compression, stretch and contusion, or transection [94]. Traumatic closed head injury affecting the third nerve tends to be more severe than in cases where the fourth or sixth cranial nerve is affected. Typically, traumatic third nerve palsy is due to motor vehicle accidents [94].

Mechanisms of Injury

The third nerve is vulnerable in the cisternal space where it passes in close proximity to the superior cerebellar artery and posterior communicating artery. Aneurysms of the respective arteries may impinge on the nerve and affect the peripheral parasympathetic fibers that run along with the nerve. Pupil involvement (mydriasis) with a third nerve palsy suggests a compressive etiology. Ruptured aneurysms can cause direct hemorrhagic damage to the nerve or lead to uncal herniation, while unruptured aneurysms are thought to cause compressive mechanical distortion, edema, and fibrosis of the nerve itself [94].

The third nerve is vulnerable to damage by mechanical stretching and contusion where it attaches to the dura near the cavernous sinus and adjacent to the posterior clinoid processes [95]. Transtentorial herniation of the uncus may also compress the third nerve. In the cav-

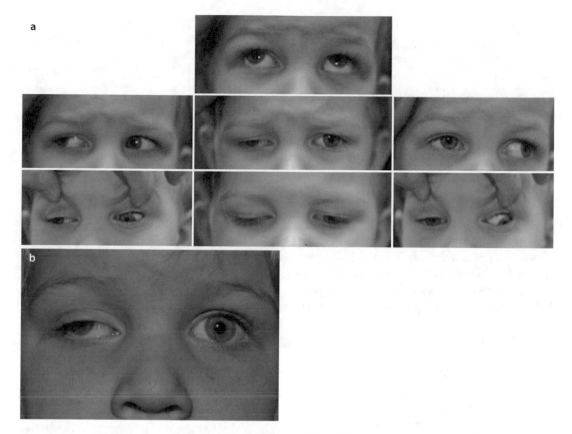

◘ **Fig. 10.11** Third nerve palsy. **a** Ocular motility showing limited supraduction, adduction, and infraduction. **b** Right ptosis and displacement of the eye down and out. The right pupil is also dilated. (Adapted from Evaluation and management of third nerve palsy in children [slides] [Neuro-Ophthalmology Virtual Education Library: NOVEL Web Site] with permission from Paul H. Phillips, M.D. Available at ▶ https://collections. lib.utah.edu/ark:/87278/s6t7749q. © North American Neuro-ophthalmology Society 2019)

ernous sinus, CN III dysfunction can be due to traumatic carotid-cavernous fistula. Both direct and indirect subtypes may involve the third, fourth, and sixth nerves and present with ophthalmoplegia and other findings such as dilated, tortuous conjunctival vessels, elevated intraocular pressure, chemosis, and proptosis [96].

Diagnosis

Traumatic third nerve palsy is primarily a clinical diagnosis with physical examination findings described above. Various etiologies may be confirmed with neuroimaging. Subarachnoid hemorrhage associated with a suspected ruptured aneurysm may easily be visualized on non-contrast head CT. Imaging with CTA or MRA may detect vascular injuries such as aneurysms or findings consistent with carotid-cavernous fistula. Fracture of the skull base may be detected with CT.

Management

The offending etiology should be promptly diagnosed and addressed, particularly in aneurysmal and vascular cases. Diplopia from traumatic third nerve palsy should be managed conservatively with monocular occlusion or prism lenses. Often the complete ptosis occludes the visual axis initially, allowing for relief of diplopia until the ptosis recovers. Partial recovery often occurs after about 5 months [97]. Overall, after 6–12 months, surgical interventions may be considered.

10.1.11 Cranial Nerve IV: The Trochlear Nerve

10.1.11.1 Anatomy

The trochlear nerve is unique among the three ocular motor cranial nerves because of its particularly long intracranial course and dorsal exit from the brainstem. The trochlear nerve originates in the midbrain at the level of the inferior colliculus, near the junction of the midbrain and pons. The trochlear nerve eventually passes into the cavernous sinus where it runs along the lateral wall close to the third nerve superiorly and the ophthalmic division of the trigeminal nerve inferiorly. The trochlear nerve then enters the orbit via the superior orbital fissure and proceeds to pass over the optic nerve before innervating the superior oblique muscle.

10.1.11.2 Traumatic Fourth Nerve Palsy

Clinical Presentation

The trochlear nerve's primary role is intorsion but also serves to abduct and depress the eye. Damage to the trochlear nerve causes excyclotorsion and limited downgaze in the adducted position, resulting in vertical binocular diplopia from elevation of the affected eye.

Pathophysiology

Physically slender with a long intracranial course, the trochlear nerve is the most common congenital cranial nerve palsy and is particularly subject to traumatic damage [98]. The trochlear nerve is vulnerable to avulsion and compression by the tentorial edge [99]. Damage to the trochlear nerve can occur with local ischemia in the setting of trauma when shearing forces damage the vulnerable paramedian branches of the basilar bifurcation [94].

Diagnosis

Since the superior oblique moves the eye down and in, the involved eye might be deviated superiorly (also called a hypertropia). The affected eye may additionally be extorted and the child may adopt a compensatory head tilt to the side opposite the paralyzed muscle. Clinical examination for suspected trochlear nerve palsy involves measuring the vertical deviation with cross-cover testing using prism lenses in all gazes including head tilt.

Management

As with other acute ocular motor cranial nerve palsies, monocular occlusion may be used in the acute setting for the relief of diplopia. Recovery occurs over the course of about 6 months. If the vertical deviation causing diplopia is less than 15 prism diopters, Fresnel prisms (flexible plastic prisms adhered to the lens in a pair of spectacle glasses) may be used. Fresnel prism correction higher than 15 prism diopters is not practical due to the degradation of visual acuity from the thicker prism. When symptomatic relief is not achieved after prism correction for larger deviations, some patients may require surgical correction.

10.1.12 Cranial Nerve VI: The Abducens Nerve

10.1.12.1 Anatomy

The abducens nucleus originates in the brainstem and follows a course similar to the oculomotor nerve with a course through the cavernous sinus. The sixth nerve has the longest subarachnoid course of all the ocular motor cranial nerves, making it particularly susceptible to damage from subarachnoid processes causing raised intracranial pressure (Fig. 10.12). In the cavernous sinus, the abducens nerve proceeds within the medial cavernous sinus, in close contact with the internal carotid artery (ICA) and the sympathetic plexus (Fig. 10.8). For this reason, sixth nerve palsy presenting with ipsilateral Horner's syndrome localizes to the cavernous sinus. The nerve then enters the orbit via the superior orbital fissure, within the annulus of Zinn, and proceeds to innervate the lateral rectus muscle.

10.1.12.2 Traumatic Sixth Nerve Palsy

Clinical Presentation

The abducens nerve allows for ipsilateral horizontal gaze. Isolated sixth nerve palsy presents with horizontal binocular diplopia, with ipsilateral impaired abduction and

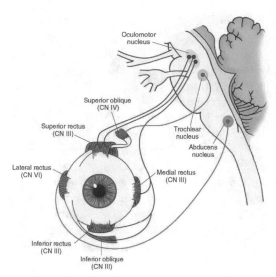

■ **Fig. 10.12** Innervation of the extraocular muscles. (Adapted from Figure 14-10 in ▶ http://what-when-how.com/neuroscience/the-cranial-nerves-organization-of-the-central-nervous-system-part-4/)

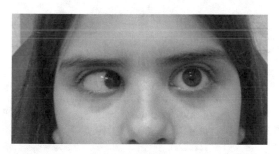

■ **Fig. 10.13** Sixth nerve palsy of the right eye demonstrating ipsilateral impaired abduction and inward deviation (esotropia). (Reproduced from Gonçalves et al. [104]. Copyright © 2017 Rita Gonçalves et al. Open access article distributed under the Creative Commons Attribution License.)

inward deviation of the affected eye. Patients will be most symptomatic in ipsilateral lateral gaze and when looking in the distance (■ Fig. 10.13).

Pathophysiology

Trauma most frequently damages the abducens nerve in cases of raised intracranial pressure or herniation. In the cavernous sinus, the sixth nerve's close relation to the internal carotid artery leaves it at risk of being involved with any extradural carotid aneurysms [96]. However, it should be noted that cavernous carotid aneurysms typically present with a constellation of cranial nerve abnormalities rather than isolated unilateral sixth nerve palsy [96].

Diagnosis

Patients may present with partial or complete limitation of abduction. In primary gaze position, there is often a large esotropia (inward deviation) initially. Patients may often rotate their head toward the paralyzed side in order to compensate for the palsy. The etiology of sixth nerve palsy can be detected with neuroimaging with CT for assessment of skull base fractures or MRI for assessment of the brain parenchyma. If there is suspicion for raised intracranial pressure as a cause for bilateral sixth nerve palsy, a proper workup must be undertaken and urgent intervention is necessary to lower the CSF pressure [96].

Management

Similar to third and fourth nerve palsy, the affected eye in sixth nerve palsy should be managed initially by monocular occlusion and prisms. If the diplopia has not recovered after 6 months, strabismus surgery may be considered for relief.

Case Presentation

An 8-year-old girl was admitted to the hospital after a severe motor vehicle accident. The patient had no specific past medical or ocular history. On examination, there was limitation of abduction of the left eye, which raised suspicion for a left 6th nerve palsy. Concurrently, the patient had decreased corneal sensation of the left eye. Neuroimaging and subsequent angiography revealed a dissecting carotid aneurysm causing compression of the 6th nerve, V1 and V2 within the cavernous sinus.

Case Presentation

A 15-year-old female with no past ocular or medical history presented to the emergency department following assault with loss of consciousness. The patient recalled that she was punched multiple times in the back of her head. At presentation, she reported acute decreased vision in the right eye and right periorbital pain. Right eye examination was significant for visual acuity of 20/40, relative afferent pupillary defect, decreased color vision, and periorbital edema and ecchymosis. Confrontation visual field testing identified an inferior altitu-dinal defect in the right eye, and full visual field in the left eye. A CT orbits without contrast did not identify any orbital fractures, there was no tenting of the right globe, and the right optic nerve was not on stretch. An MRI orbits and brain with and without contrast also did not demonstrate acute optic nerve pathology. The patient was diagnosed with indirect traumatic optic neuropathy. She was managed conservatively. Over a period of 1 month, the patient's visual acuity improved to 20/20, color vision normalized, and visual field defects resolved.

Key Points
- Traumatic optic neuropathy most often occurs due to acceleration-deceleration head injuries causing trauma to the fixed intracanalicular segment of the optic nerve where the nerve is adherent to the periosteum in the optic canal. Many cases will spontaneously improve, and there is limited evidence of steroid benefit.
- Acquired pediatric Horner syndrome presents with ipsilateral blepharoptosis, miosis, and facial anhidrosis, with anisocoria more evident in dim lighting. If acquired in early infancy, ipsilateral iris heterochromia and straight hair may also be present. Causes of acquired pediatric Horner syndrome include birth trauma, iatrogenic injury, neuroblastoma, or other malignancy.
- Intracranial hemorrhage is less common after head trauma in children compared to adults. Subdural hematoma can occur in abusive head trauma and has a higher association of intraparenchymal injury, resulting in worse prognosis.
- Ophthalmic manifestations of traumatic brain injury include photophobia, headache often causing retrobulbar pain, eye movement abnormalities, ocular motor deficits with resultant diplopia, and visual field loss.
- Ocular motor cranial nerve palsy can be caused by direct trauma, hemorrhage, or compression by vasculature or parenchyma.

❓ Review Questions
1. Which of the following studies showed that steroid use in head injury may be harmful (thus limiting the benefit in traumatic optic neuropathy)?
   (a) ONTT
   (b) IIHTT
   (c) CRASH
   (d) IONDT

2. Traumatic optic neuropathy is most often associated with a fracture of the:
   (a) Medial wall of the orbit
   (b) Frontal bone/orbital roof
   (c) Orbital floor
   (d) Lateral wall of the orbit

3. A 3-month-old boy presents with unilateral ptosis associated with a smaller pupil and lack of facial sweating. Which of the following pharmacologic pupil tests for Horner syndrome is contraindicated?
   (a) 4 or 10% Topical cocaine
   (b) hydroxyamphetamine
   (c) 1% apraclonidine

4. Which of the following are true regarding traumatic brain injury?
   (a) It is the leading cause of disability and death in children
   (b) It is more common in girls over the age of 14
   (c) Post-traumatic seizures are less common when associated with subdural hematoma
   (d) CT is the best imaging modality to identify diffuse axonal injury

5. Which of the following choices matches the ocular motor cranial nerve with its unique anatomic feature?
   (a) Trochlear nerve: longest intracranial course
   (b) Third nerve: travels in close proximity to the cavernous carotid artery
   (c) Sixth nerve: contains fibers from the Edinger-Westphal nucleus

✅ **Answer**

1. (c)
2. (b)
3. (c)
4. (a)
5. (a)

References

1. Steinsapir KD, Goldberg RA. Traumatic optic neuropathy: an evolving understanding. Am J Ophthalmol. 2011;151:928–933.e2.
2. McClenaghan FC, Ezra DG, Holmes SB. Mechanisms and management of vision loss following orbital and facial trauma. Curr Opin Ophthalmol. 2011;22:426–31.
3. Sarkies N. Traumatic optic neuropathy. Eye (Lond). 2004;18:1122–5.
4. Maegele M. Reversal of isolated unilateral optic nerve edema with concomitant visual impairment following blunt trauma: a case report. J Med Case Reports. 2008;2:50.
5. Pirouzmand F. Epidemiological trends of traumatic optic nerve injuries in the largest Canadian adult trauma center. J Craniofac Surg. 2012;23:516–20.
6. Ford RL, Lee V, Xing W, Bunce C. A 2-year prospective surveillance of pediatric traumatic optic neuropathy in the United Kingdom. J AAPOS. 2012;16(5):413–7.
7. Gise R, Truong T, Parsikia A, Mbekeani JN. Visual pathway injuries in pediatric ocular trauma-a survey of the National Trauma Data Bank From 2008 to 2014. Pediatr Neurol. 2018;85:43–50.
8. Mahapatra AK, Tandon DA. Traumatic optic neuropathy in children: a prospective study. Pediatr Neurosurg. 1993;19:34–9.
9. Goldenberg-Cohen N, Miller NR, Repka MX. Traumatic optic neuropathy in children and adolescents. J AAPOS. 2004;8:20–7.
10. Ellis MJ, Ritchie L, Cordingley D, Essig M, Mansouri B. Traumatic optic neuropathy: a potentially unrecognized diagnosis after sports-related concussion. Curr Sports Med Rep. 2016;15(1):27–32.
11. Urolagin SB, Kotrashetti SM, Kale TP, Balihallimath LJ. Traumatic optic neuropathy after maxillofacial trauma: a review of 8 cases. J Oral Maxillofac Surg. 2012;70:1123–30.
12. Lee V, Ford RL, Xing W, Bunce C, Foot B. Surveillance of traumatic optic neuropathy in the UK. Eye (Lond). 2010;24(2):240–50.
13. Sawhney R, Kochhar S, Gupta R, Jain R, Sood S. Traumatic optic nerve avulsion: role of ultrasonography. Eye (Lond). 2003;17:667–70.
14. Warner N, Eggenberger E. Traumatic optic neuropathy: a review of the current literature. Curr Opin Ophthalmol. 2010;21:459–62.
15. Wu M, Yip JLY, Kuper H. Rapid assessment of avoidable blindness in Kunming, china. Ophthalmology. 2008;115:969–74.
16. Yu-Wai-Man P, Griffiths PG. Steroids for traumatic optic neuropathy. Cochrane Database Syst Rev. 2013;6:CD006032.
17. Anderson RL, Panje WR, Gross CE. Optic nerve blindness following blunt forehead trauma. Ophthalmology. 1982;89:445–55.
18. Bracken MB, et al. A randomized, controlled trial of methylprednisolone or naloxone in the treatment of acute spinal-cord injury. Results of the Second National Acute Spinal Cord Injury Study. N Engl J Med. 1990;322:1405–11.
19. Bracken MB, et al. Administration of methylprednisolone for 24 or 48 hours or tirilazad mesylate for 48 hours in the treatment of acute spinal cord injury. Results of the Third National Acute Spinal Cord Injury Randomized Controlled Trial National Acute Spinal Cord Injury Study. JAMA. 1997;277:1597–604.
20. Levin LA, Beck RW, Joseph MP, Seiff S, Kraker R. The treatment of traumatic optic neuropathy: the International Optic Nerve Trauma Study. Ophthalmology. 1999;106:1268–77.
21. Entezari M, Rajavi Z, Sedighi N, Daftarian N, Sanagoo M. High-dose intravenous methylprednisolone in recent traumatic optic neuropathy; a randomized double-masked placebo-controlled clinical trial. Graefes Arch Clin Exp Ophthalmol. 2007;245:1267–71.
22. Roberts I, et al. Effect of intravenous corticosteroids on death within 14 days in 10008 adults with clinically significant head injury (MRC CRASH trial): randomised placebo-controlled trial. Lancet Lond Engl. 2004;364:1321–8.

23. Osborne NN, et al. Optic nerve and neuroprotection strategies. Eye (Lond). 2004;18:1075–84.

24. Zimmerer R, Rana M, Schumann P, Gellrich N-C. Diagnosis and treatment of optic nerve trauma. Facial Plast Surg FPS. 2014;30:518–27.

25. Carta A, et al. Visual prognosis after indirect traumatic optic neuropathy. J Neurol Neurosurg Psychiatry. 2003;74:246–8.

26. Wang BH, et al. Traumatic optic neuropathy: a review of 61 patients. Plast Reconstr Surg. 2001;107: 1655–64.

27. Smith SJ, Diehl N, Leavitt JA, Mohney BG. Incidence of pediatric Horner syndrome and the risk of neuroblastoma: a population-based study. Arch Ophthalmol. 2010;128(3):324–9.

28. Jeffery AR, Ellis FJ, Repka MX, Buncic JR. Pediatric Horner syndrome. J AAPOS. 1998;2(3): 159–67.

29. Robertson WC, Pettigrew LC. "Congenital" Horner's syndrome and carotid dissection. J Neuroimaging. 2003;13(4):367–70.

30. Gupta M, Dinakaran S, Chan TK. Congenital horner syndrome and hemiplegia secondary to carotid dissection. J Pediatr Ophthalmol Strabismus. 2005;42(2):122–4.

31. Bayhan Gİ, Karaca M, Yazici Ü, Tanir G. A case of Horner's syndrome after the surgical treatment of pulmonary hydatid cyst. Turkiye Parazitol Derg. 2010;34(4):196–9.

32. Demiral M, Binay C, Simsek E, Ilhan H. Horner syndrome secondary to thyroid surgery. Case Rep Endocrinol. 2017;2017:1689039.

33. Mahoney NR, Liu GT, Menacker SJ, Wilson MC, Hogarty MD, Maris JM. Pediatric horner syndrome: etiologies and roles of imaging and urine studies to detect neuroblastoma and other responsible mass lesions. Am J Ophthalmol. 2006;142(4):651–9.

34. Barrea C, Vigouroux T, Karam J, Milet A, Vaessen S, Misson JP. Horner syndrome in children: a clinical condition with serious underlying disease. Neuropediatrics. 2016;47(4):268–72.

35. Deprez FC, Coulier J, Rommel D, Boschi A. Congenital horner syndrome with heterochromia iridis associated with ipsilateral internal carotid artery hypoplasia. J Clin Neurol. 2015;11(2):192–6.

36. Ott C, Bobylev A, Holland-cunz SG, Mayr J. Unilateral straight hair-a symptom of acquired horner's syndrome in a neonate. European J Pediatr Surg Rep. 2018;6(1):e32–6.

37. Kadom N, Rosman NP, Jubouri S, Trofimova A, Egloff AM, Zein WM. Neuroimaging experience in pediatric Horner syndrome. Pediatr Radiol. 2015;45(10):1535–43.

38. Martin GC, Aymard PA, Denier C, et al. Usefulness of cocaine drops in investigating infant anisocoria. Eur J Paediatr Neurol. 2017;21(6):852–7.

39. Coulthard MG, Varghese V, Harvey LP, Gillen TC, Kimble RM, Ware RS. A review of children with severe trauma admitted to pediatric intensive care in Queensland, Australia. PLoS ONE. 2019;14(2): e0211530.

40. Karasu A, Sabanci PA, Izgi N, et al. Traumatic epidural hematomas of the posterior cranial fossa. Surg Neurol. 2008;69(3):247–51.

41. Densmore JC, Lim HJ, Oldham KT, Guice KS. Outcomes and delivery of care in pediatric injury. J Pediatr Surg. 2006;41(1):92–8.

42. Odebode TO, Ademola-Popoola DS, Ojo TA, Ayanniyi AA. Ocular and visual complications of head injury. Eye (Lond). 2005;19:561–6.

43. Samii M, Tatagiba M. Skull base trauma: diagnosis and management. Neurol Res. 2002;24:147–56.

44. Leibu S, Rosenthal G, Shoshan Y, Benifla M. Clinical significance of long-term follow-up of children with posttraumatic skull base fracture. World Neurosurg. 2017;103:315–21.

45. Yilmazlar S, et al. Cerebrospinal fluid leakage complicating skull base fractures: analysis of 81 cases. Neurosurg Rev. 2006;29:64–71.

46. Baugnon KL, Hudgins PA. Skull base fractures and their complications. Neuroimaging Clin N Am. 2014;24:439–65, vii–viii.

47. Wang H, Zhou Y, Liu J, Ou L, Han J, Xiang L. Traumatic skull fractures in children and adolescents: a retrospective observational study. Injury. 2018;49(2):219–25.

48. Bumm K, Heupel J, Bozzato A, Iro H, Hornung J. Localization and infliction pattern of iatrogenic skull base defects following endoscopic sinus surgery at a teaching hospital. Auris Nasus Larynx. 2009;36:671–6.

49. Kienstra MA, Van Loveren H. Anterior skull base fractures. Facial Plast Surg FPS. 2005;21:180–6.

50. Ziu M, Savage JG, Jimenez DF. Diagnosis and treatment of cerebrospinal fluid rhinorrhea following accidental traumatic anterior skull base fractures. Neurosurg Focus. 2012;32:E3.

51. Archer JB, Sun H, Bonney PA, et al. Extensive traumatic anterior skull base fractures with cerebrospinal fluid leak: classification and repair techniques using combined vascularized tissue flaps. J Neurosurg. 2016;124(3):647–56.

52. Schlosser RJ, Bolger WE. Nasal cerebrospinal fluid leaks: critical review and surgical considerations. Laryngoscope. 2004;114:255–65.

53. Bell RB, Dierks EJ, Homer L, Potter BE. Management of cerebrospinal fluid leak associated with craniomaxillofacial trauma. J Oral Maxillofac Surg. 2004;62:676–84.

54. Lin DT, Lin AC. Surgical treatment of traumatic injuries of the cranial base. Otolaryngol Clin North Am. 2013;46:749–57.

55. Rocchi G, et al. Severe craniofacial fractures with frontobasal involvement and cerebrospinal fluid fistula: indications for surgical repair. Surg Neurol. 2005;63:559–63.

56. Santos G, Lima T, Pereira S, Machado E. Traumatic middle cerebral artery aneurysm secondary to a gunshot wound. J Neuroimaging. 2013;23:115–7.

57. Buckingham MJ, et al. Traumatic intracranial aneurysms in childhood: two cases and a review of the literature. Neurosurgery. 1988;22:398–408.

58. Kim M, Lee HS, Lee S, et al. Pediatric intracranial aneurysms: favorable outcomes despite rareness and complexity. World Neurosurg. 2019;125:e1203–16.

59. Kieck CF, de Villiers JC. Vascular lesions due to transcranial stab wounds. J Neurosurg. 1984;60:42–6.

60. Larson PS, Reisner A, Morassutti DJ, Abdulhadi B, Harpring JE. Traumatic intracranial aneurysms. Neurosurg Focus. 2000;8:e4.

61. Zangbar B, et al. Traumatic intracranial aneurysm in blunt trauma. Brain Inj. 2015;29:601–6.

62. Parchani A, et al. Traumatic subarachnoid hemorrhage due to motor vehicle crash versus fall from height: a 4-year epidemiologic study. World Neurosurg. 2014;82:e639–44.

63. Mattioli C, et al. Traumatic subarachnoid hemorrhage on the computerized tomography scan obtained at admission: a multicenter assessment of the accuracy of diagnosis and the potential impact on patient outcome. J Neurosurg. 2003;98:37–42.

64. Compagnone C, et al. Patients with moderate head injury: a prospective multicenter study of 315 patients. Neurosurgery. 2009;64:690–696-697.

65. Boesiger BM, Shiber JR. Subarachnoid hemorrhage diagnosis by computed tomography and lumbar puncture: are fifth generation CT scanners better at identifying subarachnoid hemorrhage? J Emerg Med. 2005;29:23–7.

66. Servadei F, et al. Traumatic subarachnoid hemorrhage: demographic and clinical study of 750 patients from the European brain injury consortium survey of head injuries. Neurosurgery. 2002;50:261–7.

67. Ropper AH, Davis KR. Lobar cerebral hemorrhages: acute clinical syndromes in 26 cases. Ann Neurol. 1980;8:141–7.

68. Freeman WD, Aguilar MI. Intracranial hemorrhage: diagnosis and management. Neurol Clin. 2012;30:211–240, ix.

69. Gerlach R, Dittrich S, Schneider W, Ackermann H, Seifert V, Kieslich M. Traumatic epidural hematomas in children and adolescents: outcome analysis in 39 consecutive unselected cases. Pediatr Emerg Care. 2009;25(3):164–9.

70. Araujo JLV, Aguiar U, do P, Todeschini AB, Saade N, Veiga JCE. Epidemiological analysis of 210 cases of surgically treated traumatic extradural hematoma. Rev. Colégio Bras. Cir. 2012;39:268–71.

71. Jamous MA, Abdel Aziz H, Al Kaisy F, Eloqayli H, Azab M, Al-Jarrah M. Conservative management of acute epidural hematoma in a pediatric age group. Pediatr Neurosurg. 2009;45(3):181–4.

72. Flaherty BF, Moore HE, Riva-cambrin J, Bratton SL. Pediatric patients with traumatic epidural hematoma at low risk for deterioration and need for surgical treatment. J Pediatr Surg. 2017;52(2):334–9.

73. Champagne PO, He KX, Mercier C, Weil AG, Crevier L. Conservative management of large traumatic supratentorial epidural hematoma in the pediatric population. Pediatr Neurosurg. 2017;52(3):168–72.

74. Maugeri R, Anderson DG, Graziano F, Meccio F, Visocchi M, Iacopino DG. Conservative vs. surgical management of post-traumatic epidural hematoma: a case and review of literature. Am J Case Rep. 2015;16:811–7.

75. Melo JR, Di Rocco F, Bourgeois M, et al. Surgical options for treatment of traumatic subdural hematomas in children younger than 2 years of age. J Neurosurg Pediatr. 2014;13(4):456–61.

76. Tallon JM, Ackroyd-Stolarz S, Karim SA, Clarke DB. The epidemiology of surgically treated acute subdural and epidural hematomas in patients with head injuries: a population-based study. Can J Surg J Can Chir. 2008;51:339–45.

77. Segun Toyin Dawodu. Traumatic Brain Injury (TBI) – definition and pathophysiology: overview, epidemiology, primary injury. 2015.

78. Choi JH, et al. Multimodal early rehabilitation and predictors of outcome in survivors of severe traumatic brain injury. J Trauma. 2008;65:1028–35.

79. Bazarian JJ, Blyth B, Cimpello L. Bench to bedside: evidence for brain injury after concussion-looking beyond the computed tomography scan. Acad Emerg Med Off J Soc Acad Emerg Med. 2006;13:199–214.

80. Li X-Y, Feng D-F. Diffuse axonal injury: novel insights into detection and treatment. J Clin Neurosci. 2009;16:614–9.

81. Popernack ML, Gray N, Reuter-rice K. Moderate-to-severe traumatic brain injury in children: complications and rehabilitation strategies. J Pediatr Health Care. 2015;29(3):e1–7.

82. Araki T, Yokota H, Morita A. Pediatric traumatic brain injury: characteristic features, diagnosis, and management. Neurol Med Chir (Tokyo). 2017;57(2):82–93.

83. Faul 2010. Traumatic brain injury in the United States - Emergency Department Visits, Hospitalizations and Deaths 2002–2006. Available at: http://www.cdc.gov/traumaticbraininjury/pdf/blue_book.pdf. Accessed: 5 Apr 2019.

84. Morrissey K, Fairbrother H. Severe traumatic brain injury in children: an evidence-based review of emergency department management. Pediatr Emerg Med Pract. 2016;13(10):1–28.

85. Meythaler JM, Peduzzi JD, Eleftheriou E, Novack TA. Current concepts: diffuse axonal injury-associated traumatic brain injury. Arch Phys Med Rehabil. 2001;82:1461–71.

86. Kraus JF, Hsu P, Schafer K, Afifi AA. Sustained outcomes following mild traumatic brain injury: results of a five-emergency department longitudinal study. Brain Inj. 2014;28:1248–56.

87. Ryan LM, Warden DL. Post-concussion syndrome. Int Rev Psychiatry Abingdon Engl. 2003;15:310–6.

88. Bennett KS, Dewitt PE, Harlaar N, Bennett TD. Seizures in Children With Severe Traumatic Brain Injury. Pediatr Crit Care Med. 2017;18(1):54–63.

89. Akiyama Y, et al. Susceptibility-weighted magnetic resonance imaging for the detection of cerebral microhemorrhage in patients with traumatic brain injury. Neurol Med Chir. (Tokyo). 2009;49:97–9; discussion 99.

90. Mittenberg W, Canyock EM, Condit D, Patton C. Treatment of post-concussion syndrome following mild head injury. J Clin Exp Neuropsychol. 2001;23:829–36.

91. Belisle S, Lim R, Hochstadter E, Sangha G. Approach to pediatric traumatic brain injury in the emergency department. Curr Pediatr Rev. 2018;14(1):4–8.

92. American Academy of Ophthalmology. 2019–2020 BCSC: Basic and clinical science course. San Francisco: American Academy of Ophthalmology; 2019. Print.

93. Smith F, Rathore G, Suh D. Clinical presentations of pediatric horner syndrome. Open J Ophthalmol. 2017;7:37–43. https://doi.org/10.4236/ojoph.2017.71006.

94. Adams ME, Linn J, Yousry I. Pathology of the ocular motor nerves III, IV, and VI. Neuroimaging Clin N Am. 2008;18:261–82.

95. Miller NR, Newman NJ, Biousse V, Kerrison JB. Walsh and Hoyt's Clinical Neuro-Ophthalmology. Philadelphia: Lippincott Williams & Wilkins; 2005.

96. Elmalem VI, Palazzolo L, Akanda M. Optic nerve, visual pathways, oculomotor system, and consequences of intracranial injury. In: Kaufman S, Lazzaro D, editors. Textbook of ocular trauma. New York: Springer International Publishing; 2017.

97. Kim E, Chang H. Isolated oculomotor nerve palsy following minor head trauma: case illustration and literature review. J Korean Neurosurg Soc. 2013;54:434–6.

98. Holmes JM, Mutyala S, Maus TL, Grill R, Hodge DO, Gray DT. Pediatric third, fourth, and sixth nerve palsies: a population-based study. Am J Ophthalmol. 1999;127(4):388–92.

99. Hanson RA, Ghosh S, Gonzalez-Gomez I, Levy ML, Gilles FH. Abducens. length and vulnerability? Neurology. 2004;62:33–6.

100. Betts JG, Young KA, Wise JA, et al. Anatomy and physiology. Houston: Rice University; 2013.

101. Wilson SR, Hirsch NP, Appleby I. Management of subarachnoid hemorrhage in a non-neurosurgical centre. Anaesthesia. 2005;60:470–85.

102. Chang EF, Meeker M, Holland MC. Acute Traumatic Intraparenchymal Hemorrhage: Risk Factors for Progression in the Early Post-injury Period. Neurosurgery. 2006;58(4):647–56. https://doi.org/10.1227/01.NEU.0000197101.68538.E6.

103. Chowdhury FH, Haque MR, Hossain MZ, Sarker MH. Cavernous sinus syndrome. In: Turgut M, Challa S, Akhaddar A, editors. Fungal infections of the central nervous system. Cham: Springer; 2019. https://doi.org/10.1007/978-3-030-06088-6_24.

104. Gonçalves R, Coelho P, Menezes C, Ribeiro I. Benign recurrent sixth nerve palsy in a child. Case Rep Ophthalmol Med. 2017;2017:8276256. https://www.hindawi.com/journals/criopm/2017/8276256/.

10

Infections

Contents

Ocular Infections

Charles G. Miller and Frank Cao

Contents

© Springer Nature Switzerland AG 2021
R. Shinder (ed.), *Pediatric Ophthalmology in the Emergency Room*,
https://doi.org/10.1007/978-3-030-49950-1_11

11.1 Introduction

Ocular infections in the pediatric population can involve the conjunctiva, cornea, or entire globe. Infectious etiologies include bacteria, viruses, fungi, and atypical organisms. Prompt diagnosis and treatment are critical to prevent poor visual outcomes in this patient population.

11.2 Endophthalmitis

11.2.1 Definitions

Endophthalmitis refers to an infection of bacteria or fungi in the eye involving the vitreous and aqueous humor. The human eye contains three compartments: the anterior chamber between the iris and cornea, posterior chamber between the iris and lens, and vitreous cavity posterior to the lens containing the vitreous humor. Endophthalmitis can be categorized as exogenous or endogenous [1]. In exogenous endophthalmitis, organisms are introduced directly into the eye via trauma, surgery, or an infected cornea. In contrast, endogenous endophthalmitis is in the setting of an infection seeded to the eye via the bloodstream. Panophthalmitis is defined as endophthalmitis that also involves the sclera and choroid [1].

Patients with endogenous endophthalmitis will usually have ocular symptoms or a known diagnosis of an underlying systemic infection [1]. Endogenous endophthalmitis is rare, accounting for 2–8% of all reported cases of endophthalmitis, and occurs mostly in adults [2]. Pediatric endogenous endophthalmitis is reported to account for 0.4–1% of all cases [2]. Due to its rare nature, endogenous endophthalmitis is often misdiagnosed or diagnosed late, which can result in poor visual outcomes [3]. The most common sources of pediatric endogenous endophthalmitis include wound infection, meningitis, endocarditis, urinary tract infection, indwelling intravenous catheters, or hemodialysis fistulas [3]. The earliest symptoms of endogenous endophthalmitis in adults include pain and decreased vision,

leading these patients to seek medical care. These symptoms are difficult to elicit in pediatric patients, which can lead to misdiagnosis or diagnostic delay and potentially devastating visual outcomes. Pediatric endogenous endophthalmitis can be misdiagnosed as uveitis, persistent fetal vasculature, cataract, retinopathy of prematurity, toxocariasis, Coat's disease, retinal detachment, and retinoblastoma [3]. The most common organisms responsible for bacterial endophthalmitis are Gram-positive organisms such as *Staphylococcal* and *Streptococcal* species, accounting for 60–80% of all cases [3].

Exogenous endophthalmitis is a vision-threatening complication of ocular trauma or surgery. Approximately 3% of open globe injuries are associated with endophthalmitis [4]. Risk factors associated with exogenous endophthalmitis after pediatric open globe injury include young age, delayed presentation, delayed primary repair, incomplete history regarding the etiology of the injury, incomplete examination, injury with a contaminated object, rural setting, and retained intraocular foreign body (IOFB) [4]. Delay in primary repair of the wound is the most important risk factor [4]. The United States Eye Injury Registry recommends primary repair after open globe injury as soon as possible and preferably within 24 hours [4]. Studies have shown that delaying repair increases the risk of developing endophthalmitis [4]. However, some studies indicate that nearly half of pediatric patients with open globe injury present after 24 hours [5]. The main reasons cited for delay in seeking medical attention are distance, cost, negligence, delayed referral and no symptoms [4]. Studies have shown that many pediatric open globe injuries occur at home and are caused by sharp objects [4]. A significant percentage of injuries have been reported to be self-inflicted or bystander injuries [4]. Rural settings have higher incidences of infection compared to urban settings [5, 6]. Several studies have demonstrated an increased risk of endophthalmitis in the presence of an IOFB, particularly wooden IOFBs [4]. Factors such as traumatic lens rupture, posteriorly located wound, and intraocular tissue prolapse have not been shown to be definitive risk factors for development of endophthalmitis [4]. The most common causative organisms of pediatric post-traumatic endophthalmitis are streptococcal species and staphylococcal species, compared with *Staphylococcus epidermis* and *Bacillus* in the adult population [7]. The incidence of fungal post-traumatic endophthalmitis ranges from 0 to 15.4%, and the most common causative organisms are *Candida*, A*spergillus*, and *Fusarium* [4].

11.2.2 History and Physical Examination

Several factors make obtaining an accurate history and physical exam difficult in the setting of suspected pediatric endophthalmitis. The most important element of the history is eliciting trauma to the eye, but the patient may be afraid to admit to an injury or too young to explain the type of injury. Parents may not know about a previous injury or be afraid to reveal an injury to their child for fear of being accused of neglect or intentional abuse. In cases of endogenous endophthalmitis, patients may not admit to non-ocular pain unless specifically questioned.

The physical exam is made difficult by the presence of pain limiting the ability to perform a thorough eye examination. Some symptoms of endophthalmitis include decreased visual acuity, photophobia, and pain out of proportion to an injury [4]. Signs include severe conjunctival injection, hemorrhagic chemosis, corneal edema or infiltrates, hypopyon or fibrin in the anterior chamber, vitritis, and loss of the red reflex (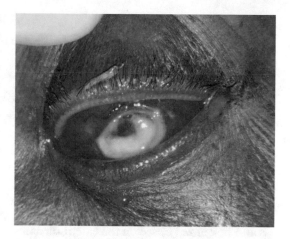 Fig. 11.1) [4]. Edema of the eyelids and decreased extraocular movements are some extraocular signs that may hint at endophthalmitis but are nonspecific [4]. In cases of uncooperative patients, an examination under anesthesia (EUA) with measurement of intraocular pressure and dilated fundus examination should be carried out [4]. If a provider suspects a case of endophthalmitis, an ophthalmologist should be consulted to perform a thorough history and eye exam. The duration between injury and onset of clinically

Fig. 11.1 Endophthalmitis depicting diffuse conjunctival injection and chemosis, dense hypopyon with corneal thinning, and obliterated anterior chamber structures

detectable signs of endophthalmitis may take anywhere from hours to weeks after injury [8]. The rapidity of the disease depends on the pathogen, with *Bacillus* progressing to panophthalmitis within hours to days while fungal infections tend to have a more indolent course [4].

Imaging can help detect IOFB and orbital fractures. A CT of the orbits is typically the study of choice in any trauma situation despite requiring possible anesthesia, and exposure to ionizing radiation [4]. MRI should be avoided in the initial trauma setting due to the possibility of metallic IOFB causing further damage [4]. In endogenous cases, scans of the body searching for a primary source of infection should be guided by a thorough history and physical examination.

Cultures can be obtained at the time of a pars plana vitrectomy (PPV) to guide treatment. Children would not cooperate for a vitreous biopsy under topical or local anesthesia, and the vitreous sample in a child would be thick and difficult to aspirate [4]. Ideally the sample should be obtained prior to treatment; however, therapy should not be delayed if endophthalmitis is strongly suspected. An initial Gram stain and KOH prep can guide therapy until definitive culture results return. A Gram stain is only positive 60% of the time even in culture positive cases [4].

11.2.3 Management

There is a lack of evidence-based guidelines for managing pediatric post-traumatic or endogenous endophthalmitis [4]. While the endophthalmitis vitrectomy study provides some guidelines regarding taking a patient to surgery or injecting the eye with antibiotics, the patient population was adults who developed endophthalmitis after cataract surgery [1]. In traumatic cases, the globe should be closed as soon as possible and repair should be attempted if at all possible [4]. Treatment should be guided based on the extent of damage, nature of injury, and presence or absence of an IOFB. Empiric therapy with systemic broad-spectrum antibiotics covering Gram-positive and Gram-negative organisms is typically administered [4]. If there is a known history of trauma involving organic material such as wood or vegetable matter, consideration should be given to add anaerobic and antifungal coverage [4]. Intravitreal antibiotics alone have questionable efficacy, and many cases will require pars plana vitrectomy (PPV) to salvage the globe [4]. Typically, the adult dosage of intravitreal antibiotics such as vancomycin or ceftazidime is given [4]. Prompt PPV should be considered in cases where there is extensive vitreous exudation and poor red reflex, retained IOFB, strong suspicion of fungal etiology, or poor response within 24 hours of primary repair and intravitreal antibiotic injection [4]. Surgery can aid in debulking vitreous toxins, microorganisms, inflammatory cells, obtaining sample for microbiological testing, and direct administration of antibiotics [4]. If an IOFB is present initially and cannot be conveniently removed at the time of initial globe repair, a second surgery to remove the IOFB can be scheduled shortly afterward. In the pediatric population, it may be difficult to surgically induce a posterior vitreous detachment (PVD) [4]. Silicone oil can be used to tamponade the retina, inhibit the growth of microorganisms by decreasing the potential culture medium, and prevent the onset of phthisis bulbi [4]. Repeat intravitreal antibiotics may be necessary under sedation or general anesthesia if there is worsening or persistent inflammation [4]. Repeat surgery should be considered if there is minimal or no improvement within 72 hours [4].

In endogenous endophthalmitis, treatment should be initiated as soon as the diagnosis is suspected with prompt intravitreal antibiotic administration, hospitalization, infectious disease consultation, and intravenous antibiotics. Vancomycin and ceftazidime are the most commonly used intravitreal antibiotics [9]. Review studies in adults indicate that eyes undergoing pars plana vitrectomy are more like to retain useful vision and less likely to undergo evisceration or enucleation [9]. Broad-spectrum intravenous antibiotics are typically used as an adjunct to local therapy and are often continued for several weeks after initiation. In cases of fungal endogenous endophthalmitis, intravitreal injection with voriconazole, or amphotericin B should be started along with intravenous amphotericin B, oral fluconazole or oral voriconazole [10]. Vitrectomy can help decrease the infectious load and provide better accessibility of antifungal therapy to intraocular structures [9]. Even with early diagnosis and treatment, the morbidity and mortality are significant [2].

11.3 Keratitis

11.3.1 Definitions

The cornea is the clear anterior most structure in the eye that is avascular and permits light to enter the eye. It contributes the majority of the focusing power of the eye [11]. Disease of the cornea is a leading cause of monocular blindness worldwide and tends to disproportionately affect marginalized populations [12]. Infection of the cornea, or infectious keratitis, is a leading cause of global blindness and affects both developed and developing countries [12]. In the United States, infectious keratitis in adults is typically associated with contact lens wear, while in developing countries it is usually a consequence of ocular trauma sustained during agricultural work [12]. In addition to these risk factors, colonization of the eyes during birth and trauma are significant risk factors [13]. Treatment of pediatric infectious keratitis is typically the same as for adults and consists of topical administration of antimicrobial agents, sometimes with co-administration of anti-inflammatory agents [13]. Challenges specific to the pediatric population include secondary amblyopia, severe inflammatory reaction, and difficulty in examining and treating patients with topical medication [13]. Microbial agents that can infect the cornea include bacteria, fungi, viruses, and atypical organisms such as acanthamoeba [13].

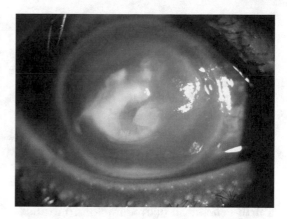

◘ Fig. 11.2 Corneal infiltrate with hypopyon in the setting of bacterial keratitis

11.3.2 **Bacterial**

While there are case reports of *Pseudomonas* keratitis in premature neonates without preceding trauma, typically bacteria cannot infect an intact corneal surface without prior damage to the corneal epithelium [13]. Once bacteria have successfully invaded the corneal surface, they can proliferate and penetrate into the corneal stroma [13]. The predominant bacteria that cause keratitis in children are similar to those found in adults [13]. *Staphylococcus aureus* and *Streptococcus pneumoniae* are the major Gram-positive microorganisms, while *Pseudomonas aeruginosa* is the major Gram-negative microorganism associated with infectious keratitis in children [13]. Coagulase-negative staphylococci such as *Staphylococcus epidermis* are typically part of the normal ocular microbiota, but they can be associated with opportunistic infection [13]. Bacteria are the second most prevalent cause of infectious keratitis in children after viruses, followed by fungi and parasites [13].

The major risk factors for bacterial keratitis in children are trauma and contact lens wear [13]. Trauma with plant material can seed bacteria or fungi [13]. Other risk factors include severe systemic illness, which is most commonly seen in those younger than 4 years of age, and congenital and acquired external ocular disease [13]. The primary symptoms of bacterial keratitis include rapid onset of pain, conjunctival injection, blurry vision, photophobia, ocular discharge, and eyelid edema [13]. The signs include a corneal infiltrate with overlying fluorescein staining (◘ Fig. 11.2) [13]. The nature of the infiltrate can be central or paracentral and is usually anterior to mid-stromal [12]. Other possible findings include hypopyon, folds in Descemet's membrane, and superficial endothelial inflammatory plaques [14]. It can be difficult to distinguish between various types of keratitis based on clinical exam, and so cultures are important to establish the causative organism and guide therapy [12].

In order to better interpret culture results, it is imperative to have a basic understanding of the normal ocular flora. In newborns, *Lactobacillus, Bifidobacterium, Corynebacterium, Peptostreptococcus*, coagulase-negative *Staphylococcus*, and *Propionibacterium* species compose the normal ocular flora [14]. In older children, Streptococci dominate the conjunctival flora, and Corynebacteria do so in adults [14]. The rate of culture positive specimens varies widely and has been reported to be 48–87% [14]. The most commonly isolated organisms in microbial keratitis in children are Gram-positive organisms *Streptococcus pneumoniae* and *Staphylococcus Aureus* and Gram-negative *Pseudomonas Aeruginosa* [14]. The responsible microorganisms vary by geographic location [14]. To obtain corneal scrapings in children, sedation or general anesthesia may be required [14].

Smears should be inoculated in blood, chocolate, Sabouraud agar, Lowenstein-Jensen agar, and thioglycolate broth [14]. Corneal scrapings and microbiological examination yield positive cultures in only 52–65% of cases [14]. Therefore, culture results should not delay therapy, nor should negative cultures prompt cessation of antibiotic therapy.

Treatment of microbial keratitis in children should be aggressive and prompt. Typically, either fortified antibiotics consisting of an aminoglycoside and cefazolin or a fourth-generation fluoroquinolone (moxifloxacin or gatifloxacin) are used [14]. Older generation fluoroquinolones may be utilized if newer generations are unobtainable, but 80% of ocular isolates of methicillin-resistant *Staphylococcus aureus* in the United States have been reported to be resistant to fluoroquinolones [12]. While following clinical progress, it is important that toxicity from antibiotic drops can delay corneal healing [12]. In some younger patients, regular topical administration may not be tolerated. In these cases, subconjunctival injection under sedation can be considered [14]. However, there are no standard guidelines regarding the dosage or amount of antibiotic injected [14]. In addition to antibiotics, anticollagenases and topical steroids are often administered [12]. While tetracyclines have been shown to inhibit collagenase and metalloproteinase, there are no high-quality randomized controlled trials in humans to guide use of doxycycline as an adjuvant treatment for corneal ulceration [12]. Topical steroids have long been proposed as adjuvant treatment for bacterial keratitis in order to decrease inflammation, scarring, neovascularization, and stromal melting [12]. While no randomized controlled trials comparing adjuvant steroids and topical antibiotics alone have shown a definitive benefit for adjuvant topical steroids, subgroup analysis within some large randomized clinical trials have suggested a benefit of steroids in certain subgroups [12]. Patients with low vision at baseline, central corneal ulcers and deep ulcers had better final vision when treated with adjuvant steroids after 2–3 days of antibiotics [12]. Importantly, ulcers caused by *Nocardia* or *Pseudomonas aeruginosa* did not

benefit from adjuvant steroids [12]. It is important to note that these are studies of adult populations and may not be directly applicable to pediatric populations.

11.3.3 Fungal

Fungal keratitis shares many similarities with bacterial keratitis and can be difficult to distinguish clinically. While fungal keratitis is classically associated with warm, humid environments, the major predisposing risk factors are agricultural associated trauma and contact lens wear [12, 14]. The incidence can vary widely by geographic location, as fungal microbial keratitis has been reported to be responsible for 18% of keratitis cases in the United States, and 48.7% of cases in China [14]. Clinically, satellite lesions have been commonly described as a characteristic feature of fungal keratitis [13]. However, satellite lesions can be found in other infections such as acanthamoeba keratitis [15]. Studies have not found any features capable of allowing differentiation of fungal from bacterial keratitis, although patients with bacterial keratitis tend to be older [15].

Antifungal treatment options are limited and can be very toxic to the cornea. Topical natamycin 5% was introduced in the 1960s and is limited by poor penetration into the corneal stroma [12]. Topical amphotericin B 0.3–0.5% can be used but requires a compounding pharmacy and is fairly toxic to the cornea [12]. Voriconazole is a newer-generation triazole which penetrates well into the cornea [12]. Large randomized controlled clinical trials comparing topical natamycin to topical voriconazole in the treatment of filamentous fungal ulcers were stopped due to worse outcomes in the topical voriconazole group [12]. These results were especially pronounced in cases of *Fusarium* keratitis [12]. Additionally, randomized, controlled trials comparing adjuvant oral voriconazole to placebo for smear-positive filamentous fungal keratitis did not find any benefit to adjuvant oral voriconazole [12]. There were significantly more adverse events in the oral voriconazole group, including elevations of aspartate aminotransferase or alanine amino-transferase and visual disturbances, compared to the placebo group [12]. Subgroup analysis did find possible benefit to adjuvant oral voriconazole in *Fusarium* ulcers [12].

11.3.4 Acanthamoeba

Acanthamoeba keratitis (AK) was first described in 1984 in the United Kingdom [16]. These ubiquitous microorganisms are opportunistic pathogens with a cyst form and a trophozoite form [17]. Acanthamoeba keratitis is typically implicated in contact lens associated keratitis in developed countries and trauma-related keratitis in developing countries [17]. The incidence of AK is higher in soft contact lens wearers than rigid gas permeable lens wearers and has been related to lens hygiene [17]. The classic symptom associated with AK is pain out of proportion to exam findings, and examination signs include a radial kerato-neuritis (inflamed corneal nerves) and ring infiltrates [17]. However, these findings do not present in all patients, and the clinical presentation of AK can be highly variable [17]. Early cases can present with punctate epithelial erosions, anterior stromal haze, nummular or coin-shaped keratitis, and stromal edema with keratic precipitates [17]. Many cases are misdiagnosed and treated as herpes simplex virus keratitis due to the similar presentations [17]. Late-stage findings include ring-shaped infiltrates, necrotizing keratitis, and diffuse infiltrative keratitis [17]. It is important to suspect AK in any presumed cases of viral, bacterial, or fungal keratitis not responding to therapy, cases of chronic keratitis especially with ring infiltrates, and patients with inflamed corneal nerves in association with corneal infiltrates [15]. In general, patients with acanthamoeba keratitis tend to be younger, have a longer duration of symptoms and have ring infiltrates and disease confined to the epithelium [15].

Diagnosis of AK should not delay therapy, and involves microscopic examination of scraped corneal specimen inoculated and grown on various culture media and smears [17]. The *Acanthamoeba* cysts appear as double-walled structures with an inner hexag-onal wall on smears stained with Calcofluor-White or Gram stain [17]. Culture confirmation can be performed on non-nutrient agar with *Escherichia coli* overlay and can take up to 1–3 days [17]. Corneal biopsy may be performed in cases of deep infiltrates and negative corneal scrapings [17]. Molecular methods of diagnosis are not currently available in most clinics but show promise in providing a rapid and accurate diagnosis of AK [17]. In vivo confocal microscopy (IVCM), a noninvasive imaging technique that allows direct visualization of pathogens in cornea tissue can aid in clinical diagnosis [17]. However, this technique is highly dependent on user experience and requires significant patient cooperation [17].

Treatment of acanthamoeba keratitis typically consists of topical biguanides such as 0.02–0.06% polyhexamethylene biguanide (PHMB) or 0.02–0.2% chlorhexidine [17]. These are the therapies that have the capability to eradicate the cyst form of acanthamoeba [17]. Drops typically need to be administered every hour for the first 48 hours, followed by hourly drops until clinical signs of resolution are observed [17]. Intensive early treatment is recommended because organisms may be more susceptible before the cyst forms have matured [17]. The average duration of medical therapy has been reported to be approximately 6 months [17]. Topical steroids may be considered if there is presence of increase in deep vascularization of the cornea, inflammatory complications such as scleritis, iridocyclitis, chronic keratitis or severe pain out of proportion to clinical findings [17]. Topical steroids should not be started until 2 weeks of biguanide treatment has been completed, and antiamoebic therapy should be continued after steroids are stopped [17]. Surgical treatment is indicated in cases of large infiltrates extending or threatening the limbus, failure of medical therapy and gross thinning or perforation of the cornea [17]. Important complications of acanthamoeba keratitis include cataract, iris atrophy and fixed dilated pupil, scleritis, and intraocular spread [17]. The prognosis of acanthamoeba keratitis is highly variable and depends on the time to diagnosis and treatment as well as the severity of the infection [17]. In general, cases diagnosed and treated promptly (typically within 3 weeks) respond well to medical therapy [17].

11.3.5 Viral (Herpes)

Herpes simplex virus (HSV) is a ubiquitous virus that is a major cause of visual morbidity in the United States and worldwide [18]. Primary ocular infection occurs in many children and manifests as blepharitis or blepharoconjunctivitis [19]. Primary herpetic keratitis is rare and is usually confined to the epithelium [19]. The virus typically establishes latency and can reactivate, causing herpetic keratitis which can manifest as blepharoconjunctivitis, epithelial keratitis, stromal keratitis, or iridocyclitis [18]. Reactivation can be triggered by fever, trauma, stress, immunosuppressant therapy, or UV radiation [20]. In US children, the median time to recurrent disease is 13 months, and the probability of recurrence during the first 18 months after primary infection is 73% [20]. Recurrent infectious HSV keratitis can present as epithelial vesicles which can coalesce to form a dendritic ulcer or geographic ulcer (◘ Fig. 11.3) [18]. It can also manifest as an immune stromal keratitis or iridocyclitis, which is thought to develop as a result of a cell-mediated immune response [18]. While in adults, the most common manifestation of HSV keratitis is dendritic keratitis; inflammation and stromal keratitis are more common in the pediatric

population [20]. Rarely, a severe HSV stromal necrotic keratitis can also develop but is caused by active viral invasion into the cornea. Disciform endotheliitis, inflammation of the corneal endothelium with stromal or epithelial edema but no stromal infiltrate has also been described [18]. Misdiagnosis rates of 30% have been reported for HSV keratitis [20]. Rates of bilateral disease in the pediatric population have been reported as high as 26%, which is higher than the adult population which is usually less than 3% [21].

Medical management of herpes simplex epithelial keratitis consists of oral acyclovir suspension dosed by weight in infants and young children or acyclovir (400 mg three times daily), valacyclovir (500 mg twice daily), or famciclovir (250 mg twice daily) pills in older children [20]. Topical therapy with 3% vidarabine ointment or 1% trifluridine drops can also be used [20]. Stromal keratitis, endotheliitis, and iridocyclitis can be treated with topical steroids such as prednisolone acetate 1% in addition to systemic antiviral treatment [20] (◘ Table 11.1).

The steroid dosage can be adjusted based on clinical response, as there are no published guidelines regarding the dosage or duration of treatment. Therapy is typically well tolerated, but acyclovir suspension can cause diarrhea, and acyclovir capsules contain lactose which may not be tolerated by lactose intolerant

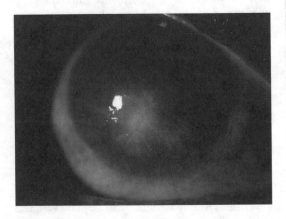

◘ **Fig. 11.3** Corneal dendrite in the setting of herpes simplex virus keratitis

◘ **Table 11.1** Treatment of different types of HSV eye disease in the pediatric population

Diagnosis	Treatment
HSV epithelial keratitis (infants and young children)	Oral acyclovir suspension dosed by weight
HSV epithelial keratitis (older patients)	Acyclovir 400 mg TID, valacyclovir 500 mg BID, or famciclovir 250 mg BID
Stromal keratitis, endotheliitis, iridocyclitis	Prednisolone acetate 1% and systemic antiviral treatment
Recurrent disease	Acyclovir 200–400 mg BID (prophylaxis)

children [20]. In patients with recurrent disease or at high risk for recurrent disease, oral acyclovir can be used prophylactically to prevent further recurrences [20]. Oral acyclovir can also be used in patients on topical corticosteroid medication for immune stromal keratitis to prevent active infection [22]. When using oral acyclovir for prophylaxis, the proper dosage can only be determined from clinical experience as there are no fixed guidelines in pediatric patients. Studies suggest starting with twice daily acyclovir dosed by weight, but due to small sample sizes, the effect of continuous prophylactic antiviral therapy has not been assessed [20].

Sequelae of HSV keratitis that can permanently decrease vision include corneal scarring, astigmatism and corneal anesthesia [20]. In some studies, over 50% of patients develop central corneal opacities, and over 8% develop irregular astigmatism greater than 2 diopters, with over 30% of patients developing amblyopia as a result [23]. Due to the high rates of amblyopia, these patients need close long-term follow-up after the acute infection has resolved. The risk of amblyopia also demonstrates the importance of timely and aggressive therapy as soon as the diagnosis is properly made. In cases requiring surgery, antiviral prophylaxis is important, with some studies advocating 6 months of oral acyclovir prior to keratoplasty and permanent acyclovir prophylaxis after surgery [24].

11.4 Conjunctivitis

11.4.1 Definitions

Conjunctivitis, inflammation of the conjunctiva, is estimated to affect six million people annually in the United States and result in hundreds of millions of dollars in annual healthcare costs. The majority of affected patients are treated by primary care physicians, as 1% of all primary care office visits in the United States are related to conjunctivitis. All patients presenting with signs and symptoms of conjunctivitis should receive an eye exam including visual acuity, type of discharge; presence of corneal opacities; eyelid

swelling; proptosis of the globe; and the size, shape, and reactivity of the pupil. Infectious conjunctivitis is typically caused by bacterial or viral organisms. Any patient with presumed infectious conjunctivitis should be referred to an ophthalmologist if there is vision loss, severe pain, purulent discharge, corneal findings, conjunctival scarring, lack of response to initial therapy after 1-week, recurrent episodes of conjunctivitis, history of herpes simplex virus eye disease, or history of contact lens wear. Additional cases that should be considered for referral include patients with photophobia or requiring steroids [25].

11.4.2 Bacterial

Bacteria are reported to account for a significant proportion of cases of acute infectious conjunctivitis, although there may be false positive bacterial cultures due to the presence of normal ocular flora. The most common causative organisms include *Staphylococcus aureus, Staphylococcus epidermidis, Streptococcus pneumoniae, Moraxella catarrhalis, Pseudomonas aeruginosa,* and *Haemophilus influenzae. Neisseria gonorrhoeae* can cause hyperacute conjunctivitis, and Chlamydia and Bartonella species may cause distinct forms of conjunctivitis [26].

Bacterial conjunctivitis typically presents with conjunctival hyperemia with mild to moderate discharge and early morning crusting in one or both eyes (◘ Fig. 11.4). While most forms of acute bacterial conjunctivitis are self-limiting, Neisseria conjunctivitis presents with hyperacute purulence with pseudomembranes and preauricular lymphadenopathy. Chlamydial conjunctivitis can present as trachoma or inclusion conjunctivitis. Trachoma, mostly seen in developing countries, is caused by chlamydial serotypes A through C. Trachoma presents as a severe follicular reaction of the superior tarsal conjunctiva. The tarsal conjunctiva can form a line of chronic scarring called Arlt's line. Follicles at the corneoscleral limbus can develop, called Herbert's pits. Trachoma can cause vision loss due to corneal cicatrization. Inclusion conjunctivitis is caused by chlamydial serotypes D through K. It is characterized by a unilateral,

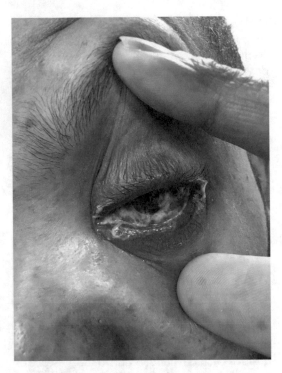

Fig. 11.4 Purulent discharge, chemosis and conjunctival injection in bacterial conjunctivitis. (Photo courtesy of Laura Palazzalo MD)

chronic follicular conjunctivitis with mucopurulent discharge commonly seen in sexually active adolescents. It can be associated with preauricular lymphadenopathy, urethritis, and vaginitis. Another condition with preauricular and submandibular lymphadenopathy is Parinaud oculoglandular syndrome, which is often caused by *Bartonella henselae*. Parinaud syndrome most commonly presents as a unilateral granulomatous conjunctivitis, which may also be accompanied by a neuroretinitis and corresponding decrease in visual acuity [26]. If suspected bacterial conjunctivitis lasts longer than 4 weeks, ophthalmic consultation should be sought for possible chronic bacterial conjunctivitis. Some common causes include *Staphylococcus aureus, Moraxella lacunata*, and enteric bacteria. Conjunctivitis that does not respond to standard antibiotic therapy in sexually active patients should prompt evaluation for chlamydia. Any patients presenting with symptoms of conjunctivitis who wear contact lenses should discontinue wearing lenses and be referred to an ophthalmologist to rule out bacterial keratitis, which can be vision threatening [25].

Diagnosis of bacterial conjunctivitis is typically made clinically, and many cases are treated empirically. Gram stain and culture are indicated if there is severe conjunctivitis with copious discharge. In severe cases, it is important to rule out Neisseria species, as *Neisseria gonorrhoeae* may raise concern for sexual abuse, and *Neisseria meningitidis* can cause meningitis. Corneal scrapings can be used to diagnose chlamydia. [26]

Treatment of bacterial conjunctivitis is not necessary in many cases due to the self-limited nature of the disease. Antibiotics have been shown to induce earlier remission of some strains of bacterial conjunctivitis [26]. Meta-analysis has shown that patients with purulent discharge or mild severity of red eye may have a small benefit from antibiotics [27]. Antibiotics seem to be more effective in patients with a positive bacterial culture result [25]. Topical antibiotics such as trimethoprim-polymyxin B, gentamicin, tobramycin, sulfacetamide, and erythromycin carry low risks and can generally be used safely [26]. Drops or ointment can be used, but ointment can blur vision and be poorly tolerated in pediatric patients. There are no significant differences in cure rates between various broad-spectrum topical antibiotics. Topical steroids should be avoided as they can prolong disease course and worsen infection. In general, antibiotics should be considered in cases of immunocompromised patients, contact lens wearers, and patients with purulent or mucopurulent discharge [25]. In cases of Neisseria and chlamydia, topical treatment is insufficient and systemic therapy should be initiated. Chlamydia can be treated with oral azithromycin 1 g or 100 mg of doxycycline twice daily for 7 days along with concurrent treatment for Neisseria. *Neisseria gonorrhoeae* can be treated with 1 g of intramuscular Ceftriaxone once, and treatment to cover chlamydia. The copious discharge of Neisseria infections may require frequent lavage to remove debris and allow for better penetration of topical therapy. Surgical intervention may be indicated to prevent cicatrization in severe cases of chlamydia [26].

Fig. 11.5 Clear left ocular discharge and conjunctival injection in viral conjunctivitis. (Photo courtesy of Laura Palazzalo MD)

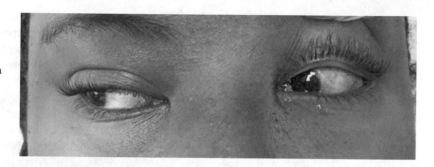

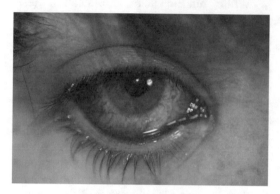

Fig. 11.6 Clear right ocular discharge and diffuse conjunctival injection in viral conjunctivitis. (Photo courtesy of Rudolph Wagner MD)

11.4.3 Viral

Viral conjunctivitis is extremely common in the pediatric population, and causative agents include adenovirus, enterovirus, coxsackievirus, and pox virus [26]. Adenovirus, the most common cause of viral conjunctivitis, is highly contagious. Adenovirus is capable of transmission via contaminated fingers, medical instruments, water, or personal items. Typical incubation time is 5 to 12 days, with an infectious window of 10–14 days [25]. Patients usually present with unilateral tearing and follicular conjunctival injection (Figs. 11.5 and 11.6). Adenovirus strains can cause various presentations such as epidemic keratoconjunctivitis (EKC), pharyngoconjunctival fever, and acute hemorrhagic conjunctivitis. EKC is caused by adenoviruses 8, 19, and 37 and is associated with preauricular lymphadenopathy and immune-mediated corneal infiltrates. Pharyngoconjunctival fever is caused by adenoviruses 3 and 7. It is characterized by subconjunctival hemorrhages, conjunctival edema, sore throat, preauricular lymphadenopathy, and fever. Acute hemorrhagic conjunctivitis is caused by enterovirus 70, coxsackievirus A2 and adenovirus 11 [26]. It is highly contagious, characterized by a rapid onset, and leads to a severely painful conjunctivitis with subconjunctival hemorrhage. It is usually a benign condition that resolves in 5–7 days [28]. Herpes simplex virus can also cause a unilateral follicular conjunctivitis, often but not always in the setting of an ipsilateral vesicular facial rash [26]. Herpetic conjunctivitis does tend to be unilateral, and corneal involvement with dendrite is seen in 50% of patients [29]. While primary infection is usually self-limited, recurrent disease can result in corneal opacification and loss of vision [29]. Pox virus, the causative virus in molluscum contagiosum, is a frequent cause of chronic unilateral follicular conjunctivitis. Close exam will reveal umbilicated lesions along the eyelid [26].

Diagnosis of viral conjunctivitis is typically clinical, although rapid immunochromatographic tests can confirm adenovirus infections in the office [26]. Treatment is usually supportive as most cases are self-limited. Topical artificial tears, topical antihistamines, and cool compresses may help alleviate some symptoms. Strict hand washing, instrument disinfection, and isolation of infected patients from other patients in the clinic are recommended to prevent transmission. Topical antibiotics are not recommended as they do not protect against secondary infections, and their use may delay diagnosis by causing allergic or toxic reactions of the conjunctiva. Additional concerns with topical antibiotics include increasing antibiotic resistance and spreading the infection to the other eye from contaminated eye drop bottles. Patients with presumed viral conjunctivitis should be referred to an ophthalmologist if symptoms do not resolve within 7–10 days because of the risk of complications. Patients should avoid other children for up to 1 week to prevent viral transmission to others [25]. In cases where herpes simplex virus (HSV) is suspected, ophthalmologic referral is recommended to rule out corneal involvement and possible sight-threatening complications [26]. HSV causes a small percentage of acute conjunctivitis cases, typically presenting as unilateral conjunctivitis with vesicular eyelid lesions. Topical and oral antivirals can shorten the course of the disease and are recommended, but topical corticosteroids should be avoided as they can potentiate the virus [25]. Molluscum contagiosum can also be spread by contact but can be cured with incision and curettage, excision, or cryotherapy of the offending eyelid lesion [26].

11.4.4 Ophthalmia Neonatorum

Conjunctivitis in the first month of life is often known as *ophthalmia neonatorum* [26]. Causes include Chlamydia, Neisseria, and herpes viruses. Risk factors include increased shedding of organisms in the vaginal tract during the third trimester, premature rupture of membranes, and prolonged labor [30]. The most frequently identified cause of neonatal conjunctivitis is *Chlamydia trachomatis* serotypes D-K, usually transmitted perinatally by infected mothers [31, 32]. The prevalence of chlamydia in pregnant women is as high as 18% [31]. While infected mothers transmit the infection to babies born vaginally 50% of the time, babies born by cesarean section with intact membranes can also be infected. Among perinatally infected infants, 25–50% goes on to develop conjunctivitis [31]. Patients present with conjunctival edema, hyperemia, and watery or mucopurulent discharge. Symptoms typically start 5–14 days after birth and can last over 2 weeks [31]. Silver nitrate, erythromycin, or tetracycline, which is often given as prophylaxis for gonococcal conjunctivitis, reduces the incidence of *Chlamydia trachoma-*

tis, but do not prevent colonization in the nose and throat. It is important to emphasize that screening pregnant women at high risk for disease can be a highly successful strategy for prevention, allowing some countries to dismiss universal ocular prophylaxis [32]. At the time of diagnosis, the infant's mother and sexual partners must be tested. Untreated infections may result in chronic corneal and conjunctival scarring and long-term vision loss [31].

While nucleic acid amplification tests (NAATs) have largely replaced culture for diagnosing chlamydial infection in adults, the gold standard for diagnosing *C. trachomatis* is still culture, which is also approved by the Food and Drug Administration (FDA) for conjunctival use. Culture is the preferred method for confirming diagnosis in all medicolegal cases. Specimens must contain epithelial cells because chlamydia species are obligate intracellular organisms. Specimens should be obtained using an aluminum-shafted Dacron-tipped swab and transported and processed under specified temperature guidelines. Wooden or calcium alginate swabs are not recommended because they may inhibit the growth of the organism. Culture is 98–100% specific and also highly sensitive but is labor-intensive and expensive, and the test requires incubation for 48–72 hours which delays diagnosis. Other tests for chlamydial conjunctivitis include enzyme-linked immunosorbent assay, nucleic acid probe, and direct fluorescent antibody tests. These tests are generally not as sensitive as culture, but do have a rapid turnaround time [31].

Treatment for chlamydia conjunctivitis is typically oral erythromycin 50 mg/kg per day in four divided doses for 14 days [31]. Topical erythromycin can be added as an adjunct [30]. Many cases are mild and self-limited, but severe cases with eyelid swelling, chemosis, papillary conjunctival reaction, pseudomembrane formation, peripheral pannus, or corneal involvement require treatment [32]. Other options include 150 mg/kg sulfisoxazole orally per day divided every 4–6 hours [31]. Approximately 10–20% of infants diagnosed with chlamydial conjunctivitis require retreatment. WHO guidelines recommend treating *N. gonorrhoeae* at the same time.

Gonococcal conjunctivitis, caused by *Neisseria gonorrhoeae*, is typically more severe than chlamydial conjunctivitis. It had been eradicated in the United States in the 1950s; however, it resurfaced following an increasing incidence of adult gonococcal infections and development of antimicrobial resistance. Gonococcal conjunctivitis is typically severe and bilateral, with an incubation period of 2–5 days. Symptoms include hyperacute purulent discharge, eyelid edema, and chemosis. Screening for gonococci is important because the organism can penetrate intact corneal epithelium and cause corneal ulceration, perforation, and endophthalmitis. Additionally, systemic complications such as stomatitis, arthritis, rhinitis, septicemia, and meningitis can arise [30]. The 2019 updated United States Preventive Services Task Force (USPSTF) recommendation on ocular prophylaxis for gonococcal ophthalmia neonatorum is to use 0.5% erythromycin ophthalmic ointment in all newborns [33].

Diagnosis of gonococcal conjunctivitis can be made by detection of intracellular Gram-negative diplococci on blood agar, chocolate agar, or Thayer-Martin media. Treatment consists of intravenous penicillin G 100,000 units/kg/day for 1 week. In areas where penicillinase-producing strains of *N. gonorrhoeae* are endemic, a third-generation cephalosporin drug should be used for 7 days. Alternatively, the WHO recommends a single dose of ceftriaxone 50 mg/kg. Alternative options include a single dose of intramuscular spectinomycin 25 mg/kg or kanamycin 25 mg/kg. Infected mothers should be given a single dose of ceftriaxone (25–50 mg/kg). Frequent normal saline lavage of the infant's eyes may also be necessary to eliminate all discharge. Again, all neonates treated for gonococcal conjunctivitis should be treated concomitantly for chlamydia due to the high co-infection rates [30].

A less common infectious cause of neonatal conjunctivitis is herpes simplex virus, which usually presents in an infant with generalized herpes infection. Common signs include vesicles around the eye and corneal involvement [30]. These infants require a diagnostic lumbar puncture and ophthalmology assessment [34]. Treatment consists of low-dose intravenous acyclovir (30 mg/kg/day in divided doses) or vidarabine (30 mg/kg/day in divided doses) for at least 2 weeks [30]. Supplementation with topical vidarabine ointment or trifluridine drops can be added.

Case Presentation

A 17-year-old male presented to the emergency department with a 1-week history of worsening irritation, redness, swelling, and copious mucopurulent discharge from his right eye associated with eye pain and photophobia. He had no past ocular or medical history and initially denied any systemic symptoms. Upon further questioning including a thorough review of systems, the patient ultimately endorsed pain with urination and urethral discharge. He also reported having multiple unprotected sexual encounters.

On examination, his visual acuity unaided was decreased to 20/100 in the right eye, no improvement with pinhole, and 20/20 in the left eye. External examination of the right eye revealed significant eyelid edema and erythema with profuse mucopurulent discharge at the

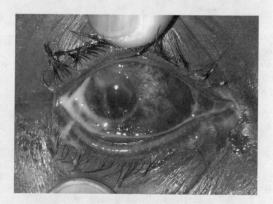

☐ **Fig. 11.7** Diffuse mucopurulent discharge and conjunctival injection in the setting of gonococcal conjunctivitis.

eyelid margin (☐ Fig. 11.7). The ocular surface was coated with discharge, and there was significant conjunctival injection and chemosis. The corneal exam was significant for a peripheral crescentic stromal infiltrate extending from the 10 o'clock to 3 o'clock positions, with a surrounding 1 mm wide band of 70% thinning. The left anterior segment was normal. Conjunctival surface samples for bacterial culture were obtained from the right eye with sterile swabs. The ocular surface was then copiously irrigated with sterile saline to clear away the discharge. This material rapidly reaccumulated within minutes. The emergency department also obtained urethral swabs for gonococcal and chlamydial testing. The patient was commenced on topical moxifloxacin drops to the right eye hourly. Based on a high clinical sus-picion for gonococcal disease, the patient received 1 g of ceftriaxone intramuscularly and azithromycin 1 g orally for treatment of possible chlamydial co-infection. Gram stain ultimately revealed Gram-negative intracellular diplococci, and in the context of corneal involvement, the patient was admitted for continued systemic treatment, which consisted of ceftriaxone 1 g intravenously every 24 hours. The patient's condition steadily improved after initiation of systemic treatment with his vision returning to 20/20 in the affected right eye by day 10 of his hospital stay. He was tapered off of the topical antibiotics. A residual stromal scar outside of the visual axis remained after treatment.

Key Points

- Endophthalmitis is a vision-threatening emergency frequently precipitated by trauma that should warrant an ophthalmology consultation.
- Keratitis can be caused by bacteria, viruses, fungi, or atypical organisms.
- The treatment of viral herpes keratitis in the pediatric population is different from that of adults.
- Most cases of bacterial conjunctivitis are self-limited and do not require treatment.
- Bacterial conjunctivitis caused by Neisseria or chlamydia requires systemic treatment.
- Conjunctivitis in the first month of life is known as ophthalmia neonatorum and can be caused by Chlamydia, *Neisseria*, and herpes viruses. Treatment is organism specific.

❓ Review Questions

1. All of the following are signs of possible endophthalmitis EXCEPT
   (a) 360 degrees of hemorrhagic chemosis
   (b) vitritis
   (c) hypopyon
   (d) iris nodules

2. Which of the following is a major risk factor for bacterial keratitis?
   (a) eye rubbing
   (b) contact lens wear
   (c) playing outdoors
   (d) intense screen time

3. What is recommended for prophylaxis of gonococcal ophthalmia neonatorum in all newborns?
   (a) Ceftriaxone
   (b) Clarithromycin
   (c) Erythromycin
   (d) Doxycycline

✓ Answers

1. (d)
2. (b)
3. (c)

References

1. Durand ML. Endophthalmitis. Clin Microbiol Infect. 2013;19:227–34.
2. Murugan G, Shah PK, Narendran V. Clinical profile and outcomes of pediatric endogenous endophthalmitis: a report of 11 cases from South India. World J Clin Pediatr. 2016;5(4):370–3.
3. Chaudhry IA, Shamsi FA, Al-Dhibi H, Khan AO. Pediatric endogenous bacterial endophthalmitis: case report and review of the literature. J AAPOS. 2006;10(5):491–3. Epub 2006 Sep 7.

11

4. Bansal P, Venkatesh P, Sharma Y. Posttraumatic endophthalmitis in children: epidemiology, diagnosis, management, and prognosis. Semin Ophthalmol. 2018;33(2):284–92.

5. Narang S, Gupta V, Simalandhi P, Gupta A, Raj S, Dogra MR. Paediatric open globe injuries. Visual outcome and risk factors for endophthalmitis. Indian J Ophthalmol. 2004;52(1):29–34.

6. Boldt HC, Pulido JS, Blodi CF, Folk JC, Weingeist TA. Rural endophthalmitis. Ophthalmology. 1989; 96:1722–6.

7. Alfaro DV, Roth DB, Laughlin RM, Goyal M, Liggett PE. Pediatric posttraumatic endophthalmitis. Br J Ophthalmol. 1995;79:888–91.

8. Affeldt JC, Flynn HW, Forster R, Mandelbaum S, Clarkson JG, Jarus GD. Microbial endophthalmitis resulting from ocular trauma. Ophthalmology. 1987;94:407–13.

9. Jackson TL, Paraskevopoulos T, Georgalas I. Systematic review of 342 cases of endogenous bacterial endophthalmitis. Surv Ophthalmol. 2014;59: 627–35.

10. Riddell J, Comer GM, Kauffman CA. Treatment of endogenous fungal endophthalmitis: focus on new antifungal agents. Clin Infect Dis. 2011;52(5):648–53. Pub 2011 Jan 16.

11. Facts about the Cornea and Corneal Disease. National Eye Institute. https://nei.nih.gov/health/cornealdisease. Accessed 18 Feb 2019.

12. Austin A, Lietman T, Rose-Nussbaumer J. Update on the management of infectious keratitis. Ophthalmology. 2017;124(11):1678–89 https://doi.org/10.1016/j.ophtha.2017.05.012.

13. Stretton S, Gopinathan U, Willcox MD. Corneal ulceration in pediatric patients: a brief overview of progress in topical treatment. Paediatr Drugs. 2002;4:95–110.

14. Al-Otaibi AG. Non-viral microbial keratitis in children. Saudi J Ophthalmol. 2012;15:191–7. https://doi.org/10.1016/j.sjopt.2011.10.002.

15. Mascarenhas J, Lalitha P, Prajna NV, et al. Acanthamoeba, fungal, and bacterial keratitis: a comparison of risk factors and clinical features. Am J Ophthalmol. 2014;157(1):56–62. https://doi.org/10.1016/j.ajo.2013.08.032.

16. Jones DB, Visvesvara GS, Robinson NM. *Acanthamoeba polyphaga* keratitis and A*centhamoeba* uveitis associated with fatal meningoencephalitis. Trans Ophthalmol Soc UK. 1975;95:221–32.

17. Garg P, Kalra P, Joseph J. Non-contact lens related *Acanthamoeba* keratitis. Indian J Ophthalmol. 2015;65(11):1079–86.

18. Azher TN, Yin XT, Tajfirouz D, Huang AJ, Stuart PM. Herpes simplex keratitis: challenges in diagnosis and clinical management. Clin Ophthalmol. 2017;11:185–91. https://doi.org/10.2147/opth.s80475.

19. Poirier RH. Herpetic ocular infections of childhood. Arch Ophthalmol. 1980;98:704–6.

20. Liu S, Pavan-Langston D, Colby KA. Pediatric herpes simplex of the anterior segment. Ophthalmology. 2012;119:2003–8.

21. Chong EM, Wilhelmus KR, Matoba AY, et al. Herpes simplex virus keratitis in children. Am J Ophthalmol. 2004;138:474–5.

22. Schwartz GS, Holland EJ. Oral acyclovir for the management of herpes simplex virus keratitis in children. Ophthalmology. 2000;107:278–82.

23. Sema-Ojeda JC, Ramirez-Miranda A, Navas A, Jimenez-Corona A, Graue-Hernanadez EO. Herpes simplex virus disease of the anterior segment in children. Cornea. 2015;34(Suppl 10):S68–71.

24. Sema-Ojeda JC, Loya-Garcia D, Navas A, Lichtinger A, Ramirez-Miranda A, Graue-Hernandez EO. Long-term outcomes of pediatric penetrating keratoplasty for herpes simplex virus keratitis. Am J Ophthalmol. 2017;173:139–44.

25. Azari AA, Barney NP. Conjunctivitis: a systematic review of diagnosis and treatment. JAMA. 2013; 310(16):1721–9.

26. LaMattina K, Thompson L. Pediatric conjunctivitis. Dis Mon. 2014;60(6):231–8.

27. Jefferis J, Perera R, Everitt H, van Weert H, Rietveld R, Glasziou P, et al. Acute infective conjunctivitis in primary care: who needs antibiotics? An individual patient data meta-analysis. Br J Gen Pract. 2011;61(590):e542–8.

28. Wright PW, Strauss GH, Langford MP. Acute hemorrhagic conjunctivitis. Am Fam Physician. 1992; 45(1):173–8.

29. Wagner RS, Aquino M. Pediatric ocular inflammation. Immunol Allergy Clin N Am. 2008;28(1):169–88–vii.

30. Mallika P, Asok T, Faisal H, Aziz S, Tan A, Intan G. Neonatal conjunctivitis – a review. Malays Fam Physician. 2008;3(2):77–81.

31. Chandran L, Boykan R. Chlamydial infections in children and adolescents. Pediatr Rev. 2009;30(7): 243–50.

32. Zuppa AA, D'Andrea V, Catenazzi P, Scorrano A, Romagnoli C. Ophthalmia neonatorum: what kind of prophylaxis? J Matern Fetal Neonatal Med. 2011; 24(6):769–73.

33. US Preventive Services Task Force, Curry SJ, Krist AH, Owens DK, Barry MJ, Caughey AB, et al. Ocular prophylaxis for gonococcal ophthalmia neonatorum: US preventive services task Force reaffirmation recommendation statement. JAMA. 2019; 321(4):394–8.

34. Matejcek A, Goldman RD. Treatment and prevention of ophthalmia neonatorum. Can Fam Physician. 2013;59(11):1187–90.

Extraocular Infections

Liza M. Cohen and Daniel B. Rootman

Contents

© Springer Nature Switzerland AG 2021
R. Shinder (ed.), *Pediatric Ophthalmology in the Emergency Room*,
https://doi.org/10.1007/978-3-030-49950-1_12

12.1 Introduction

Infections of the ocular adnexa are common among children and often present to the emergency room. The variation in both presentation and management depends on the anatomical structures affected and etiology of the infectious process. In this chapter, the relevant anatomical, clinical, and management considerations for the most common extraocular infections in the pediatric population will be addressed. These include hordeolum, molluscum contagiosum, dacryoadenitis, preseptal cellulitis, and orbital cellulitis.

12.2 Hordeolum

12.2.1 Case Presentation

A 4-year-old girl presented with right lower eyelid redness, swelling, and pain. On examination, there was an elevated erythematous, tender lesion on the right lower eyelid with surrounding eyelid edema and erythema (■ Fig. 12.1). Visual function and extraocular motility were intact, and the globe appeared normal. The diagnosis of hordeolum was made, and she was treated with warm compresses and erythromycin ointment with resolution of symptoms.

12.2.2 Relevant Anatomy

The upper and lower tarsal plates are comprised of dense connective tissue and provide structural support to the eyelids. The upper tarsal plate contains approximately 25 meibomian

glands and lower tarsal plate 20 meibomian glands. These are modified holocrine sebaceous glands which secrete lipids that contribute to the tear film (■ Fig. 12.2) [1]. The meibomian glands can become obstructed, resulting in a buildup of oils and an inflammatory reaction to the foreign substance in the subcutaneous tissues. Whether the inciting event or a secondary process, infection of the meibomian glands is referred to as an internal hordeolum.

The eyelids also contain the glands of Zeis, which are sebaceous glands located at the base of the eyelash follicles. The lashes originate on the anterior aspect of the eyelid margin. There are approximately 100 eyelashes on the upper eyelid and 50 on the lower eyelid [1]. Blockage and subsequent infection of the glands of Zeis is referred to as an external hordeolum.

12.2.3 Clinical Presentation

Hordeola typically develop over the course of a few days and present with an elevated lesion on the eyelid margin associated with localized eyelid edema, erythema, and tenderness. Purulent material drains from the eyelashes in the case of external hordeola or through the

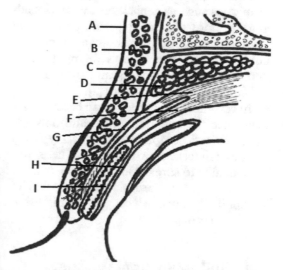

■ Fig. 12.2 Cross-section of the upper eyelid. A. Eyelid skin. B. Orbicularis oculi muscle. C. Orbital septum. D. Preaponeurotic orbital fat. E. Levator palpebrae superioris muscle. F. Müller's muscle. G. Levator aponeurosis. H. Palpebral conjunctiva. I. Tarsus containing meibomian glands. (photo courtesy of Roman Shinder, MD)

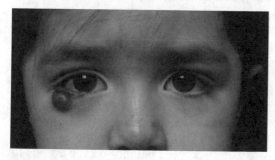

■ Fig. 12.1 External photograph of right lower eyelid hordeolum

tarsal conjunctiva for internal hordeola. There may be evidence of predisposing factors such as meibomian gland dysfunction, blepharitis, or acne rosacea. The remainder of the ophthalmic examination, including visual function, globe appearance, and extraocular motility is typically unremarkable. A history of previous episodes is common.

12.2.4 Investigations

The diagnosis of hordeolum is made clinically, and work-up is typically not required. The infection is usually caused by gram-positive skin flora, most commonly Staphylococci or Streptococci [1].

12.2.5 Treatment

Hordeola often resolve spontaneously without treatment. Conservative management with warm compresses with gentle massage several times daily can hasten drainage of the lesion. Topical antibiotic therapy that provides gram-positive coverage, such as erythromycin or bacitracin ointment, may also aid in resolution [1]. Systemic therapy with oral antibiotics such as cephalexin can be considered for hordeola not responding to topical treatment. Oral doxycycline can be used in children older than 8 years for multiple or recurrent hordeola for its antibacterial and anti-inflammatory properties [2].

In certain cases, hordeola can become chalazia once the infection clears, and only the inflammatory component remains, typically without tenderness or discharge. These may be amenable to surgical intervention.

In rare cases, hordeola may progress to preseptal cellulitis, which will be discussed later in this chapter.

12.3 Molluscum Contagiosum

12.3.1 Case Presentation

A 9-year-old boy presented with left periocular lesions as well as irritation, redness, and

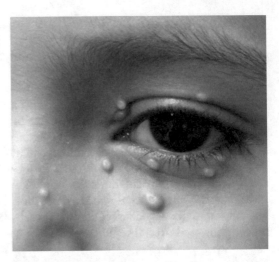

Fig. 12.3 External photograph of left periocular molluscum contagiosum lesions. (photo courtesy of Roman Shinder, MD)

foreign body sensation of the left eye. On examination, there were multiple elevated flesh-colored waxy nodules with central umbilication on the left eyelids and nasal skin (Fig. 12.3). Slit lamp examination revealed follicular conjunctivitis. The diagnosis of molluscum contagiosum was made, and he was treated with incision and curettage of the lesions with resolution of symptoms.

12.3.2 Relevant Anatomy

Molluscum contagiosum is an infection of the epidermis that often involves the eyelid in children and can lead to a secondary follicular conjunctivitis. This is an inflammatory response due to the release of toxic viral particles from an eyelid margin lesion onto the conjunctival surface [1].

12.3.3 Clinical Presentation

Molluscum contagiosum is an infection with the molluscum contagiosum virus, which is a double-stranded DNA poxvirus. It most commonly occurs in children and typically presents with multiple 1–5 mm dome-shaped, waxy, flesh-colored papules on the eyelids or eyelid margins with central umbilication. These lesions may cause pruritis or irritation.

12

There may be a secondary follicular conjunctivitis resulting in foreign body sensation and conjunctival injection. Corneal pannus and superficial punctate keratitis can also occur. Immunocompromised patients may have larger and more numerous lesions with less conjunctival reaction [1]. There may be a history of atopic dermatitis, as there is an increased incidence of molluscum contagiosum infection in this population [3]. Molluscum infection is very contagious and can be spread via direct skin contact, autoinoculation, or fomites [1].

12.3.4 Investigations

Molluscum contagiosum is a clinical diagnosis based on the characteristic appearance of lesions and typically does not require work-up. While the presence of many lesions is common in young children due to autoinoculation, in older patients it may warrant systemic testing for immunocompromised states such as HIV, AIDS, and Wiskott-Aldrich syndrome [1]. The diagnosis can be confirmed by excisional biopsy, with the typical appearance being a nodular proliferation of epithelium with central focus of necrotic cells and intracytoplasmic inclusions called molluscum bodies.

12.3.5 Treatment

Many lesions resolve spontaneously and do not require treatment; however this can take months or years [1]. Lesions causing conjunctivitis can be treated by incision and curettage of the central core of the lesion. One technique involves utilizing a chalazion curette [4]. Follicular conjunctivitis typically resolves with removal of the lesion [1].

Other treatment modalities are utilized for lesions found elsewhere on the body but carry risks when used in the periocular region. Surgical excision of the entire lesion may cause unacceptable scarring. Cryotherapy, ablative laser therapy, and cautery can cause loss of eyelashes and/or pigmentary skin changes. Topical chemical agents (e.g., cantharidin, potassium hydroxide, podophyllotoxin, benzoyl peroxide, tretinoin, trichloroacetic acid, lactic acid, glycolic acid, salicylic acid), immune-modulating agents (e.g., imiquimod, interferon-alpha, cimetidine), and anti-viral agents (e.g., cidofovir) can risk injury to the ocular surface [5–7].

12.4 Infectious Dacryoadenitis

12.4.1 Case Presentation

An 13-year-old girl presented with right periorbital edema of the lateral right upper lid for one day that coincided with an upper respiratory illness. Examination revealed edema and tenderness of the lacrimal fossa and an enlarged and hyperemic right lacrimal gland (◘ Fig. 12.4a,b). CT scan of the orbits showed an enlarged enhancing right lacrimal gland (◘ Fig. 12.4c). She was diagnosed with viral dacryoadenitis and treated with a conservative regimen of oral NSAIDS, showing resolution within 1 week (◘ Fig. 12.4d).

12.4.2 Relevant Anatomy

The lacrimal gland is an exocrine gland located in the superolateral orbit. It resides within a shallow concave depression in the orbital process of the frontal bone, known as the lacrimal fossa. The gland is divided by the lateral horn of the levator aponeurosis into an orbital lobe superiorly and palpebral lobe inferiorly. Approximately 8–12 major ducts secrete tears into the superior cul-de-sac 5 mm above the lateral superior tarsal border after passing through Müller's muscle and conjunctiva [1]. Since the lacrimal excretory ducts pass through the palpebral lobe, removal of the palpebral lobe can reduce secretion from the entire gland. Thus, biopsy of the orbital lobe is preferred when biopsy is warranted.

12.4.3 Clinical Presentation

Dacryoadenitis refers to inflammation of the lacrimal gland and can occur with infectious, inflammatory, or less frequently neoplastic etiologies. Infectious dacryoadenitis presents

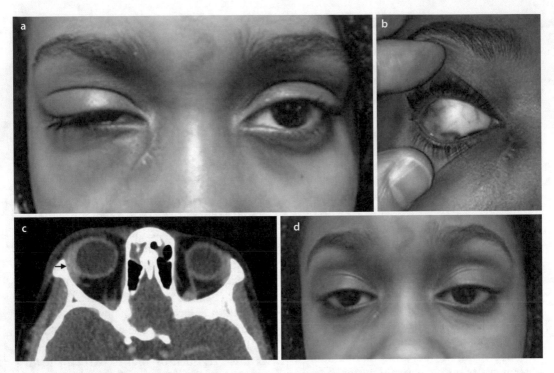

◘ Fig. 12.4 a External photograph showing lateral right upper lid edema and "S" shaped ptosis. **b** Injection and inflammation of the lacrimal gland noted during lid retraction. **c**. Axial orbital CT with contrast showing enlargement and enhancement of the right lacrimal gland (arrow). **d**. External photograph showing clinical resolution at 1 week. (Photos courtesy of Roman Shinder, MD)

most acutely, is more common in children/young adults, and is typically unilateral. It presents with erythema, edema, and tenderness over the lateral upper eyelid, which can result in a "S-shaped" ptosis [1]. There can be associated tearing or discharge. Pus in the lateral conjunctival fornix with pouting ductules can be a clue to a bacterial infectious etiology. The palpebral lobe of the lacrimal gland may appear enlarged and hyperemic. Ipsilateral conjunctival chemosis, preauricular lymphadenopathy (particularly in viral dacryoadenitis), fever, and elevated white blood cell count are also characteristic. Upper respiratory symptoms may be present. The parotid glands can be enlarged in mumps and syphilis.

12.4.4 Investigations

Infectious dacryoadenitis in children is most commonly caused by a virus, with the principal etiologies being Epstein-Barr virus, cytomegalovirus, herpes simplex virus, varicella zoster virus, influenza, and mumps [8–12]. Bacterial dacryoadenitis is rare in children but typically caused by gram-positive cocci such as Staphylococci, Streptococci, and Neisseria; however, gram-negative bacteria such as *Haemophilus*, *Moraxella*, and *Pseudomonas* have also been identified [8, 13]. Rare cases have been associated with Brucellosis, tuberculosis, syphilis, lyme disease, and cysticercosis [14–17].

Although the diagnosis can often be made clinically based on characteristic presentation and signs, orbital imaging is useful in confirming the diagnosis and ruling out alternative etiologies such as preseptal or orbital cellulitis, ruptured dermoid cyst, or neoplasm. CT or MRI of the orbits, preferably with contrast, can be used to image the lacrimal gland. The advantages of CT are that it provides superior detail of adjacent bony anatomy, is time-efficient in acquisition, and may avoid the need for general anesthesia in children. However, CT exposes children to ionizing radiation, whereas MRI does not. On imaging, dacryoadenitis

12

appears as diffuse enlargement and enhancement of the lacrimal gland that tends to mold around the globe (▣ Fig. 12.4c). A lack of discrete mass, bony remodelling of the lacrimal fossa, indentation of the globe, and intraconal soft tissue stranding help distinguish dacryoadenitis from other entities.

Laboratory work-up can help determine the etiology when infectious dacryoadenitis is suspected. If the patient is febrile, a complete blood count with differential and blood cultures should be obtained to assess for sepsis. Viral serologies can also be useful. Though uncommon, if conjunctival discharge is present, it could be sampled for gram stain and bacterial/viral cultures.

12.4.5 Treatment

If the specific etiology is unclear, one typically treats empirically with systemic antibiotics for 36–48 hours. Reassessment for clinical response at this time point can guide further management. In mild-to-moderate cases, oral antibiotics with good gram-positive coverage such as amoxicillin/clavulanate or cephalexin can be used. In moderate-to-severe cases, hospital admission for treatment with intravenous antibiotics and close monitoring may be necessary. If there is clinical improvement with antibiotics, a bacterial etiology is likely, and the course of antibacterial treatment should be continued. If cultures are positive, coverage can be tailored to the specific pathogen and susceptibility.

If there is no improvement in clinical status after a 36–48-hour trial of systemic antibiotics, a viral or inflammatory etiology may be suspected. Viral dacryoadenitis is best treated with supportive measures including cool compresses and oral analgesics as needed. A non-viral inflammatory dacryoadenitis is treated with steroids, which will be discussed in a later chapter.

If symptoms worsen or become associated with signs of orbital involvement such as decreased vision, extraocular motility limitation, or proptosis, repeat imaging for assessment of abscess formation and admission for intravenous antibiotics should be considered.

Rarely, bacterial dacryoadenitis may result in a lacrimal gland abscess. The characteristic radiographic sign is a rim-enhancing lesion located within the lacrimal gland. Early surgical drainage via orbitotomy through a lateral upper eyelid crease incision often leads to complete recovery; [18] however these often resolve with antibiotic therapy alone [19].

12.5 Preseptal Cellulitis

12.5.1 Relevant Anatomy

The distinction between preseptal and orbital cellulitis is based on whether the infection involves the periorbital tissues anterior to the orbital septum (preseptal cellulitis) or orbital tissues posterior to the septum (postseptal/orbital cellulitis). The septum is a thin, multilayered sheet of fibrous tissue, which arises from the periosteum of the superior and inferior orbital rims at the arcus marginalis and defines the anterior boundary of the orbit (▣ Fig. 12.2) [1]. In the upper eyelid, the septum fuses with the levator aponeurosis approximately 2–5 mm above the superior border of the tarsus [20]. In the lower eyelid, the septum fuses with the capsulopalpebral fascia either at or just below the inferior tarsal border [1]. Although the orbital septum defines preseptal versus orbital cellulitis, these two conditions often represent a continuum with overlapping underlying causes requiring similar treatments.

12.5.2 Clinical Presentation

The clinical manifestations of preseptal cellulitis are consistent with its localization anterior to the orbital septum. It presents with acute onset of unilateral eyelid edema, erythema, warmth, and tenderness (▣ Fig. 12.5). Preseptal cellulitis is typically more rapidly progressive and severe in children than in adults [1]. The eyelid edema is often worse than in orbital cellulitis, although this is an unreliable sign as the two may coexist. Fluctuance of skin and soft tissue may indicate an abscess.

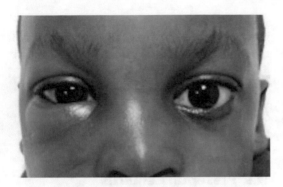

Fig. 12.5 External photograph of a child with right lower lid preseptal cellulitis showing erythema and edema of the lid. (photo courtesy of Roman Shinder, MD)

Distinctively, the orbit is uninvolved, and therefore measures of optic nerve function including visual acuity, pupillary reactions, color vision, and optic nerve appearance are normal. As well, extraocular motility is intact and without pain. Chemosis and proptosis are characteristically absent. Fever and elevated white blood cell count can occur in more severe infections. It is important to inquire about and examine the patient for potential sources of infection, such as sinusitis, trauma, or insect bites.

12.5.3 Investigations

Preseptal cellulitis in the pediatric population is caused by bacterial infection in the vast majority of cases. The infection can originate from three sources: spread from contiguous structures (sinuses, lacrimal sac, lacrimal gland, hordeola), direct inoculation (insect bite, laceration, surgery), and hematologic spread from a distant focus (bacteremia, otitis media, pneumonia). The most common etiology in children is underlying sinus infection due to gram-positive cocci such as *Staphylococcus aureus*, *Staphylococcus epidermidis*, *Streptococcus pyogenes*, and *Streptococcus pneumonia*. *Haemophilus influenza* should be considered in nonimmunized children. Anaerobes should be suspected if there is a history of animal or human bite, foul-smelling discharge, or necrosis [1]. Although rare, necrotizing fasciitis can occur in the pediatric population, with associated morbidity.

Imaging of the brain, orbits, and sinuses via CT with contrast may be obtained in severe cases, if the etiology is unclear (e.g., no direct inoculation site identified), or sinusitis is suspected. If there are any orbital signs such as decreased vision, proptosis, or extraocular motility limitation, imaging is necessary to exclude orbital involvement. On imaging, preseptal cellulitis is characterized by soft tissue stranding anterior to the orbital septum.

In patients with moderate-to-severe preseptal cellulitis and/or fever, systemic work-up with a complete blood count with differential and blood cultures is warranted. If an abscess is present, it should be drained and gram stain/cultures sent to identify the causative organism.

12.5.4 Treatment

Empiric antibiotics should be initiated upon making the diagnosis of preseptal cellulitis. Mild-to-moderate cases in which the patient is not systemically ill and can reliably follow up may be treated with oral antibiotics as an outpatient. Broad-spectrum antibiotics that provide good gram-positive coverage, including cephalosporins for purely anterior preseptal cellulitis and amoxicillin/clavulanate for infection originating in the sinuses, are commonly prescribed. If there is suspicion for community acquired MRSA, trimethoprim-sulfamethoxazole, clindamycin, or doxycycline can be considered [1].

In all infants <1 year of age as well as children with moderate-to-severe disease, signs of systemic illness, and/or if there is no clinical improvement after 48 hours of outpatient therapy, admission to the hospital for close monitoring, imaging, cultures, and treatment with intravenous antibiotics is appropriate. Consultation with an infectious disease specialist can aid in selection of intravenous antibiotics, which typically include ampicillin-sulbactam, piperacillin-tazobactam, or a third-generation cephalosporin, plus vancomycin or clindamycin for MRSA coverage [1]. After significant improvement is observed, intravenous antibiotics can be de-escalated to oral antibiotics for the remainder of the course.

12

If a localized abscess is present, incision and drainage can facilitate resolution of the infection. Care should be taken to avoid opening the orbital septum, as this can facilitate spread of the infection into the orbit. Patients with an abscess may require stronger initial treatment with trimethoprim-sulfamethoxazole or clindamycin to provide coverage for MRSA [1]. Nasal decongestants in cases with concurrent sinusitis can also provide relief of symptoms.

Prognosis is typically good with prompt and appropriate treatment. However, posterior extension of the infection can result in orbital cellulitis.

12.6 Bacterial Orbital Cellulitis

12.6.1 Case Presentation

A 13-year-old girl presented with fever, redness, swelling, and pain of the left eye. Examination revealed erythema and edema of the eyelids, chemosis, left-sided proptosis, and limitation of extraocular motility (◻ Fig. 12.6a, b, c). Visual function was intact. CT scan of the orbits revealed left medial orbital cellulitis extending from adjacent ethmoid sinusitis (◻ Fig. 12.6d, e). The diagnosis of orbital cellulitis was made, and she was admitted to the hospital for treatment with intravenous ampicillin-sulbactam and vancomycin. With clinical improvement, antibiotics were de-escalated to oral clindamycin, and she was discharged home.

12.6.2 Relevant Anatomy

The orbit is an anatomically complex space that contains the globe, extraocular muscles, nerves, blood vessels, and fat. Its boundaries are defined by four walls comprised of seven bones as well as the orbital septum anteriorly. The periosteum of the orbital bones is contiguous with the orbital septum anteriorly and dura mater of the optic nerve posteriorly (◻ Fig. 12.7). Pus can accumulate in the space between the bone and periosteum, with a characteristic radiographic appearance (◻ Fig. 12.8). The orbit can be subdivided into intraconal and extra-

conal compartments (◻ Fig. 12.7), although this distinction may be artificial in cases of a diffuse infective process.

Adjacent to the superior (anteriorly), medial, and inferior boundaries of the orbit are the paranasal sinuses. The close proximity of the sinuses to the orbit is relevant to the disease process in orbital cellulitis, as orbital cellulitis in children tends to arise from the adjacent sinuses.

12.6.3 Clinical Presentation

The clinical findings of orbital cellulitis are consistent with its location posterior to the orbital septum. Characteristic nonspecific signs include eyelid erythema, edema, and tenderness, much like preseptal cellulitis. Additional features of an orbital process are characteristically present and include proptosis, chemosis, limitation of and pain with extraocular movements, and/or signs of optic neuropathy including decreased visual acuity, color vision, visual fields, and a relative afferent pupillary defect, with or without optic disc edema. Fever and leukocytosis are also typical. Nasal congestion, rhinorrhea, and headache are common if there is concurrent sinusitis. A history of frequent sinus infections may be elicited. Tooth pain can indicate dental infection as the source. Severe or delayed cases may proceed to manifestations of central nervous system infection including changes in mental status and headache.

12.6.4 Investigations

Like preseptal cellulitis, orbital cellulitis is caused by three primary mechanisms: spread from contiguous structures (sinuses, teeth, lacrimal sac, lacrimal gland, preseptal cellulitis, hordeola), direct inoculation (penetrating injury, surgery), and hematologic spread (bacteremia, otitis media, pneumonia). Also similar to preseptal cellulitis, the most common etiology in children is contiguous spread from bacterial sinusitis, with the ethmoid sinuses being most frequently affected.

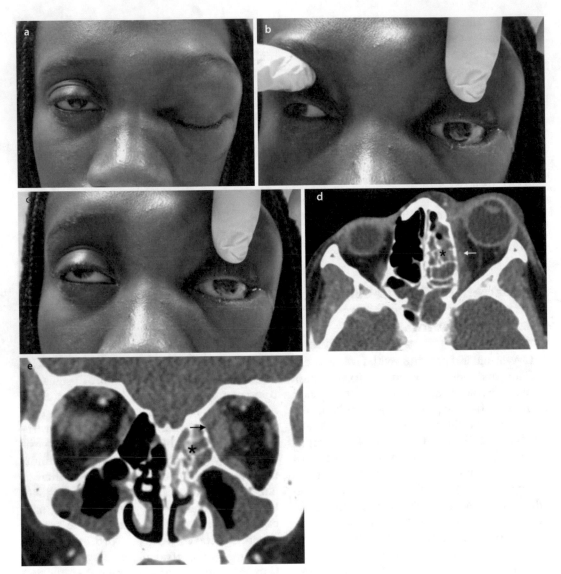

Fig. 12.6 Orbital cellulitis. **a**. External photograph showing left periorbital edema and complete mechanical ptosis. Extraocular movements disclosed decreased adduction **b** and supraduction **c**. Axial **d** and coronal **e** CT showing medial orbital cellulitis (arrows) extending from ethmoid sinusitis (asterisks). (Photo courtesy of Roman Shinder, MD)

The etiologic organisms responsible for orbital cellulitis vary with age. In general, children younger than 9 years have infections caused by a single aerobic organism, whereas children older than 9 years are more likely to have polymicrobial infections [21]. Gram-positive cocci are usually involved, typically *Staphylococcus* and *Streptococcus* species. In nonimmunized children, *Haemophilus influenza* should be considered. Gram-negative pathogens are generally found in immunosup-pressed patients [1]. Polymicrobial infections from a combination of aerobes and anaerobes can be related to a dental abscess.

If orbital cellulitis is suspected based on clinical presentation, imaging of the brain, orbits, and sinuses via CT scan with contrast is indicated. Imaging may demonstrate non-specific inflammatory signs such as proptosis and orbital fat stranding. Sinusitis of the adjacent sinuses is typical. Abscess formation may occur, commonly in the medial orbit (**Fig. 12.8**).

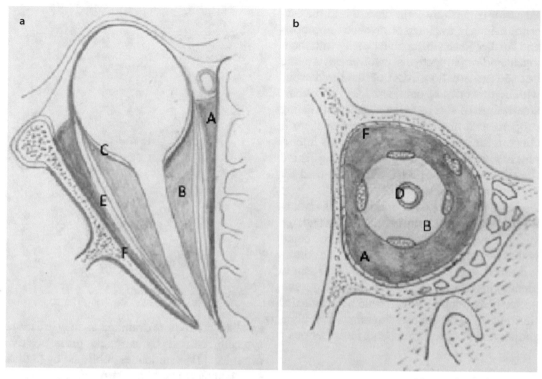

Fig. 12.7 **a** Axial and **b** Coronal view of the orbital spaces: A. Extraconal space, B. Intraconal space, C. Sub Tenon space, D. Subarachnoid space, E. Extraocular Muscle, F. Subperiosteal space. (Photo courtesy of Roman Shinder, MD)

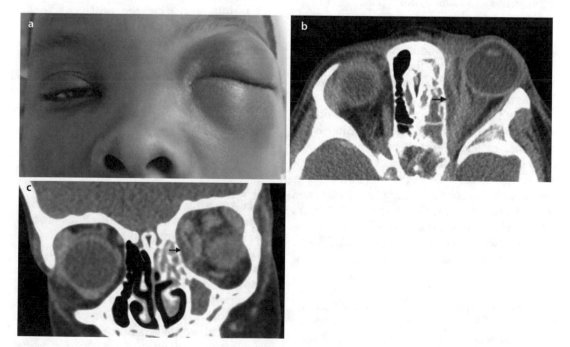

Fig. 12.8 **a** Clinical photograph of a child showing extensive left periorbital edema and complete mechanical ptosis. Axial **b** and coronal **c** CT orbits with contrast showing medial orbital subperiosteal abscess (arrows) from adjacent ethmoid sinusitis. (Photo courtesy of Roman Shinder, MD)

Posterior extension of the disease into the cavernous sinus in the form of mycotic thrombosis and further to the intracranial cavity with meningeal and/or parenchymal involvement is a rare but serious situation. MRI of the brain/orbits with contrast can be considered for better characterization of soft tissue involvement including subperiosteal abscess, especially when there is concern for intracranial extension. It is important to note that imaging findings can lag behind the clinical picture and should not be used for monitoring disease course [22].

Once the diagnosis of orbital cellulitis is confirmed with imaging, the patient should undergo systemic evaluation with a complete blood count with differential and blood cultures. If an abscess is drained, gram stain/cultures should be sent to identify the causative organism. Spread by a suspected hematologic source should be investigated thoroughly with echocardiogram, liver ultrasound, and/or other appropriate investigations.

12.6.5 Treatment

Orbital cellulitis requires prompt and aggressive management in order to avoid potential complications. The mainstay of treatment is hospitalization with intravenous antibiotics. Empiric broad-spectrum antibiotics with ampicillin-sulbactam, pipercillin-tazobactam, or a third-generation cephalosporin plus either vancomycin or clindamycin for MRSA coverage may be used initially. This should be narrowed based on culture results. Antibiotics can be transitioned to oral therapy once clinical improvement is noted. In a cohort study of 42 patients with nonsurgical subperiosteal abscess, the mean duration of intravenous antibiotic therapy was 4 days and post-discharge oral antibiotic therapy 2–3 weeks [23]. An infectious disease specialist may be consulted to aid in choosing appropriate antibiotics. Decongestant nasal spray can improve sinus congestion if there is concurrent sinusitis.

If a subperiosteal abscess is present, it may or may not require surgical drainage. This represents a difference in management between pediatric and adult orbital cellulitis. Whereas most adult subperiosteal abscesses should be drained because infections are usually polymicrobial, pediatric subperiosteal abscesses are

Table 12.1 List of criteria for surgical drainage of pediatric subperiosteal abscess per Garcia and Harris [24]

Age greater than 9 years-old
Frontal sinusitis
Nonmedial subperiosteal abscess
Large subperiosteal abscess
Suspicion of anaerobic infection
Recurrence of subperiosteal abscess after prior drainage
Evidence of chronic sinusitis (nasal polyps)
Acute optic nerve or retinal compromise
Infection of dental origin (anaerobic infection likely)

less likely to require drainage, as they are more typically caused by a single gram-positive organism [21]. Guidelines published by Garcia and Harris suggest that surgical drainage of pediatric subperiosteal abscess is not necessary unless any of the following criteria are present [24] (Table 12.1).

Consultation with an otolaryngologist may be sought if there is concurrent sinusitis, as combined sinus with subperiosteal abscess drainage has been associated with improved outcomes compared to subperiosteal abscess drainage alone [25]. Intraconal orbital abscesses are much less common in children and require urgent surgical drainage [1].

Adjunctive use of steroids in addition to antibiotic therapy remains controversial. Small studies have shown it may hasten recovery while posing a low risk of exacerbating infection [26, 27]. However, the risk of immunosuppression in the presence of an unknown infectious process must be weighed with the potential benefits [28].

While the majority of patients with orbital cellulitis respond well to medical/surgical management, infection can occasionally spread posteriorly and lead to cavernous sinus thrombosis. The valveless venous drainage system of the eyelids, sinuses, and orbit via the superior and inferior ophthalmic veins can facilitate this spread of infection. Cavernous sinus thrombosis typically presents as worsening proptosis, ophthalmoplegia, and hypesthesia in the distributions of V1 and V2. Bilateral orbital involvement and superior ophthalmic vein engorgement are highly suggestive of cavernous sinus thrombosis [1]. Intracranial extension of infection can occur and manifest as meningitis or brain abscess. Consultation with neurosurgery and infectious disease in these cases is advised.

Key Points
- Extraocular infections in the pediatric population have varying presentation and management depending on the anatomical structures affected and etiology of the infectious process.
- Hordeolum is an infection of eyelid sebaceous glands presenting as an elevated erythematous tender lesion on the eyelid and often resolves with conservative measures such as warm compresses.
- Molluscum contagiosum is a viral infection that frequently affects the eyelid skin in children, may result in a secondary follicular conjunctivitis, and can be treated with incision and curettage of lesions.
- Infectious dacryoadenitis is an infection of the lacrimal gland and most commonly results from viral or bacterial infection. Clinical history, examination, and laboratory investigations can guide appropriate therapy.
- Preseptal cellulitis is an infection of the periorbital soft tissues anterior to the orbital septum, and thus the orbit is uninvolved. Identification of the source of the infection can often guide therapy with oral and/or intravenous antibiotics.
- Orbital cellulitis is an infection posterior to the orbital septum and therefore may present with orbital signs including proptosis, extraocular motility limitation, and decreased visual function. Orbital imaging is necessary to evaluate for sinusitis and the extent of infection and may demonstrate a subperiosteal abscess. Treatment consists of prompt initiation of intravenous antibiotics and in some cases surgery.

❓ Review Questions

1. In the pediatric population, infectious dacryoadenitis is most commonly caused by which type of infection?
   (a) Viral
   (b) Bacterial
   (c) Fungal
   (d) Parasitic

2. The distinction between preseptal and orbital cellulitis is made by which anatomical structure?
   (a) Tarsal plate
   (b) Septum
   (c) Conjunctiva
   (d) Extraocular muscles

3. A 7-year-old boy presents with pain, erythema, proptosis, and extraocular motility limitation of the right eye, and CT imaging confirms orbital cellulitis. Treatment is initiated with intravenous ampicillin-sulbactam and vancomycin. After 48 hours, he is not improving clinically and his proptosis has worsened. What should be the next step in management?
   (a) Continue intravenous antibiotic therapy.
   (b) Repeat CT imaging to assess for worsening of disease such as subperiosteal abscess and/or cavernous sinus thrombosis.
   (c) De-escalate treatment to oral antibiotics.
   (d) Take the patient to the operating room for surgery.

✅ Answers

1. (a)
2. (b)
3. (b)

References

1. Orbit, eyelids, and lacrimal system. Basic and clinical science course 2016–2017. San Francisco: American Academy of Ophthalmology. 2016; Section 7.
2. Gonser LI, Gonser CE, Deuter C, Heister M, Zierhut M, Schaller M. Systemic therapy of ocular and cutaneous rosacea in children. J Eur Acad Dermatology Venereol. 2017;31(10):1732–8.

3. Seize MB, Ianhez M, Cestari Sda CP. A study of the correlation between molluscum contagiosum and atopic dermatitis in children. An Bras Dermatol. 86(4):663–8.

4. Gonnering RS, Kronish JW. Treatment of periorbital Molluscum contagiosum by incision and curettage. Ophthalmic Surg. 1988;19(5):325–7.

5. Serin Ş, Bozkurt Oflaz A, Karabağlı P, Gedik Ş, Bozkurt B. Eyelid Molluscum Contagiosum lesions in two patients with unilateral chronic conjunctivitis. Turkish J Ophthalmol. 2017;47(4):226–30.

6. Khare S, Dubey S, Nagar R. A new method for removal of eyelid margin molluscum. J Am Acad Dermatol. 2018;78(6):e151–2.

7. Leung AK, Barankin B, Hon KL. Molluscum Contagiosum: An Update. Recent Patents Inflamm Allergy Drug Discov. 2017;11(1):22–31.

8. Rhem MN, Wilhelmus KR, Jones DB. Epstein-Barr virus dacryoadenitis. Am J Ophthalmol. 2000; 129(3):372–5.

9. Foster WJ, Kraus MD, Custer PL. Herpes simplex virus dacryoadenitis in an immunocompromised patient. Arch Ophthalmol. 2003;121(6):911–3.

10. Obata H, Yamagami S, Saito S, Sakai O, Tsuru T. A case of acute dacryoadenitis associated with herpes zoster ophthalmicus. Jpn J Ophthalmol. 2003; 47(1):107–9.

11. Galpine JF, Walkowski J. A case of mumps with involvement of the lacrimal glands. Br Med J. 1952;1(4767):1069–70.

12. Krishna N, Lyda W. Acute suppurative dacryoadenitis as a sequel to mumps. AMA Arch Ophthalmol. 1958;59(3):350–1.

13. Mawn LA, Sañon A, Conlon MR, Nerad JA. Pseudomonas dacryoadenitis secondary to a lacrimal gland ductule stone. Ophthal Plast Reconstr Surg. 1997;13(2):135–8.

14. Bekir NA, Güngör K. Bilateral dacryoadenitis associated with brucellosis. Acta Ophthalmol Scand. 1999;77(3):357–8.

15. Nieto JC, Kim N, Lucarelli MJ. Dacryoadenitis and orbital myositis associated with Lyme disease. Arch Ophthalmol. 2008;126(8):1165–6.

16. Sen DK. Tuberculosis of the orbit and lacrimal gland: a clinical study of 14 cases. J Pediatr Ophthalmol Strabismus. 1980;17(4):232–8.

17. Sen DK. Acute suppurative dacryoadenitis caused by a cysticercus cellulosa. J Pediatr Ophthalmol Strabismus. 1982;19(2):100–2.

18. Lai THT, Lai FHP, Chan TCY, Young AL, Chong KKL. Lacrimal gland abscess in children: two case reports and literature review. Orbit. 2017;36(6): 468–72.

19. Liu W, Rootman DB, Berry JL, Hwang CJ, Goldberg RA. Methicillin-resistant Staphylococcus aureus dacryoadenitis. JAMA Ophthalmol. 2014;132(8): 993–5.

20. Meyer DR, Linberg JV, Wobig JL, McCormick SA. Anatomy of the orbital septum and associated eyelid connective tissues. Implications for ptosis surgery. Ophthal Plast Reconstr Surg. 1991;7(2): 104–13.

21. Harris GJ. Subperiosteal abscess of the orbit. Age as a factor in the bacteriology and response to treatment. Ophthalmology. 1994;101(3):585–95.

22. Harris GJ. Subperiosteal abscess of the orbit: computed tomography and the clinical course. Ophthal Plast Reconstr Surg. 1996;12(1):1–8.

23. Emmett Hurley P, Harris GJ. Subperiosteal abscess of the orbit. Ophthalmic Plast Reconstr Surg. 2012;28(1):22–6.

24. Garcia GH, Harris GJ. Criteria for nonsurgical management of subperiosteal abscess of the orbit: analysis of outcomes 1988–1998. Ophthalmology. 2000;107(8):1454–8.

25. Dewan MA, Meyer DR, Wladis EJ. Orbital cellulitis with subperiosteal abscess: demographics and management outcomes. Ophthalmic Plast Reconstr Surg. 2011;27(5):330–2.

26. Pushker N, Tejwani LK, Bajaj MS, Khurana S, Velpandian T, Chandra M. Role of oral corticosteroids in orbital cellulitis. Am J Ophthalmol. 2013;156(1):178183.e1.

27. Chen L, Silverman N, Wu A, Shinder R. Intravenous steroids with antibiotics on admission for children with orbital cellulitis. Ophthal Plast Reconstr Surg. 2018;34(3):205–8.

28. Campbell AA, Harris GJ, Neu N, Kazim M. Re: intravenous steroids with antibiotics on admission for children with orbital cellulitis. Ophthal Plast Reconstr Surg. 2017;33(5):389.

12

Inflammations

Contents

Ocular Inflammation

Levon Djenderedjian and David Mostafavi

Contents

© Springer Nature Switzerland AG 2021
R. Shinder (ed.), *Pediatric Ophthalmology in the Emergency Room*,
https://doi.org/10.1007/978-3-030-49950-1_13

13.1 Introduction

Uveitis in children and adolescents include a range of inflammatory or infectious causes that are isolated to the eye or associated with systemic disease. The incidence of uveitis is less frequent in children than adults; however, the overall prognosis is worse because of delayed diagnosis [1]. Issues like exam difficulty, history obtainment, and lack of expected ocular symptoms like pain as seen in juvenile idiopathic arthritis (JIA) uveitis, delay the diagnosis, and potentially cause permanent ocular damage. Often, presenting symptoms can be strabismus or leukocoria which are first noticed by parents. Diagnosis delay can eventually lead to amblyopia in children under 8 years old [2].

13.2 Anatomy and Definition

The uvea consists of the iris, ciliary body, and choroid (■ Fig. 13.1). The iris is responsible for the amount of light entering the eye by constricting or dilating. The ciliary body produces aqueous fluid and is also responsible for accommodation. The choroid is comprised of blood vessels which supply the outer retina and retinal pigment epithelium. Uveitis is the inflammation of any of these aforementioned structures due to an abnormal or excessive inflammatory response mediated by macrophages, neutrophils, and lymphocytes. The inflammation can

become chronic and lead to ocular damage [2]. The eye has three main compartments: anterior, intermediate (vitreous), or posterior (retina/choroid). The term iritis is generally used to describe inflammation seen anteriorly or in the aqueous humor (■ Table 13.1).

13.3 Causes and Symptoms

The two possible causes of inflammation are either infectious or noninfectious. Masquerade syndromes like retinoblastoma can mimic uveitis and should always be ruled out first. Infectious causes are often related to congenital exposure of TORCH infections like toxoplasmosis, HIV, rubella, cytomegalovirus, herpes simplex, or zoster. Noninfectious causes are autoimmune mediated and can either be localized to the eye or associated with a systemic autoimmune process.

As mentioned earlier, most children with uveitis will be asymptomatic making diagnosis challenging. Other signs and symptoms

■ **Table 13.1**   Uveitis Subtypes

Type	Affected structures
Anterior	Iris
Intermediate	Ciliary body and vitreous
Posterior	Retina and/or choroid

■ **Fig. 13.1** Sagittal drawing of the eye. (Image courtesy of Erin Harpur, designer)

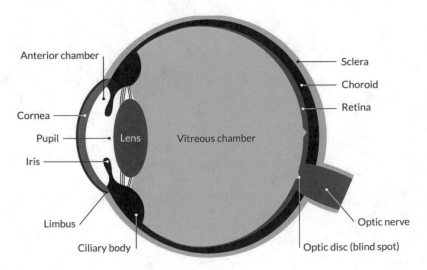

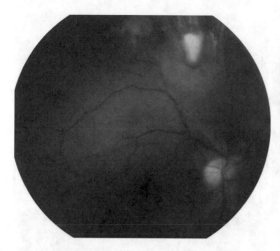

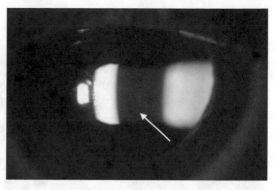

◼ Fig. 13.3 Slit lamp photograph at high magnification showing white blood cells floating in the aqueous humor (arrow, photo courtesy of Sanjay Kedhar MD)

◼ Fig. 13.2 Fundus photograph of toxoplasmosis chorioretinitis. The white lesion superior to the optic nerve is the site of active infection with inflamed retinal vasculature. The adjacent dark lesion is inactive scar tissue from prior infection. (Photo courtesy of Sanjay Kedhar MD)

can include a red eye, photophobia, decreased visual acuity, or unusual behavior [1].

The location of the primary source of inflammation (anterior, intermediate, posterior) can help determine the etiology of inflammation. For example, JIA remains the most common cause of anterior uveitis in children, while toxoplasmosis (◼ Fig. 13.2) is the most common posterior uveitis. Intermediate uveitis, accounting for 25% of uveitis in the pediatric age group can be caused by Lyme disease, sarcoidosis, or tuberculosis; however, it is largely idiopathic [2].

13.4 Juvenile Idiopathic Arthritis Uveitis

Juvenile idiopathic arthritis (JIA) is a systemic autoimmune disease affecting 70,000 children in the United States [2]. The peak onset is between 6 months and 4 years and is subdivided into six groups: systemic, polyarticular, oligoarticular, psoriatic, enthesitis-related, and undifferentiated [3]. Oligoarthritis, which is defined as persistent arthritis which affects four or fewer joints (usually large joints like knees, ankles and elbows), is the most frequent type of JIA and also has the highest

likelihood of associated uveitis with 10–30% involvement [3]. Children of this subtype are usually positive for antinuclear antibodies (ANA) and negative for rheumatoid factor. JIA uveitis is usually silent and can present prior to the joint inflammation making diagnosis challenging. Uveitis associated with JIA is also more common among females [3].

JIA associated uveitis is bilateral, anterior, and usually nongranulomatous with associated small keratic precipitates [3]. White blood cells will be present in the aqueous humor (◼ Fig. 13.3) and can be graded in intensity depending on the amount seen at the slit lamp. The eye will look quiet with an absence of conjunctival injection. If the child is old enough to complain of blurry vision, then distance visual acuity in the emergency room should be taken with an occluder (◼ Fig. 13.4a). The pinhole feature (◼ Fig. 13.4b) will often correct a refractive error (myopia or hyperopia), and absence of 20/20 vision can signify an anatomic determent such as band keratopathy, cataract, or cystoid macular edema. However, children with JIA uveitis can remain 20/20. Band keratopathy (calcium on the cornea) can be seen with penlight and signifies chronic inflammation (◼ Fig. 13.5). Posterior synechia represents scarring of the iris at the pupillary border with the anterior lens capsule. It is another sign of chronic inflammation that can be observed by penlight exam (◼ Fig. 13.6) and can cause the pupil to look irregular or be nonreactive to light. Lack of a red reflex with a direct ophthalmoscope can signify a dense

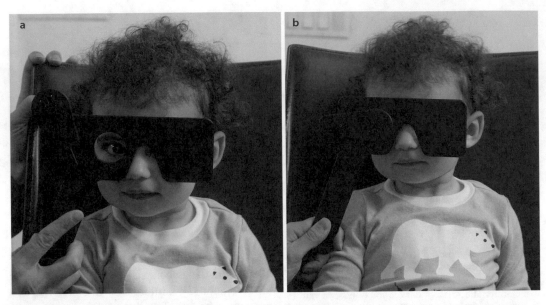

Fig. 13.4 Vision checked with an occluder **a** and using pinhole function **b** to help reduce refractive error

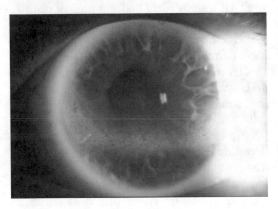

Fig. 13.5 Slit lamp photograph showing band keratopathy, or calcium deposition on the cornea, which can be a sign of chronic ocular inflammation. (Photo courtesy of Sanjay Kedhar MD)

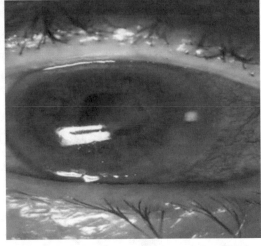

Fig. 13.6 Slit lamp photograph of posterior synechia causing an irregularly shaped pupil. (Photo courtesy of Scott Richter OD)

cataract. There should be low threshold to place an ophthalmology consult in children with known JIA who have ocular complaints.

Treatment of JIA uveitis ranges from topical steroids, localized steroid injections, systemic immunosuppression such as oral steroids, and immune modulators like methotrexate and adalimumab [4]. Follow-up should be guided by the degree of disease activity and the intensity of therapy. Weekly visits may be appropriate initially, followed by more extended intervals based on disease response. Quiescent patients may be followed every

3–6 months [3]. A typical steroid drop treatment regimen is prednisolone acetate 1% given four times per day, though higher initial doses may be used based on the degree of inflammation. Systemic steroids like prednisone are typically started at a dose of 1 mg/kg body weight, followed by a slow taper. While systemic corticosteroids may be a reasonable initial therapy, extended use is discouraged given their unfavorable systemic side effect profile [3]. Clinicians should also be mindful of the

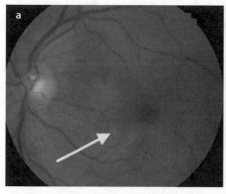

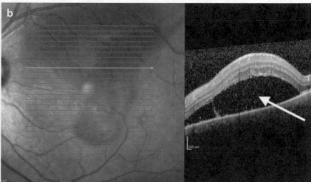

◨ **Fig. 13.7** **a** Fundus photograph of a patient presenting with sympathetic ophthalmia in his sympathizing eye. Notice yellow subretinal lesions (arrow). **b** Macular OCT displaying subretinal fluid causing retinal elevation (arrow)

risk of cataract formation and glaucoma with continued steroid use, especially with topical formulations. Those patients requiring continued systemic therapy should be transitioned to steroid-sparing immunomodulating therapy. Systemic steroids or immmunomodulators such as methotrexate should be managed in accordance with a pediatric rheumatologist.

Approximately 30% of eyes effected by JIA present with vision of 20/50 or worse, while 20% present with 20/200 or worse vision [5]. Thirty percent of effected eyes will progress to vision of 20/50 or worse and 20% of eyes will progress to 20/200 or worse [5]. The most common causes of severe vision loss are cataract formation and band keratopathy [5]. Risk of progression to severe vision loss has been shown to be significantly reduced with immunosuppressive therapy [5]. Poor prognosticators for vision loss are persistent anterior segment reaction and posterior synechia [5].

13.5 Sympathetic Ophthalmia

Sympathetic ophthalmia (SO) is a rare, bilateral granulomatous panuveitis (affecting all three chambers of eye) which occurs after ocular trauma from either penetrating accidental injuries or surgical procedures to one eye [6]. Trauma to one eye (referred to as the exciting eye) will cause an inflammatory response in the contralateral eye (referred to as the sympathizing eye). This response can occur days to years after the initial injury [7]. The cause is theorized to be an autoimmune reaction to uveal antigens which are normally sequestered in the uvea but are exposed to the immune system after trauma. Incidence of SO is low but ranges from 0.1% to 0.3% in traumatized eyes, with a possibly higher incidence in children due to their increased risk of accidental trauma [6]. Enucleation of the injured eye prior to inflammation in the sympathizing eye has been generally thought to prevent the occurrence of SO [8].

13.6 Clinical Presentation and Diagnosis

The clinical presentation of SO is variable but always bilateral, with the exciting eye usually being more symptomatic and showing more inflammation than the sympathizing eye. Diagnosis is made on history and clinical exam, therefore careful attention to a history of trauma to one eye with associated symptoms of pain, redness, decreased vision, or photophobia in both eyes warranting an urgent ophthalmology consult [8, 9]. On slit lamp exam, there will be cells in the anterior chamber with likely mutton-fat keratic precipitates on the inferior cornea. Posterior synechia can be present. Intraocular pressure will be generally normal or low due to ciliary body shutdown from inflammation. There generally is a vitritis accompanied by yellow-white subretinal lesions in the posterior pole or mid-periphery called Dalen-Fuchs nodules (◨ Fig. 13.7a) [9]. Further testing in the office with ocular coherence tomography (OCT) can show retinal elevation from subretinal fluid (■ Fig. 13.7b).

13.7 Treatment

The initial treatment of SO is almost always systemic corticosteroids given at a dose of 1 to 1.5 mg/kg of prednisone. Given SO's disease course, oral steroids generally need to be tapered slowly based on disease activity. Relapses are still common and in patients who can't tolerate corticosteroids or don't adequately respond, long-term immunomodulatory agents like methotrexate, myocophenolate, and adalimumab have been shown to be effective [8–10]. Enucleation of the exciting eye upon onset of SO has not been shown to reduce disease severity in the sympathizing eye [8].

13.8 Episcleritis and Scleritis

13.8.1 Anatomy

The sclera is a fibrous, relatively avascular structure that encloses the posterior four-fifths of the eye. It is situated in between the conjunctiva and the uveal layers. It is composed mainly of type I collagen, gylcosaminoglycans, and fibroblasts. It fuses with the optic nerve sheath posteriorly and the corneal limbus anteriorly. It ranges in thickness from 1 mm at its posterior apex to 0.3 mm just posterior to the insertion sites of the extraocular muscles. The episclera is a loose layer of fibrovascular tissue that covers the outer sclera and is deep to the bulbar conjunctiva [11].

13.8.2 Episcleritis

Episcleritis is an inflammation of the episclera that is relatively uncommon in the pediatric age group. The two forms of episcleritis are simple and nodular, with the latter exhibiting localized injection clustering around nodules with the former being

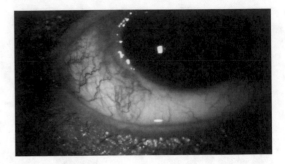

■ **Fig. 13.8** Slit lamp photograph of episcleritis showing episcleral sectoral injection of the ocular surface. (Photo courtesy of Scott Richter OD)

localized to a small area [2, 12]. It is characterized by sectoral redness overlying the sclera (■ Fig. 13.8) which will blanch with topical phenelyephrine 2.5%. Patients usually are asymptomatic or complain of minimal discomfort. Vision will not be affected. Hyperemic vessels will be mobile with a cotton tip applied over the underlying sclera in episcleritis, which helps distinguish this entity from scleritis where the injected vessels are immobile. Another difference is the injected area will be nontender in episcleritis while there is marked tenderness in scleritis. It is also easy to confuse episcleritis with conjunctivitis (viral, bacterial, or allergic). However, no conjunctival papillae or follicles will be present in episcleritis which can help distinguish it from conjunctivitis.

13.8.3 Workup and Management

Most cases of episcleritis do not require a workup; however, a thorough review of systems (ROS) should be done to help assess a possibility of a systemic autoimmune disease like juvenile idiopathic arthritis, lupus, or inflammatory bowel disease [13]. Joint pain or swelling, morning stiffness, rashes, cold sores, shortness of breath, diarrhea, constipation, or a strong family history of autoimmune disease should warrant a systemic workup. Infectious etiologies, although rare, include herpetic (HSV, VZV), lyme disease, syphilis, and tuberculosis. Cases have been reported in children younger than 5 years old following an upper respiratory illness [14].

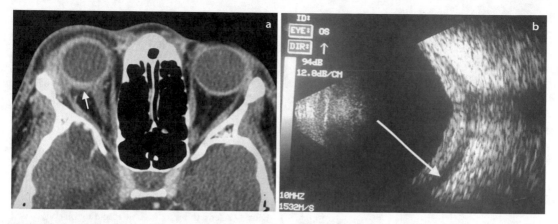

Fig. 13.9 **a** Axial CT showing right posterior scleral inflammation denoted by increased thickness and enhancement (arrow). **b** B-scan ultrasound of the eye showing classic T-sign in posterior scleritis (arrow)

In the absence of systemic disease, episcleritis is usually self-limited. Treatment with cold artificial tears four times daily can alleviate some of the signs and symptoms. It is important to avoid topical steroids, even though very effective, as the inflammation can become recalcitrant once the steroid is tapered and ultimately become a chronic process. Topical nonsteroidal anti-inflammatories (NSAIDs) are usually not effective. Oral NSAIDs can be used in cases of known systemic disease [2]. Consider a viral cause if a patient presents to the ER with chronic inflammation that has not responded to oral NSAIDs.

13.8.4 Scleritis

Scleritis is inflammation of the sclera and occurs rarely in the pediatric population. It affects either the anterior sclera where redness will be visible to the examiner or the posterior sclera which will not have visible redness. Both forms are associated with pain. Scleritis is often found in patients with known autoimmune conditions like rheumatoid arthritis (RA), systemic lupus erythematosus (SLE), inflammatory bowel disease, sarcoidosis, and granulomatous with polyangiitis (GPA) to name a few. Infectious etiology from lyme, syphilis, TB, and herpes are also possible [2]. Anterior scleritis is sub-divided into diffuse, nodular, and necrotizing [12].

13.8.4.1 Posterior Scleritis

Multiple case series have shown a predominance of the posterior form in the pediatric age group. In isolated posterior scleritis, anterior injection is either absent or mild. Presentation is bilateral in about 50 percent of cases and pain increases with extraocular movement [15]. Patients may also have diminished extraocular motility and proptosis [15]. Many clinicians regard this disease as a variant of idiopathic orbital inflammation given the proximity to the orbit. Accompanying intraocular findings can include serous retinal detachments, choroidal folds and optic nerve head edema, all of which may cause vision loss. Imaging will demonstrate a thickened posterior sclera on CT (**□** Fig. 13.9a) or MRI, while ultrasound will show a classic "T-sign," (**□** Fig. 13.9b) characterized by a layer of fluid behind the thickened sclera. Systemic disease associations with posterior scleritis in the pediatric population are uncommon [15].

13.8.4.2 Anterior Scleritis: Diffuse or Nodular

Diffuse scleritis is the most common type of scleritis and involves either a small or large area of continuous sclera [2]. It will present with injection of the deeper scleral vessels, with variable amounts of edema or scleral thickening (**□** Fig. 13.10). Nodular scleritis will also present with pain and redness centered on 1 or 2 raised nodules usually close to

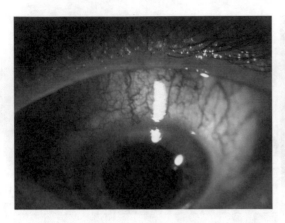

Fig. 13.10 Anterior segment photograph of diffuse anterior scleritis involving the superior sclera. (Photo courtesy of Sanjay Kedhar MD)

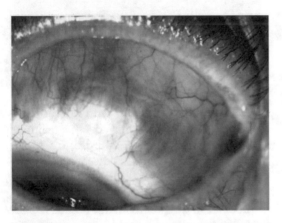

Fig. 13.11 Chronic scleritis can eventually thin the sclera, allowing the underlying uvea to be shown. (Photo courtesy of Sanjay Kedhar MD)

the limbus. Care must be taken to differentiate scleritis from episcleritis and conjunctivitis due to differences in treatment. Scleral injection from scleritis will have a violaceous hue which will not blanch with topical phenylephrine. Slit lamp examination may show thickening of the underlying sclera, and inflamed scleral vessels will have a crisscross pattern, as opposed to the radial pattern of episcleral vasculature. A cotton tip applicator can be used to displace more superficial episcleral vessels in order to more clearly differentiate which layers are affected. Complications of anterior scleritis include peripheral ulcerative keratitis (PUK), anterior uveitis, and scleral thinning in the chronic phase (Fig. 13.11) [12].

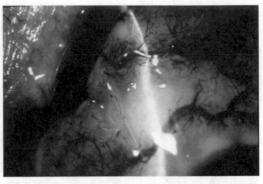

Fig. 13.12 Necrotizing scleritis with inflammation causing scleral thinning with surrounding marked scleral injection. (Photo courtesy of Sanjay Kedhar MD)

13.8.4.3 Anterior Necrotizing Scleritis

The necrotizing forms of scleritis are associated with areas of scleral thinning and may be inflammatory or non-inflammatory. The inflammatory form presents with significant pain and areas of avascular necrosis surrounded by redness (Fig. 13.12) [2]. This is associated with systemic disease in the majority of cases and usually requires immunosuppressive treatment. The non-inflammatory form, known as scleromalacia perforans, is not painful but causes severe scleral thinning that results in visualization of dark underlying uveal tissue. These necrotizing forms are more commonly associated with systemic rheumatologic disease and often necessitate long term immunomodulatory therapy. There have also been cases reports of necrotizing scleritis following pediatric strabismus surgery [16]. While spontaneous globe rupture is rare, effected eyes are more susceptible to rupture with minimal trauma

13.8.4.4 Workup

Approximately 50% of scleritis cases are associated with systemic autoimmune disease in the adult age group. While the association with systemic disease with anterior scleritis is not as clearly defined in the pediatric group, workup and referral to a pediatric rheumatologist is usually recommended. Less than 10% of cases are associated with infection, the leading cause of which is VZV, with syphilis, lyme, and TB being less common [12]. A careful clinical history should include inquiry into joint pains, gastrointestinal complaints, and ophthalmic history (surgery, prior inflammatory episodes). In the pediatric age group, isolated posterior scleritis is rarely associated with systemic disease [17]. Workup should be tailored to the history and physical but should generally include blood count (CBC) with differential, erythrocyte sedimentation rate (ESR), antinuclear antibodies, rheumatoid factor, antineutrophil cytoplasmic antibodies, syphilis serology, and lyme screen with Western blot reflex [18].

13.8.4.5 Treatment

Treatment of scleritis is always systemic. With anterior scleritis, therapy proceeds in a stepwise fashion with NSAIDS being first line in uncomplicated cases, and systemic steroids or immunomodulatory therapy reserved for severe or recurrent cases. A typical regimen is prednisone with an initial dose of 1 mg/kg followed by a slow taper over a few months once scleral inflammation is controlled [15]. Local therapy with periocular steroid injections are effective in some cases [2]. Immunomodulatory therapy options include methotrexate, cyclophosphamide, and anti-TNFa agents which should be administered in collaboration with a pediatric rheumatologist [12].

13.8.5 Allergic Conjunctivitis

13.8.5.1 Acute Allergic Conjunctivitis

Acute allergic conjunctivitis may occur in isolation or as part of a more systemic allergic response. The pathogenesis is a type I, IgE-mediated allergic response with mast cells and histamine release playing a pivotal role. Symptoms develop shortly after exposure to an allergen and include significant chemosis, eyelid edema, itching, and tearing (◘ Fig. 13.13) [18]. While the exam is often impressive, the condition usually resolves with conservative therapy. Topical and systemic antihistamines are recommended, and avoidance of the allergen is encouraged. Allergic conjunctivitis should be distinguished from infectious conjunctivitis (bacterial or viral), as the management of these entities is very different. Infectious conjunctivitis usually presents over one to 2 days with more impressive

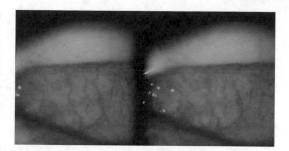

◘ **Fig. 13.13** Inferior palpebral conjunctival chemosis with follicles in acute allergic conjunctivitis. (Photo courtesy of Scott Richter OD)

injection and, in the case of bacterial infections, thick mucopurulent discharge. A history of sick contacts and recent upper respiratory infections is common. Viral conjunctivitis usually starts unilaterally before effecting the fellow eye and is usually a self-limited infection. Bacterial conjunctivitis more commonly remains unilateral, and responds to topical antibiotics. Both types of infections may form pseudomembranes on the palpebral conjunctiva, a feature uncommon to allergic conjunctivitis.

13.8.5.2 Chronic Allergic Conjunctivitis

These entities represent immune hypersensitivity reactions and are subdivided into perennial allergic conjunctivitis (PAC), seasonal allergic conjunctivitis (SAC), vernal keratoconjunctivitis (VKC), and atopic keratoconjunctivitis (AKC). The first two are more common and are usually less severe than the latter two. While SAC and PAC are both mediated by more straightforward IgE mechanisms, VKC and AKC are now thought to be mediated by more complex hypersensitivity processes [20].

13.8.5.3 Perennial and Seasonal Allergic Conjunctivitis

These common conditions are characterized by persistent conjunctival chemosis, hyperemia, itching, and mucoid discharge. Affected children often have a history of atopy, including asthma, eczema, allergic rhinitis, and chronic eyelid skin changes such as allergic shiners. The pathophysiology is a type I hypersensitivity reaction mediated by mast cells and

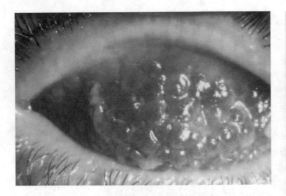

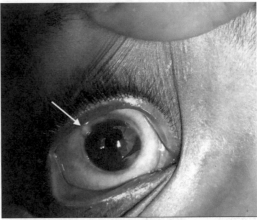

Fig. 13.14 Giant papillae seen involving the superior palpebral conjunctiva in vernal conjunctivitis. (Photo courtesy of Scott Richter OD)

Fig. 13.15 Single Horner-Trantas' dot at 11 o'clock (arrow) in vernal keratoconjunctivitis. There is mild conjunctival injection. (Photo courtesy of Maxine Miller, MD)

IgE. The attacks usually occur in the spring and fall in the seasonal variant and are caused by airborne outdoor allergens. The perennial variant is thought to be caused by household allergens, including dust mites and pet material [21]. Allergen avoidance should be encouraged and referral to an allergy specialist should be made when appropriate. Topical treatment options include antihistamine and mast cell stabilizing eye drops. The former provides relatively acute relief, while the latter requires several days for therapeutic effect [19]. Combination drops containing both antihistamine and mast cell stabilizing medications (e.g., ketotifen) are also available over-the-counter and frequently prescribed for this condition. Steroid and NSAID drops should be used sparingly given their respective side effect profiles.

13.8.5.4 Vernal Conjunctivitis

Vernal conjunctivitis (VKC) represents a distinct entity from perennial or seasonal conjunctivitis. It is now thought to be mediated by a complex, multifactorial immune process which includes Th2 cells, eosinophils, Il-4, and Il-5 [20]. It usually develops within the first decade of life and resolved by age 20. Males are more commonly affected. Symptoms include itching, burning, tearing, and mucoid discharge. Distinguishing signs include prominent papillae on the superior palpebral conjunctiva (Fig. 13.14) and

Horner-Trantas' dots (Fig. 13.15), which are raised white lesions along the limbus consisting of eosinophils and neutrophils. Additionally, affected patients may develop characteristic shield ulcers, which are sterile non-healing corneal erosions usually found in the superior cornea. A minority of patients may develop vision changes secondary to corneal scarring and induced astigmatism. Treatment is similar to the perennial and seasonal forms. Antibiotic drops may be added for epithelial defects. Topical cyclosporine drops may be tried in severe or refractory cases [22].

13.8.5.5 Atopic Keratoconjunctivitis (AKC)

AKC usually begins during the late teenage years and usually persists past early adulthood. A history of atopy is common [23]. Signs and symptoms are similar to VKC; however, the inferior palpebral conjunctiva is more commonly involved (Fig. 13.16) [19]. Eczematous periocular skin changes are commonly seen and may include prominent lower lid folds called Dennie-Morgan lines on the lower lid. AKC has also been associated with early cataract formation [23]. Treatment is similar to VKC.

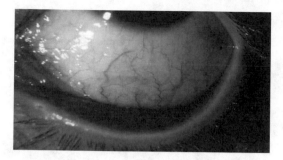

Fig. 13.16 Inferior palpebral conjunctival papillae. (Photo courtesy of Scott Richter OD)

Case Presentation

A 9-year-old female presented to the ER with blurry vision in both eyes. She denies light sensitivity or pain but complained of knee pain on review of systems. Her distance visual acuity was 20/80 in the right eye and 20/40 in the left eye with no improvement on pinhole. Pen light exam showed a fixed, small pupil in the right eye and a reactive response on the left. On further examination, she had 2+ graded white cells anteriorly in both eyes with posterior synechia in the right eye. (■ Fig. 13.17) Given her history of knee pain and iritis, a presumed diagnosis of JIA-mediated uveitis was made. She was started on topical steroids in both eyes and referred to both an ophthalmologist and pediatric rheumatologist for further workup and treatments.

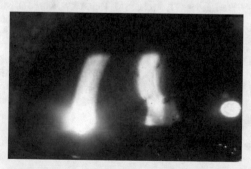

Fig. 13.17 Anterior uveitis secondary to JIA with white cells in the anterior chamber and posterior synechia. (Photo courtesy of Scott Richter OD)

Key Points
- Uveitis secondary to JIA can be relatively asymptomatic but can lead to significant ocular complications if not treated in a timely manner.
- Sympathetic ophthalmia should be considered in bilateral uveitic presentations after penetrating ocular trauma or surgery.
- It is important to distinguish scleritis from episcleritis, as the former is more likely to be secondary to a systemic inflammatory disease and requires systemic treatment.
- Posterior scleritis may present similarly to idiopathic orbital inflammation (IOI).
- Ocular allergy ranges from mild to severe and may lead to secondary ocular complications if not controlled.

❓ Review Questions
1. What subtype of JIA is most prone to developing anterior uveitis?
   (a) Oligoarticular, ANA negative
   (b) Oligoarticular, ANA positive
   (c) Polyarticular, ANA negative
   (d) Polyarticular, ANA positive

2. Which of the following findings is more typical of episcleritis as opposed to scleritis?
   (a) Association with systemic disease
   (b) Prominent dilated subconjunctival vessels in crisscross configuration that cannot be displaced with a cotton tip
   (c) Boring pain that worsens with palpation
   (d) Injection that blanches with topical phenylephrine 2.5%

3. If no specific allergen is identified, what is the most reasonable first-line therapy for seasonal allergic conjunctivitis?

(a) Artificial tear drops
(b) Systemic steroids
(c) Prednisolone acetate 1% drops
(d) Ketotifen drops

✅ **Answers**
1. (b)
2. (d)
3. (d)

References

1. BenEzra D, Cohen E, Maftzir G. Uveitis in children and adolescents. Br J Ophthalmol. 2005;89:444–8.
2. Gaudio P, Huang J. Ocular inflammatory and uveitis Manuel. Philadelphia: Lippincott Williams; 2002.
3. Raab EL, Aaby AA, Bloom JN, et al. Uveitis in pediatric age group. In: Pediatric ophthalmology and strabismus. San Francisco: American Academy of Ophthalmology; 2010. p. 267–78.
4. Smith JA, Mackensen F, Sen N, Leigh J, Watkins AS, Pyatetsky D, Tessler H, Nussenblatt R, Rosenbaum JT, Reed GF, Vitale S, Smith JR, Goldstein D. Epidemiology and course of disease in childhood uveitis. Ophthalmology. 2009;116(8):1544–51.
5. Thorne J, Woreta F, Kedhar S, Dunn J. Juvenile idiopathic arthritis-associated uveitis: incidence of ocular complications and visual acuity loss. Am J Ophthalmol. 2007;143(5):840–6.
6. Kilmartin DJ, Dick AD, Forrester JV. Prospective surveillance of sympathetic opthalmia in the UK and Replublic of Ireland. Br J Ophthalmol. 2000;84:259–63.
7. Galor A, Davis JL, Flynn HW, Feuer WJ, Dubovy SR, Setlur V, Kesen MR, Goldstein DA, Tessler HH, Ganelis IB, Jabs DA, Thorne JE. Sympathetic ophthalmia: incidence of ocular complications and vision loss in the sympathizing eye. AJO. 2009; 148(5):704–10.
8. Nussenblatt RB, Whitecup SM. Uveitis: fundamentals and clinical practice. Philadelphia: Elsevier; 1996.
9. Moorthy RS, Davis J, Foster SC, Lowder CY, Vitale AT, Lopatynsky M, Bodaghi B, Bora NS. Intraocular inflammation and uveitis. San Francisco: American Academy of Ophthalmology; 2010. p. 204–9.
10. Chang GC, Young LH. Sympathetic ophthalmia. Semin Ophthalmol. 2011;26(4–5):316–20.
11. Rose RH, Bloomer MM, Gombos DS, Milman T, et al. Sclera. In: Rose RH, Bloomer MM, editors. Ophthalmic pathology and intraocular tumors. San Francisco: American Academy of Ophthalmology; 2017. p. 107–8.
12. Weisenthal RW, Daly MK, Feder RS, Orlin SE, et al. Diagnosis and management of immune-related disorders of the external eye: immune mediated diseases of episclera and sclera. In: Weisenthal RW, Daly MK, editors. External disease and cornea. San Francisco: American Academy of Ophthalmology; 2017. p. 318–24.
13. Read RW, Weiss AH, Sherry DD. Episcleritis in childhood. Ophthalmology. 1999;106(12):2377–9.
14. Shah SA, Kazmi HS, Awan AA, Khan J. Recurrent episcleritis in children less than 5 years of age. J Ayub Med Coll Abbottabad. 2006;18(4):69–70.
15. Cheung CMG, Chee S-P. Posterior scleritis in children: clinical features and treatment. Ophthalmology. 2012;119(1):59–65.
16. Kearne FM, Blaikie AJ, Gole GA. Anterior necrotizing scleritis after strabismus surgery in a child. J AAPOS. 2007;11(2):197–8.
17. Okhravi N, Odufuwa B, McCluskey P, Lightman S. Scleritis. Surv Ophthalmol. 2005;50:351–63.
18. Akpek EK, Thorne JE, Qazi FA, Do DV, Jabs DA. Evaluation of patients with scleritis for systemic disease. Ophthalmology. 2004;111:501–6.
19. Weisenthal RW, Daly MK, Feder RS, Orlin SE, et al. Diagnosis and management of immune-related disorders of the external eye: immune mediated disorders of the conjunctiva. In: Weisenthal RW, Daly MK, editors. External disease and cornea. San Francisco: American Academy of Ophthalmology; 2017. p. 285–94.
20. La Rosa M, Lionetti E, Reibaldi M, Russo A. Allergic conjunctivitis: a comprehensive review of the literature. Ital J Pediatr. 2013;39(18)
21. Lueder GT, Archer SM, Hered RW, Karr DJ, et al. External diseases of the eye: inflammatory disease. In: Lueder GT, Archer SM, Hered RW, Karr DJ, editors. Pediatric ophthalmology and strabismus. San Francisco: American Academy of Ophthalmology; 2017. p. p270–3.
22. Bonini S, Coassin M, Aronni S, Lambiase A. Vernal keratoconjunctivitis. Eye (Lond). 2004;18(4):345–51.
23. Bielory B, Bielory L. Atopic dermatitis and keratoconjunctivitis. Immunol Allergy Clin N Am. 2010;30:323–36.

13

Extraocular Inflammation

Valerie H. Chen and Edward J. Wladis

Contents

© Springer Nature Switzerland AG 2021
R. Shinder (ed.), *Pediatric Ophthalmology in the Emergency Room*,
https://doi.org/10.1007/978-3-030-49950-1_14

14.1 Introduction

Pediatric patients often present in the acute setting with signs and symptoms of extraocular inflammation. While there is a wide differential that may produce a similar constellation of findings, we will focus on a number of non-infectious entities in this chapter. The presentation, pathology, evaluation, and treatment of idiopathic orbital inflammation, ocular rosacea, contact dermatitis, and chalazion are reviewed here.

14.2 Idiopathic Orbital Inflammation

14.2.1 Background

Idiopathic orbital inflammation (IOI), or nonspecific orbital inflammation, is a benign nonspecific, non-neoplastic inflammatory condition of the orbit without identifiable local or systemic cause. It was first described as a distinct entity by Birch-Hirschfeld in 1905 who presented a lecture on "orbital pseudotumor" diagnosed in four patients with exophthalmos [1]. In 1923, Benedict and Knight introduced "inflammatory pseudotumor" based on their experience of six patients who were believed to have a neoplasm but found to have lymphocytic infiltration of the soft tissue on surgical exploration [2].

In adults, it comprises 6–16% of all orbital lesions and accounts for up to 10% of orbital biopsies [3]. Further, it is the second most common cause of proptosis following thyroid eye disease and the third most common orbital disorder following thyroid eye disease and lymphoproliferative disease.

14.2.2 Presentation

While idiopathic orbital inflammation typically presents in the third to sixth decades, it can rarely occur in children though the actual incidence is unknown. Historically, there has been no gender predilection [4] though more recently a female predilection has been

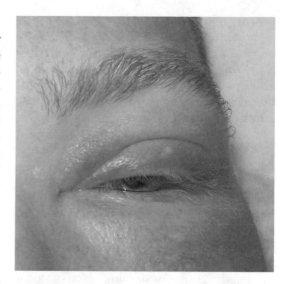

☐ **Fig. 14.1**   Left dacryoadenitis presenting as upper lid edema

suggested [5]. This disease can be either a focal or diffuse process. Focal involvement may manifest as an orbital mass, myositis (extraocular muscle, most often the medial rectus [5, 6]), dacryoadenitis (lacrimal gland) (☐ Fig. 14.1), perineuritis (optic nerve), posterior scleritis, and Tolosa-Hunt syndrome (orbital apex); the first three are the most common presentations in the pediatric population [7]. Of note, idiopathic orbital inflammation may present in several disparate anatomic areas simultaneously.

Clinical manifestation can vary widely depending on the orbital tissue involved and the degree of inflammation. In children, the most common ophthalmologic symptoms reported are periorbital swelling, orbital pain, blepharoptosis, palpable mass, proptosis, and extraocular motility dysfunction [7, 8]. Mottow et al. [8] found that the periorbital swelling was characteristically worse upon arising in the morning with improvement throughout the day. Orbital pain is more common in older children and can vary from mild discomfort or tenderness to severe boring pain [7]. The myositic variant is more commonly associated with pain which is further exacerbated by eye movement. Pain and proptosis may be less prevalent in children compared to adults [7]. In adults, idiopathic orbital inflammation is generally a unilateral process; however, bilateral involvement occurs in up to one third of children and may be more commonly seen in African Americans [7]. While systemic symptoms are rare in adults, over half of children will complain of headache, nausea, vomiting, abdominal pain, anorexia, lethargy, malaise, and fever [7, 8].

14.2.3 Differential Diagnosis

By definition, idiopathic orbital inflammation has no identifiable cause and is a diagnosis of exclusion. In the pediatric population, there is a wide differential diagnosis. Infectious etiologies may include acute orbital cellulitis, chalazion, or infectious dacryoadenitis. Noninfectious inflammatory causes may include ruptured dermoid cyst, mucocele, orbital foreign body, thyroid ophthalmopathy, sarcoidosis, or granulomatosis with polyangiitis. Neoplastic causes may be benign like Langerhans cell histiocytosis, lymphatic malformations, and optic nerve glioma or malignant like rhabdomyosarcoma, metastatic neuroblastoma, and lymphoproliferative disorders.

14.2.4 Work-Up

Any child presenting with the above symptoms needs a detailed history and full eye examination. Further work-up involves serologic testing and imaging to exclude the aforementioned etiologies. Laboratory testing depends on the presentation, clinical history, and tissues involved but often includes CBC, TFTs, ACE, lysozyme, ESR, CRP, ANA, RF, anti-CCP, ANCA, HLA-B27, RPR, FTA-Ab, Lyme, quantiferon gold, and IgG4. While they are often normal, a mild leukocytosis, peripheral eosinophilia, and elevated inflammatory markers are not uncommon. Computerized tomography (CT) is a rapid and readily available modality that does not require sedation but exposes the child to radiation. Magnetic resonance imaging (MRI) provides excellent soft tissue detail without radiation exposure but may require sedation due to the length of study. Contrast enhancement and fat suppression techniques can help show subtle areas of inflammation or enhancement that may otherwise be masked by the high intensity signal of orbital fat. Again, depending on the location as well as degree and chronicity of inflammation, the pathology may appear in a variety of ways [5]. Often, it can be seen as a diffuse orbital mass with indistinct margins. Dacryoadenitis may appear as enlargement of the lacrimal gland with adjacent fat stranding (◘ Fig. 14.2). Myositis shows diffuse involvement of the extraocular muscle including its tendon insertion giving it a tubular-like appearance; this is in contrast to the tendon-sparing muscle involvement seen in thyroid eye disease (◘ Figs. 14.3 and 14.4). Perineuritis reveals optic nerve

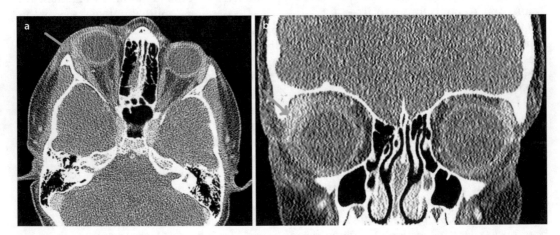

◘ **Fig. 14.2** Right dacryoadenitis. Axial **a** and Coronal **b** CT demonstrating an enlarged right lacrimal gland with indistinct margins

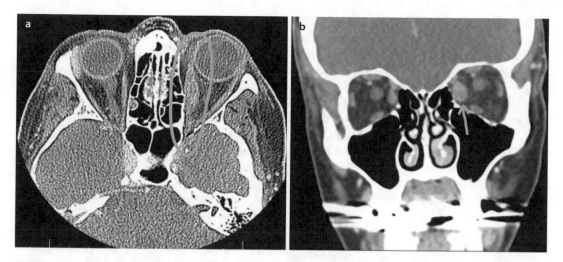

◘ Fig. 14.3   Left medial rectus myositis. Axial **a** and Coronal **b** CT demonstrating a diffusely enlarged left medial rectus muscle. Note involvement of the tendinous insertion giving a tubular-like appearance to the rectus muscle

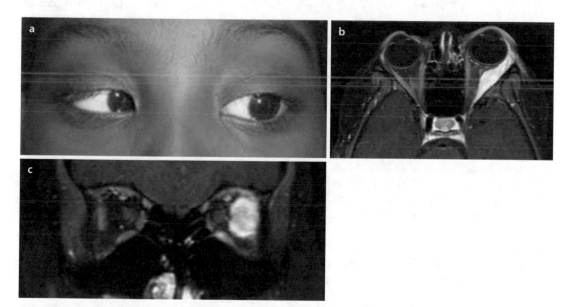

◘ Fig. 14.4   Left lateral rectus myositis. **a** Clinical photograph showing decreased left abduction. Axial **b** and coronal **c** MRI orbits with contrast and fat suppression depicting enlarged left hyperintense lateral rectus muscle

enhancement and thickening of the optic nerve sheath which can appear as a "tram-track" on axial view and "doughnut" on coronal view. Bone involvement is quite rare and prompts further evaluation for an underlying etiology [7].

There is some debate regarding biopsy. Mottow et al. [8] studied 29 cases of pediatric idiopathic orbital inflammation and found that those who underwent biopsy were more likely to suffer sequelae regardless of initial degree of severity or pattern of involvement. As such, biopsy may be reserved for patients with atypical presentation, poor response to steroids, or recurrence to rule out other causes. Particularly in patients with primary isolated myositis or optic perineuritis, the risks of induced strabismus or vision loss may outweigh the benefits of the procedure. Nonetheless, given improvements in histopathologic analysis and increased recognition that patients with idiopathic orbital inflammation may not fully respond to corticosteroids, several authorities have recommended biopsy in cases of non-myositic disease [9]. When biopsy is done, histopathology shows a nongranulomatous inflammation of plasma cells, macrophages, lymphocytes, polymorphonuclear cells with eosinophils and varying degrees of reactive fibrovascular stroma. More chronic forms have an increased amount of collagenous connective tissue.

> Idiopathic orbital inflammation is a diagnosis of exclusion. Consider the following work-up:
> — Serology: CBC, TFTs, ACE, lysozyme, ESR, CRP, ANA, RF, anti-CCP, ANCA, HLA-B27, RPR, FTA-Ab, Lyme, quantiferon gold, and IgG4
> — Orbital imaging (CT or MRI)
> — Possible biopsy

14.2.5 Pathogenesis

Several theories postulate that a triggered immune dysregulation after infections, minor trauma, or surgery may play a role in developing this nonspecific orbital inflammation [10–12]. Wladis et al. [13] found that there was significantly increased cytokine expression in IOI orbits compared to controls, in particular IL-12, TNF-α, and IFN-γ, suggesting that this disorder may represent an aberrant innate immune response. Additional studies document the presence of toll-like receptors which further support this link [14]. An autoimmune component may also be implicated given observed associations with a number of rheumatologic conditions, including Crohn's disease, systemic lupus erythematosus, rheumatoid arthritis, ankylosing spondylitis, and myasthenia gravis [15–19]. Further, Atabay et al. [20] discovered circulating serum antibodies against eye muscle membrane antigen in idiopathic orbital myositis.

14.2.6 Treatment

For mild cases of inflammation, observation or non-steroidal anti-inflammatory drugs may be acceptable. Still, the mainstay of treatment is systemic corticosteroids with a classic rapid response within 24–48 hours. Dosing is 1.0–1.5 mg/kg/day of oral steroids with a slow taper over months as premature cessation of medication may result in an incomplete response with recurrence. The myositic variant may require an even slower taper. Steroid response may be limited in more chronic forms of idiopathic orbital inflammation. Adverse events such as premature atherosclerosis, osteoporosis, diabetes, and growth retardation may limit long-term use in the pediatric group, especially in the setting of multiple recurrences. Children and their families should be counseled on the importance of strict medication compliance and the risk of sudden cessation of corticosteroids.

In adults, orbital radiation (e.g., 1500–2500 Gy over 10–15 days) has been used as a second-line treatment with good results; however there is some hesitation regarding this modality in patients younger than 20 years due to concern for an increased risk of induced malignancy. More recently, attention has turned to immunomodulators and biologic therapies. There is currently no consensus on these treatment protocols, and this should be undertaken in conjunction with a pediatric rheumatologist.

Methotrexate interferes with folic acid synthesis via inhibition of dihydrofolate reductase, resulting in suppression of both B- and T-cells. Smith et al. [21] instituted a methotrexate regimen beginning with 7.5 mg for the first week then increasing to 15 mg weekly, increasing at monthly intervals up to a maximum of 25 mg/week depending on clinical response and side effects. Of seven patients >18 years old with nonspecific orbital inflammation, four demonstrated a clinical benefit, one failed to respond, and two discontinued treatment for undisclosed reasons prior to completion of the 4-month trial. Shah et al. [22] reported five of six adult patients with steroid-intolerant or refractory idiopathic orbital inflammation responded well to 12.5 mg weekly of oral methotrexate. Adverse effects of methotrexate include hepatotoxicity, gastrointestinal disturbance, fatigue, hair loss, and neutropenia. Mycophenolate mofetil is another antimetabolite that inhibits purine synthesis and, as a result, B- and T-cell replication. Hatton et al. [23] treated five patients (ages 28–48 years) with mycophenolate mofetil, four of whom had previously experienced multiple recurrent episodes on alternative therapies and as an initial treatment for one patient with poorly controlled type 1 diabetes mellitus. Four patients responded with complete resolution of inflammation, three of whom were able to discontinue corticosteroids altogether. One discontinued the therapy due to severe nausea. The treatment dose of mycophenolate mofetil was titrated to achieve resolution, and the average maintenance dose in these patients was 2.2 g/day. Patients may complain of gastrointestinal disturbance, hypertension, peripheral edema, headache, and fever. Cyclosporine inhibits T-cell synthesis of IL-2 and related cytokines. Several case reports have shown efficacy, especially in cases of adults with uncontrolled or recalcitrant IOI [24–26]. Side effects of liver and bone marrow toxicity and pulmonary fibrosis must be monitored.

Rituximab is a chimeric mouse-human monoclonal antibody against CD20 protein and causes a selective, temporary depletion of CD20+ B-cell populations. Schafranski [27] reported a case of idiopathic orbital inflammation refractory to azathioprine therapy in a 66-year-old patient with diabetes mellitus who had marked improvement in signs and symptoms after two 1 g infusions of rituximab. Others have also reported successful treatment of IOI in the adult population with rituximab [28–30]. Reported side effects of rituximab include infusion reaction (including fevers, chills, rigors, nausea, dizziness, rash, and bronchospasm), pulmonary toxicity, cardiac toxicity, and immunosuppression. In an effort to reduce systemic side effects, Savino et al. [31] performed weekly 10 mg intraorbital rituximab injections in IOI adults refractory to corticosteroid treatment. The site of

injection was planned according to the clinical situation and imaging results. One patient experienced complete resolution after 2 months of treatment, the other two had improvement of symptoms as well as exam, radiologic, and histologic findings after 1- and 2-month cycles. The injections were tolerated well by all patients.

Infliximab is an intravenous chimeric monoclonal antibody against TNF-α. An increasing body of literature supports the use of infliximab as a steroid-sparing agent in recalcitrant IOI. The usual dosing schedule is 3–5 mg/kg of body weight given at baseline, week 2, week 6, and every 4–8 weeks thereafter. In rheumatoid arthritis, infliximab is more effective when given with methotrexate. Garrity et al. [32] presented a retrospective case series of seven patients (age 27–46 years) who were treated with infliximab after failure of traditional therapy. All patients had a favorable response, and those without other systemic conditions were able to discontinue all corticosteroid treatment. Wilson et al. [33] presented a 15-year-old patient with bilateral idiopathic orbital inflammation refractory to corticosteroid and methotrexate treatment that was started on infliximab (5 mg/kg at baseline, week 2, week 6, and then every 8 weeks thereafter) for a total of six infusions. He was successfully tapered off of steroids without any further relapse 2 years after his initial diagnosis. Miquel et al. [34] treated two adult patients with steroid-dependent IOI with eight cycles of infliximab (initially 3–5 mg/kg per month extending to 5 mg/kg every 6 weeks). Both patients demonstrated a rapid and dramatic improvement, enabling a reduction in corticosteroid dosage. These patients continued to receive infliximab and remained free of orbital manifestations after >20 months of follow-up. Sahlin et al. [35] presented a 15-year-old female with idiopathic sclerosing orbital myositis that could not be satisfactorily treated with corticosteroids, azathioprine, and methotrexate. Infliximab treatment was started at 3 mg/kg administered at weeks 0, 2, 4, and then every 8 weeks with clinical improvement noted within 3 days of the first infusion. The infusions were discontinued after the sixth dose for factors unrelated to the disease or treatment. The methotrexate was continued, but steroid treatment was tapered and discontinued. The patient remained free of disease at final follow-up. Side effects of infliximab include reactivation of latent tuberculosis, drug-induced lupus, increased risk of lymphoma, pancytopenia, severe infection, and demyelinating disease.

Adalimumab is a fully humanized IgG1 monoclonal antibody to TNF-α and may be safer than infliximab. Adams et al. [36] reported two pediatric patients with refractory, steroid-dependent, recurrent, nonspecific orbital myositis that could not be controlled with standard immunosuppressive therapies, including methotrexate, mycophenolate mofetil, and cyclophosphamide. Adalimumab was started at 40 mg subcutaneous injection weekly with prompt, long-lasting improvement; corticosteroid dosage was reduced and all other medications were discontinued. Both patients have remained in remission without recurrence. Adverse effects of adalimumab are similar to those of infliximab.

Complete surgical excision of the involved areas is typically neither possible nor indicated. Surgical approach is reserved primarily for biopsy for diagnostic purposes only. The approach varies with the area of involvement. A lacrimal gland biopsy is typically performed via an upper lid crease incision under local anesthesia in addition to sedation for older children or general anesthesia for younger children. The septum is incised and the orbital lobe of the gland is approached just inferior to the lateral superior orbital rim. Care is taken to avoid the palpebral lobe of the gland which can damage its excretory ducts and leads to dry eye. To access the inferior orbit for biopsy, a transconjunctival approach inferior to the tarsus under general anesthesia can be utilized. The surgeon must remain aware of the position of the globe as well as the inferior oblique muscle which resides between the nasal and central fat pads. The medial orbit can be readily accessed through a transcaruncular incision. By staying posterior to the posterior lacrimal crest, one can avoid injury to the medial canthal tendon and lacrimal drainage system.

Ultimately, recurrence rates in the pediatric population have been reported as high as 76% and families should be counseled to this possibility. Some studies have found that females are more likely to recur with recurrence manifesting on average 1.7 years later [7]. Those who present with bilateral disease are also more prone to recurrence [8]. Children with bilateral disease, including recurrent alternating episodes, are more likely have to have a severe degree of visual loss, greater degree of residual proptosis, papilledema, and iritis [7]. Iritis appeared to be the most telling single finding with respect to long-term sequelae [8].

14.3   Ocular Rosacea

14.3.1   Background

Acne rosacea, also known as rosacea, is a chronic inflammatory disorder that primarily affects the skin of the central face and periorbital region characterized by intermittent remissions and exacerbations. According to the National Rosacea Society, the presence of one or more of the following features is indicative of rosacea: flushing or transient erythema, nontransient erythema, inflammatory papules or pustules, and telangiectasias. Secondary features that often appear include burning and stinging sensation, elevated red plaque, dry appearance, edema, ocular manifestation, and phymatous changes [37]. These symptoms are often exacerbated by hot liquids, spicy foods, alcohol, caffeine, and environmental stimuli such as sun and wind exposure. Patients may also report an increased sensitivity to topical products such as cleansers or soaps [38].

14.3.2   Classification

In 2002, the National Rosacea Society developed a classification system consisting of four main subtypes [39]: erythematotelangiectatic, papulopustular, phymatous, and ocular. In addition, granulomatous rosacea is recog-

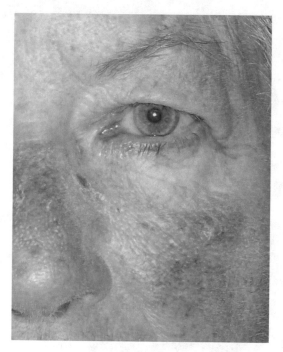

Fig. 14.5 Acne rosacea, erythematotelangiectatic subtype demonstrating bed of facial erythema and telangiectasias over the cheek and nose

nized as a variant. Erythematotelangiectatic rosacea is marked by persistent facial erythema with episodic flushing with or without telangiectasias (**Fig. 14.5**). Papulopustular is the most common subtype and presents as inflammatory papules and/or pustules on a bed of facial erythema. In the phymatous subtype, the skin thickens and becomes irregular and bumpy in texture with rhinophyma being the most common presentation. Ocular rosacea signs and symptoms include conjunctival injection, foreign body sensation, burning or stinging, dryness, itching, photophobia, vision changes, lid margin telangiectasias, and lid and periocular edema. Granulomatous rosacea is a noninflammatory variant characterized by hard yellow, brown, or red papules or nodules on the normal-appearing cheek or periorificial skin that can lead to scarring [37].

Given growing insights into the pathogenesis and pathophysiology of the disease as well as the frequent overlap of subtypes, the National Rosacea Society gave an updated classification system based on phenotype in 2017 in an attempt to unify rosacea as a single clinicopathologic entity with multiple pre-

sentations [40]. A diagnosis of rosacea may be made if either "fixed centrofacial erythema in a characteristic pattern that may periodically intensify" or phymatous changes are present. While major cutaneous signs often occur in the setting of the above phenotype diagnostic features, the presence of two or more of the following alone may also be considered diagnostic of rosacea: flushing, papules and pustules, telangiectasias, or ocular manifestations. Secondary signs and symptoms may appear with one or more diagnostic or major phenotypes: burning or stinging, facial edema, or dry appearance. As the disease progresses, it may increase not only in severity but also in the number and variety of manifestations [40].

A standard grading system has been proposed to more accurately assess and monitor disease state: mild (<10 papules/pustules, mild erythema, with or without symptoms), moderate (10–19 papules/pustules, moderate erythema, with or without symptoms), and severe (>20 papules/pustules, severe erythema, with or without symptoms). In addition, one should note the severity and frequency of flushing and telangiectasias [41]

Criteria for Rosacea Diagnosis

In order to make a diagnosis of rosacea, a patient must have:
- One diagnostic phenotype
- Two or more major cutaneous signs
- Either a diagnostic phenotype or major cutaneous sign PLUS secondary sign or symptom

Diagnostic phenotypes:
- Fixed centrofacial erythema in a characteristic pattern that may periodically intensify
- Phymatous changes

Major cutaneous signs: flushing, papules and pustules, telangiectasias, or ocular manifestations

Secondary signs and symptoms: burning or stinging, facial edema, or dry appearance

Grading

Mild: <10 papules/pustules, mild erythema, with or without symptoms

Moderate: 10–19 papules/pustules, moderate erythema, with or without symptoms

Severe: >20 papules/pustules, severe erythema, with or without symptoms

14.3.3 Presentation

Acne rosacea most commonly affects adults in their third to fifth decades [42]. Rosacea is considered to be rare in children and adolescents, but it is likely underreported due in part to a lack of awareness and misdiagnosis. Children often have a long history of symptoms and multiple visits to various specialists before the correct diagnosis is made [43]. There is no clear gender predilection in adults [42], but it may be more common in girls. Rosacea occurs more frequently in light-skinned individuals but can occur in darker-skin types, including Asians and African-Americans [44]. Pediatric patients typically have clinical features similar to that seen in adults with the exception of phymatous rosacea which has not yet been reported in children [45]. Many will report a positive family history [43].

While they can each occur independently, 58–72% cutaneous rosacea patients will also suffer from ocular rosacea [46, 47]. Patients will often report eye redness, burning, tearing, dryness, foreign body sensation, or photosensitivity. Exam findings may include blepharitis, meibomian gland dysfunction, lid margin telangiectasias, conjunctivitis, episcleritis, keratitis, iritis, recurrent chalazia (■ Fig. 14.6), and edema of the lids and periocular region. In severe cases, this can progress to corneal neovascularization, ulceration, thinning, and perforation that can result in severe visual impairment or blindness [48]. Ocular disease is most often bilateral and symmetric. Flares in ocular disease is typically independent of the activity and severity of cutaneous disease. In children, ocular symptoms tend to predominate and can precede cutaneous symptoms in up to 50% [49], compared to 20% in adults [50].

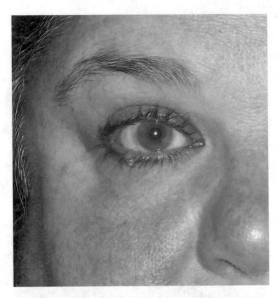

■ **Fig. 14.6**   Right lower lid chalazion in setting of ocular rosacea

14.3.4 Differential Diagnosis

In the pediatric population, the differential diagnosis for acne rosacea may include steroid rosacea, granulomatous periorificial dermatitis, sarcoidosis, systemic lupus erythematosus, acne vulgaris, and demodicosis. Steroid rosacea is a rosacea-like condition precipitated by the use of topical or inhaled steroids or their rapid withdrawal. Granulomatous periorificial dermatitis, also known as facial Afro-Caribbean childhood eruption or Gianotti-type perioral dermatitis, represents a less common variant of perioral dermatitis where monomorphic pink to yellow-brown papules are seen in the perioral, perinasal, and periocular skin of prepubertal children with darker skin types. Erythema and telangiectasias are uncommon [51]. Childhood sarcoidosis is rare but may present in a similar manner clinically and histologically to granulomatous variant rosacea. Sarcoidosis, however, tends to have systemic findings including fatigue, weight loss, and pulmonary symptoms as well as abnormal lab findings (positive angiotensin-converting enzyme and lysozyme) and radiography (bilateral hilar lymphadenopathy on chest X-ray). The malar rash of systemic lupus erythematosus can be mistaken for centrofacial erythema in rosa-

14

cea. Systemic complaints (including fatigue, arthralgia, and myalgia), serologic work-up (positive anti-nuclear antibody), and biopsy with direct immunofluorescence can help to distinguish the conditions. Acne vulgaris can appear quite similar to the papulopustular subtype of acne rosacea but has comedones as a distinguishing characteristic from the latter; of note, acne vulgaris and acne rosacea co-exist in some patients. Patients with demodicosis can also have a facial eruption with erythema associated with papules and pustules; however it is rare in immunocompetent children. Further, skin scrapings will typically show an abundance of the demodex mites [38].

14.3.5 Pathogenesis

The underlying cause of rosacea is unknown; however several pathophysiologic pathways have been investigated. The innate immune system provides constant surveillance and upon detecting an offending agent initiates a rapid but nonspecific response. It has been suggested that dysregulation of this innate immune system leads to the cutaneous inflammation seen in rosacea. Wladis et al. [52] sought to characterize the molecular biologic environment of pathological skin in ocular rosacea and found significantly increased concentrations of five specific molecules compared to normal controls: IL-1β, IL-16, monokine induced by IFN-γ, monocyte chemotactic protein-1, and stem cell factor. Increased leukocytes, in particular helper T cells, and cytokine levels are also a common feature [53]. In addition, acne rosacea is thought to be due in part to vascular hyperactivity and instability [54]. Studies have identified increased levels of cathelicidin and kallikrein 5 [55, 56], endoglin (CD105) and intercellular adhesion molecule expression in arterioles [57], and number of toll-like receptors [57, 58]. Rosacea has a well-described association with facial demodex colonization, but its significance and pathophysiology in the disease is unclear [59, 60]. A link with *H. pylori* has also been suggested [61].

14.3.6 Treatment

As there currently is no cure for rosacea, treatment is aimed at control of symptoms and prevention of complications. Treatment is based on phenotype rather than subtype. Furthermore, response to a given intervention tends to be highly idiosyncratic.

The first step entails baseline skin care and lifestyle modification. A gentle facial cleanser and moisturizer/barrier repair product is an important component to the overall management of the disease [39]. Minimizing exposure to alcohol, caffeine, chocolate, spicy foods, and hot beverages may decrease potential triggers. Broad-spectrum sunscreens and protective clothing can be used to block sunlight and weather exposures. Physical and emotional stress may aggravate the disease. Green-tinted makeup can help conceal erythema.

Sodium sulfacetamide 10%-sulfur 5% (available as a cleanser, cream, gel, and topical suspension), metronidazole (0.75% and 1% formulations available as gel, cream, and lotion) [62], and azelaic acid 15% gel [63, 64] are all FDA-approved topical agents in the treatment of cutaneous rosacea with overall favorable safety and tolerability profiles [65, 66]. These have been well-established to reduce the inflammatory lesions in papulopustular rosacea. Various studies have reported the use of other non-FDA-approved topical therapies, including tacrolimus 0.1% ointment [67], benzoyl peroxide with and without antibiotic [68, 69], and retinoid therapy [70, 71], with a range in efficacy. More recently, attention has turned to α-adrenergic receptor agonists, specifically brimonidine tartrate [72] and oxymetazoline [73], to treat diffuse centrofacial erythema, or background vascular erythema [74, 75].

The literature regarding systemic therapy of pediatric ocular rosacea is sparse. There is no established therapy regimen; dosing and duration is custom based on patient age and clinical status. Children tend to respond well to systemic antibiotics; however relapses can occur upon discontinuation. This may be blunted by gradual tapering of therapy over months.

Tetracyclines appear to be safe and effective in pediatric ocular rosacea in children over 8 years of age. It exhibits both antibacterial and anti-inflammatory effects. These medications accumulate in sebum and decrease bacterial lipase production and free fatty acid concentration. It may also decrease microbial inflammatory mediators via inhibition of protein synthesis. The second-generation tetracyclines, including doxycycline and minocycline, have longer half-lives, increased bioavailability, and decreased gastrointestinal side effects as they can be taken with food, but there is no increased efficacy compared to tetracycline. These medications should be avoided below 8 years of age as it can permanently stain teeth, interfere with tooth enamel development, and deposit in bones, causing temporary retardation in skeletal growth. As such, some authorities advocate withholding these agents until the teenage years. Dose-related phototoxicity, cutaneous hyperpigmentation, acute vestibular side effects, drug-induced lupus-like syndrome, and autoimmune hepatitis have also been reported as side effects. These are almost exclusively due to minocycline. Of note, the only systemic agent approved by the FDA is modified-release oral doxycycline 40 mg daily for the treatment of inflammatory papules and pustules [76]. When used with topical therapies, it induces a more rapid and greater therapeutic effect [77].

In children younger than 8 years of age or with an allergy to tetracyclines, oral erythromycin, metronidazole, or second-generation macrolides (e.g., azithromycin, clarithromycin) may be used. Erythromycin is typically given at a dose of 20–40 mg/kg/day. Treatment for at least 3 months is recommended for relapsing or persistent disease [49]. Erythromycin improves meibomian gland function and, consequently, lengthens tear breakup time and improves punctate keratopathy. Side effects include gastrointestinal and hepatic toxicity. Some have found increased efficacy in achieving and maintaining complete remission with metronidazole compared to erythromycin [49]. Metronidazole (dosing 250 mg daily) was once a popular treatment for rosacea in Europe, but data is limited regarding its use. Side effects include peripheral neuropathy and seizures. Patients must also avoid alcohol ingestion during treatment due to a disulfiram-like reaction. While the macrolides, specifically azithromycin, have been shown to have immunomodulatory and anti-inflammatory effects, there are no large-scale randomized controlled trials regarding use in rosacea. Side effects may include gastrointestinal intolerance, metallic taste, drug interactions, and QT prolongation. Patients are often required to take the medication (250–500 mg) 3 days per week, and many patients find adherence to such a dosing pattern to be difficult. Oral isotretinoin (0.3–1 mg/kg daily divided into BID dosing) is thought to work by decreasing sebum production and sebaceous follicles. It has been reported to be effective in severe and/or refractory cases as well as phymatous rosacea. Side effects include dry eyes, intracranial hypertension, and birth defects; as such, appropriate precautions for avoiding pregnancy in reproductive-age females must be taken. In cases of rosacea or rosacea-form facial eruptions induced by demodicosis, oral ivermectin with or without topical permethrin may be an effective treatment [76].

Ocular treatment often begins with warm compresses and eyelid hygiene to soften thick stagnant secretions, increase meibomian gland turnover, remove debris, and keep meibomian gland orifices open. Meibomian gland dysfunction-associated dry eye management focuses on lubrication with artificial tears as well as fatty acid nutritional supplementation with fish oil and flax seed. Topical ophthalmic cyclosporine 0.05% is a well-established treatment for chronic dry eye but has also been shown to improve tear quality and corneal staining specifically in ocular rosacea [78]. Tea tree oil scrubs can decrease demodex counts as well as inflammation. Topical antibiotics such as ophthalmic erythromycin or bacitracin can reduce bacterial flora, particularly *S. aureus* and *P. acnes* whose lipases may contribute to increased free fatty acids and instability of the tear film. A limited course of corticosteroids at the lowest concentration possible may be necessary to treat episcleritis or sterile keratitis.

Further ocular interventions may include punctal occlusion for refractory dry eye. Meibomian gland probing can be performed to manually open cicatrized orifices to improve outflow of contents and stabilize the tear film [79]. Recurrent chalazia that do not resolve may require incision and drainage with or without intralesional steroids.

The natural progression of the various subtypes of rosacea is not well understood. Long-term management balancing control of disease and extended exposure to treatments requires the clinical judgment of the physician as well as patient motivation and adherence [80].

14.4   Contact Dermatitis

14.4.1   Background

Contact dermatitis is an umbrella term that describes an inflammatory skin reaction caused by contact with an external substance. It manifests with varying degrees of pruritus, erythema, and edema that may be accompanied by scaling, vesicles, and bullae. Response is dependent on the causative agent, duration of contact, location of contact, and the individual patient characteristics. In chronic cases, the skin may undergo lichenification in which it becomes leathery and thickened. There are two primary types of contact dermatitis: irritant and allergic [81].

14.4.2   Irritant Contact Dermatitis

Irritant contact dermatitis is the most common type in the adult and pediatric populations and represents a general inflammatory response to a noxious substance. This subtype does not require a specific antigen-primed immune response to initiate a reaction. Mild irritants such as saliva, urine, feces, diapers, cleaning products, sanitizers, and certain insects will cause signs and symptoms with continued contact over time. It typically begins as dry, chapped skin that then progresses to itchy, red, swollen, and scaly skin with repeated exposures. If exposure contin-

ues, the skin fissures and develops sores and blisters. Diaper rash and excessive handwashing with harsh soaps are a frequent cause of mild irritant contact dermatitis [82]. Strong irritants such as fiberglass, turpentine, pepper spray, and bleach may show signs and symptoms quickly upon contact or within a few hours. Mutation in the filaggrin gene results in loss of filaggrin protein production that may alter the skin barrier and is associated with increased susceptibility to chronic irritant contact dermatitis [83].

14.4.3   Allergic Contact Dermatitis

Allergic contact dermatitis is a delayed cell-mediated type IV hypersensitivity reaction that requires a prior sensitization followed by a secondary exposure to elicit a response. This reaction is driven by T lymphocytes, particularly helper T cells [84, 85]. True prevalence is difficult to estimate as allergic contact dermatitis in children is often undiagnosed or misdiagnosed. Though the clinical relevance is still unclear, positive patch testing was found to be positive in 13.3–24.5% of healthy children [86–89]. Sensitization rates are rising with reports of sensitization beginning as early as 6 months of age [87, 90]. Females are more frequently affected [89]. Metals, in particular nickel and cobalt, are the most common allergens. They are found throughout our environment in a wide range of daily items such as jewelry, keys, clothing, electronics, and toys. Reportedly up to 10% of users can develop allergic contact dermatitis after using neomycin [81]. Bacitracin and corticosteroids are other common medical allergens (Fig. 14.7). Paraphenylenediamine (PPD) is a strong sen-

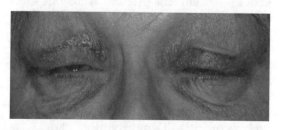

 Fig. 14.7 Allergic contact dermatitis on bilateral upper lids after using bacitracin ointment

sitizer that has been banned from skin care products since 1938 but is still found in hair dye and temporary tattoo dyes. Balsam of Peru was originally discovered in Peru from the bark of the *Myroxylon balsamum* tree. Nowadays, it is often used as a fragrance in personal toiletries, flavoring in food and drink, and mild antiseptic in medicinal products [91, 92]. *Rhus* family plants, including poison ivy and poison oak, contain urushiol and are common causes of allergic contact dermatitis. The erythematous eruption often presents in a classic geometric or linear pattern matching the contact sites of the allergen. This can provide a useful clue to identify the inciting allergen [93]. A history of allergic rhinitis or asthma may increase the risk of allergic contact dermatitis, although further investigation is needed to clarify the role of atopy [94].

Types of Contact Dermatitis

- Irritant: general inflammatory response to a noxious substance
- Allergic: delayed cell-mediated type IV hypersensitivity reaction that requires a prior sensitization followed by a secondary exposure to elicit a response

---

14.4.4   Differential Diagnosis

The differential diagnosis is wide, but one must primarily rule out other types of eczematous and noneczematous dermatitis, including atopic dermatitis, drug eruption, scabies, and seborrheic dermatitis [95]. Atopic dermatitis is an endogenous inflammatory skin condition that typically occurs before 5 years of age and can present similarly with dry, scaly skin and prominent pruritus. It may be difficult to differentiate between atopic dermatitis and contact dermatitis clinically, though the former tends to be symmetric and the latter correlating with exposure pattern. Because atopic dermatitis also causes a skin barrier dysfunction, it may actually predispose to easier hapten exposure and elicitation of contact dermatitis. Drug eruption should be considered if a patient suddenly develops a symmetric systemic cutaneous reaction after beginning a medication. Scabies is an intensely pruritic rash characterized by burrows, or serpiginous, gray, linear elevations in the superficial epidermis, frequently found in the webbed spaces between the fingers, flexor surfaces of the wrist, and palms and soles. Seborrheic dermatitis is a common skin condition that presents as greasy-appearing, scaly, red patches in sebaceous gland-rich areas. One may also consider infectious etiologies for an inflammatory skin reaction. Cellulitis can present with areas of erythema and edema; however it is typically accompanied by systemic signs such as fever and leukocytosis. If blistering lesions are present, herpetic infection or impetigo should also be on the differential.

14.4.5   Work-Up

Diagnosis of both types of contact dermatitis is typically suspected based on detailed patient clinical history, including personal products as well as home and school exposures. The diagnosis is often made on purely clinical grounds. However, epicutaneous patch testing remains the gold standard to confirm the diagnosis of allergic contact dermatitis [96]. Patch testing involves application of standardized concentrations of allergens directly to the skin, usually on the back, for 48 hours and then grading a response at multiple intervals after initial placement [97, 98]. Still, clinical correlation remains critical as patch testing has a reported sensitivity of 70% and specificity of 80% [99]. Of note, there are no FDA-approved patch testing devices currently available to those under 18 years of age. Removing the suspected offending agent can be both diagnostic as well as therapeutic. Skin biopsy is not a routine part of the diagnostic work-up, but may be performed in cases of unusual or recalcitrant cases where patch testing is negative. Histology demonstrates epidermal spongiosis and is frequently nonspecific [81].

14.4.6　Treatment

The mainstay of treatment is identification and avoidance of the suspected offending substance. Supportive therapy includes restoration of the skin barrier function with emollient moisturizers. Systemic antihistamines, cool compresses, and oatmeal baths can soothe acute symptoms and relieve discomfort. When these are not sufficient, topical corticosteroids work through various mechanisms to decrease proliferation of lymphocytes and production of cytokines to hasten resolution of clinical symptoms and cutaneous signs. There is a well-established benefit in allergic contact dermatitis, but its role in irritant contact dermatitis is more controversial [82]. The optimal steroid selection, strength (classified grades 1 through 7), and vehicle is typically adjusted according to involved location and severity of the condition. For example, lower-potency (group 7) steroids are typically applied to areas with thinner skin, whereas mid- or high-potency topical steroids may be used elsewhere on the body. While duration of treatment also varies, topical application is typically continued for a few weeks to avoid any rebound. Topical corticosteroids should be used with caution as they can become a source of sensitization. Chronic use can result in cutaneous atrophy, hirsutism, folliculitis/acne, and systemic absorption [82]. Oral corticosteroids can be used in cases of high severity, notable facial swelling, or diffuse rash covering much of the body.

Utilizing the intrinsic immunosuppressive properties of UV light, phototherapy (oral psoralens plus UVA, narrow-band UVB), is another treatment option for patients with contact dermatitis that is refractory or unresponsive to topical or systemic corticosteroids. Topical calcineurin inhibitors (Tacrolimus 0.03% and 0.1% ointment, Pimecrolimus 1% cream) inhibit the signal transduction pathway in T cells and subsequently block production of inflammatory cytokines. They have shown good success in dampening chronic cutaneous inflammation, particularly in atopic dermatitis [95, 100]. A recent study showed similar efficacy of topical tacrolimus 0.1% ointment and mometasone furoate 0.1% ointment in a randomized study of patients with allergic contact dermatitis of the hands [101]. Of note, the FDA issued a warning regarding a possible link between topical calcineurin use and malignancy in children and adults; while there was a trend toward increased risk of lymphoma and leukemia, it was not statistically significant and no definite causal relationship has been established thus far [102]. They should not be used in children under 2 years of age. Systemic treatment with immunomodulators, such as methotrexate, cyclosporine, and azathioprine, may be a second-line option for patients with chronic dermatitis that does not respond to conventional therapy. More recently, trials of ctanercept and infliximab have been used to inhibit TNF-α and diminish cytokine inflammation in the skin, though their role in contact dermatitis is not well-studied [82].

This disease persists into and throughout adulthood, necessitating continued avoidance of allergens and management of the inflammatory response [103].

14.5　Chalazion

14.5.1　Background and Presentation

Chalazia are noninfectious inflammatory lesions caused by inspissation of the meibomian glands resulting in trapping of sebaceous material and subsequent leakage into the surrounding tissue. They are the most common inflammatory lesion of the eyelid, occurring in all ages, races, and genders [104]. It typically presents as rapid onset of an erythematous eyelid lesion associated with mild focal edema and tenderness (◘ Fig. 14.8). Spontaneous resolution often occurs within 1–2 weeks, although a chronic form may develop (◘ Fig. 14.9). Patients typically present in the chronic phase weeks to months after initial onset with a persistent painless localized eyelid nodule. On exam, it is essential to evert the affected lid to examine the conjunctival surface (◘ Fig. 14.10). Diagnosis is made

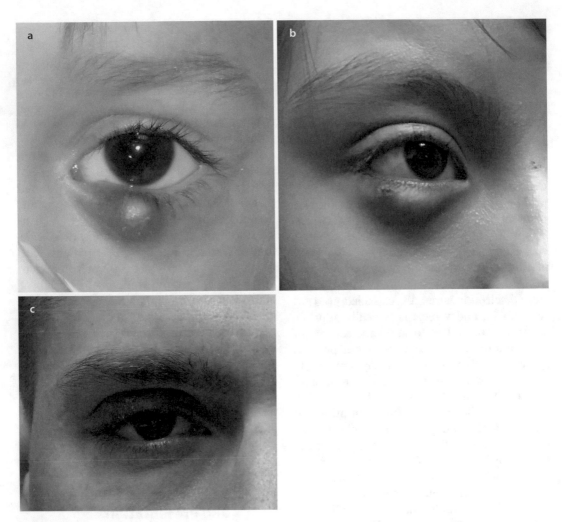

14

◘ Fig. 14.8 Single acute chalazion on **a** left lower lid (note prominent anterior presentation) and **b** right lower lid. **c** Multiple acute chalazia on right upper lid

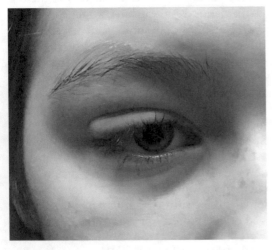

◘ Fig. 14.9 Right upper lid chronic chalazion. (Image courtesy of Tal J. Rubinstein, MD)

based on history and clinical findings. Biopsy is not routinely performed and is reserved for atypical, persistent, or recurrent lesions. Histology shows a chronic granulomatous reaction with a mixed inflammatory infiltrate including multinucleated giant cells and lipid-laden epithelioid cells [105].

14.5.2   Associations and Risk Factors

Chalazion is often associated with ocular rosacea and chronic posterior blepharitis [106]. Demodex is more prevalent in patients with chalazia, and these patients tend to have multiple chalazia and higher recurrence. The

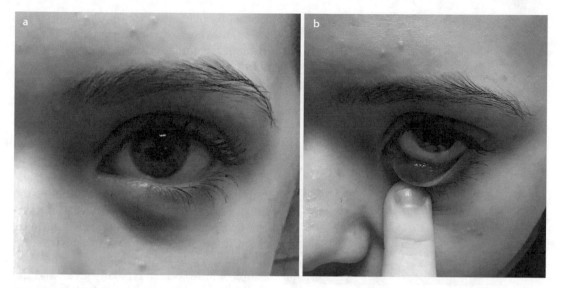

◻ Fig. 14.10 Left lower lid chalazion **a**. View with left lower lid eversion **b**. (Images courtesy of Tal J. Rubinstein, MD)

exact role of Demodex infestation in pathogenesis, however, remains unclear [107]. Gastritis, lower serum vitamin A levels, and smoking have also been reported as risk factors [106, 108].

14.5.3 Differential Diagnosis

In children, the differential diagnosis may include hordeolum, juvenile xanthogranuloma, epidermal inclusion cyst, Molluscum contagiosum, and idiopathic facial aseptic granuloma. A hordeolum is an acute purulent infection, often staphylococcal, of the meibomian gland (internal hordeolum) or gland of Zeis (external hordeolum or stye). This can progress to preseptal or orbital cellulitis in which systemic treatment and possible surgical incision and drainage is required. Juvenile xanthogranuloma is a form of histiocytosis that can present with a solitary reddish or yellow skin lesion on the head or trunk, including the eyelid. While the skin lesion tends to spontaneously regress over time, the disease can have other extracutaneous (e.g., liver, lung, spleen, lymph node, bones, and gastrointestinal tract) and ocular involvement [109]. An epidermal inclusion cyst forms after epithelial cells from the surface have been implanted into the dermis, often after trauma

or surgery. It appears as an elevated, round white-yellow lesion with a central pore that indicates the remaining pilar duct. Molluscum contagiosum is a viral infection that typically presents with multiple umbilicated, dome-shaped, waxy papules. This may be associated with a chronic follicular conjunctivitis caused by the pox virus being shed onto the eye surface [110]. Idiopathic facial aseptic granuloma is a rare pediatric dermatologic disorder characterized by painless violaceous nodules on the cheeks or eyelids that spontaneously resolve [111].

14.5.4 Complications

Complications of chalazia may include unacceptable aesthetic appearance and mechanical ptosis. These lesions can also induce refractive visual changes such as irregular astigmatism and optical aberrations, particularly when larger in size [112–114]. Pyogenic granuloma, which may be associated with bleeding and further aesthetic dissatisfaction, is often found in the setting of a chronic chalazion. A study by Fukuoka et al. found that chalazia and their excision were linked to shortening and dropout of Meibomian glands on meiboscopy which may contribute to tear film instability [91]. Similar to horde-

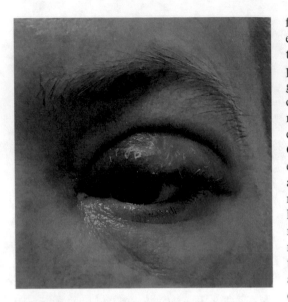

Fig. 14.11 Left upper lid chalazion complicated by secondary bacterial infection and preseptal cellulitis. (Image courtesy of Tal J. Rubinstein, MD)

ola, chalazia can become infected, and patients may present with erythema and discomfort secondary to preseptal cellulitis (■ Fig. 14.11). In such cases, oral antibiotics should be initiated to cure the infection. Ultimately, drainage of the chalazion may facilitate more rapid healing and prevent recurrence.

14.5.5 Treatment

Up to 25–43% of acute chalazia may spontaneously self-resolve [115]. Treatment often begins with conservative management including hot compresses, digital massage, and eyelid hygiene such as baby shampoo scrubs, tea tree oil, and dilute hypochlorous spray. Success of this regimen varies widely from 25–87%, heavily dependent on whether treatment is initiated during the acute or chronic stage as well as patient education and compliance [115–117]. If the lesion persists despite conservative management, incision and curettage, intralesional steroid injection, or a combination of the two can be performed. After local anesthesia is infiltrated into the affected eyelid, incision and curettage is per-

formed by placing a clamp and everting the eyelid, making a vertical or cruciate incision through the conjunctiva and posterior tarsal plate, followed by curettage to remove the gelatinous mucoid contents. In more chronic cases, the lesion may be composed predominantly of fibrotic tissue and one may need to excise this tissue and its surrounding capsule. Caution should be taken with lesions at the eyelid margin or adjacent to the punctum to avoid lid notching and damage to the lacrimal system, respectively. Occasionally, the lesion may be more prominent from the anterior aspect of the lid and the incision can be made through the skin and orbicularis into the tarsus. Following incision and curettage, a topical antibiotic is typically given and the eyelid may or may not be patched depending on physician and patient preference. Intralesional steroids can be injected (typically 0.05–0.15 ml) either transcutaneously or transconjunctivally into the chalazion. Triamcinolone acetonide (available in 10 mg/ml and 40 mg/ml concentrations) is the most widely used intralesional corticosteroid, but triamcinolone diacetate, dexamethasone, and betamethasone have also been used. Triamcinolone is a suspension of small corticosteroid crystals that functions as a depot, storing in the tissue and slowly releasing over weeks [118]. Though the anterior approach is associated with less discomfort for the patient, it may predispose to injection site depigmentation [119] and, rarely, embolization of the steroid to retinal and/or choroidal vasculature that can lead to retinal vascular occlusive events and loss of vision [120, 121]. Reported recurrence rates range from 0 to 16% for incision and curettage and 0 to 27.3% for intralesional steroids. When only one procedure is done, incision and curettage is generally more effective than intralesional steroids, however that superiority diminishes after repeated treatments [122]. Incision and curettage is often associated with greater discomfort and inconvenience than intralesional steroids though similar satisfaction scores were reported with both procedures [123, 124].

14

> **Step-by-Step Incision and Drainage of Chalazion**
>
> Step-by-step incision and drainage of chalazion:
> 1. Anesthetize the lid (e.g., subcutaneous 2% lidocaine with epinephrine).
> 2. Place chalazion clamp.
> 3. Evert the lid.
> 4. Use an #11 blade to create a vertical (or cruciate incision) through the conjunctiva and tarsus overlying the lesion.
> 5. Perform curettage to remove gelatinous inner contents.
> 6. Excision of the capsule (often in more chronic cases).
> 7. +/− intralesional steroid injection.
> 8. Removal of chalazion clamp.
> 9. Application of antibiotic or antibiotic-steroid ointment to surgical site.

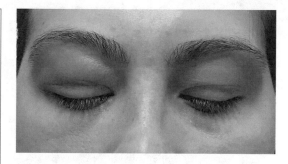

Fig. 14.12 Clinical photograph of a young female who presented with right upper lid edema. (Image courtesy of Tal J. Rubinstein, MD)

Topical antibiotics have no role in the treatment of chalazia, but can treat associated staphylococcal blepharitis. Acute secondary infection may require treatment with systemic antibiotics directed against skin flora. Tetracyclines may be indicated for recurrent or multiple chalazia or accompanying rosacea. As described previously, these medications accumulate in sebum and decrease bacterial lipase production, free fatty acid concentration, and microbial inflammatory mediators. Dosing is typically oral doxycycline 50–100 mg once or twice a day. Side effects include permanent staining of teeth, interference with tooth enamel development, deposition in bones causing temporary retardation of skeletal growth, and photosensitivity. The medication should be reserved for patients over 8 years of age and avoided in pregnancy. If unable to take tetracyclines, erythromycin or metronidazole may be an acceptable alternative.

14.5.6 Sample Case

A 16-year-old girl presented with a five-day history of right upper eyelid edema. She reported notable itching and burning. On exam, the right upper lid was noted to be diffusely edematous (Fig. 14.12). She was found to have a mild papillary conjunctivitis with chemosis and trace superficial punctate keratitis. On further questioning, the patient denied any history of trauma or sinusitis but reported a visit to Urgent Care 1 week previously where she was diagnosed with "conjunctivitis" and started on an "antibiotic eye drop." She was diagnosed with likely allergic contact dermatitis, but patch testing was deferred. The ophthalmic drop was discontinued, and the patient was instructed to use artificial tears and cool compresses with complete resolution of symptoms.

> **Key Points**
> - Idiopathic orbital inflammation can affect any tissue in the orbit; it most commonly presents as an orbital mass, myositis, or dacryoadenitis.
> - Bilateral involvement, recurrence, and systemic symptoms are more common in pediatric idiopathic orbital inflammation.
> - The mainstay of IOI treatment is systemic corticosteroids with a classic response within 24–48 hours; this is tapered slowly over several months.
> - Rosacea is likely a single clinicopathologic entity with various presentations characterized by erythema, telangiectasias, and papules or pustules. Ocular involvement is common and can have serious sequelae.

— History regarding possible exposures and pattern of involvement on physical exam are helpful clues in diagnosis (and treatment) of contact dermatitis.

— Chalazia are benign inflammatory lesions representing blocked meibomian glands, often in the setting of blepharitis and ocular rosacea. These lid nodules commonly self-resolve but may require further intervention, such as incision and drainage and/or intralesional steroid injection.

? Review Questions

1. An otherwise healthy 11-year-old girl presents with right upper lid edema and erythema. Visual acuity, pupil exam, and intraocular pressure are normal, but there is mild limitation of extraocular motility. On exam, she has ptosis as well as temporal conjunctival injection. An orbital CT scan reveals an enlarged lacrimal gland with adjacent fat stranding. All of the following would be an acceptable step in the evaluation and treatment *except*:
   (a) Excisional biopsy of the lacrimal gland
   (b) Initiation of steroid therapy
   (c) A serologic work-up
   (d) Referral to a pediatric rheumatologist

2. Rosacea may be exacerbated by all of the following *except*:
   (a) Hot and spicy food
   (b) Alcohol
   (c) Doxycycline
   (d) Sun and wind exposure

3. Contact dermatitis often presents as a pruritic, erythematous rash. The severity is dependent on all of the following *except*:
   (a) Causative agent
   (b) Ultraviolet (UV) light exposure
   (c) Duration of contact
   (d) Individual patient characteristics

4. Intralesional steroids are commonly used in the treatment of chalazia. Complications may include all of the following *except*:
   (a) Skin depigmentation
   (b) Vaso-occlusive event
   (c) Intraocular pressure (IOP) elevation
   (d) Lid notching

✓ Answers

1. (a)
2. (c)
3. (b)
4. (d)

References

1. Birch-Hirschfeld A. Zur Diagnostik und Pathologie der Orbitaltumoren. Ber 32 Versamm Ophthal Ges Heidelberg. 1906;32:127–35.
2. Benedict WLKM. Inflammatory pseudotumor of the orbit. Arch Ophthalmol. 1923(52):582–93.
3. Shields JA, Shields CL, Scartozzi R. Survey of 1264 patients with orbital tumors and simulating lesions: the 2002 Montgomery Lecture, part 1. Ophthalmology. 2004;111(5):997–1008.
4. Kitei D, DiMario FJ Jr. Childhood orbital pseudotumor: case report and literature review. J Child Neurol. 2008;23(4):425–30.
5. Yuen SJ, Rubin PA. Idiopathic orbital inflammation: distribution, clinical features, and treatment outcome. Arch Ophthalmol. 2003;121(4):491–9.
6. Mombaerts I, Koornneef L. Current status in the treatment of orbital myositis. Ophthalmology. 1997;104(3):402–8.
7. Spindle J, Tang SX, Davies B, Wladis EJ, Piozzi E, Pellegrini M, et al. Pediatric idiopathic orbital inflammation: clinical features of 30 cases. Ophthal Plast Reconstr Surg. 2016;32(4):270–4.
8. Mottow LS, Jakobiec FA. Idiopathic inflammatory orbital pseudotumor in childhood. I. Clinical characteristics. Arch Ophthalmol. 1978;96(8):1410–7.
9. Mombaerts I, Bilyk JR, Rose GE, McNab AA, Fay A, Dolman PJ, et al. Consensus on diagnostic criteria of idiopathic orbital inflammation using a modified delphi approach. JAMA Ophthalmol. 2017;135(7):769–76.
10. Guerriero S, Di Leo E, Piscitelli D, Ciraci L, Vacca A, Sborgia C, et al. Orbital pseudotumor in a child: diagnostic implications and treatment strategies. Clin Exp Med. 2011;11(1):61–3.
11. Yuen SJ, Rubin PA. Idiopathic orbital inflammation: ocular mechanisms and clinicopathology. Ophthalmol Clin N Am. 2002;15(1):121–6.

14

12. Espinoza GM. Orbital inflammatory pseudotumors: etiology, differential diagnosis, and management. Curr Rheumatol Rep. 2010;12(6):443–7.

13. Wladis EJ, Iglesias BV, Gosselin EJ. Characterization of the molecular biologic milieu of idiopathic orbital inflammation. Ophthal Plast Reconstr Surg. 2011;27(4):251–4.

14. Wladis EJ, Iglesias BV, Adam AP, Nazeer T, Gosselin EJ. Toll-like receptors in idiopathic orbital inflammation. Ophthal Plast Reconstr Surg. 2012;28(4):273–6.

15. Sobrin L, Kim EC, Christen W, Papadaki T, Letko E, Foster CS. Infliximab therapy for the treatment of refractory ocular inflammatory disease. Arch Ophthalmol. 2007;125(7):895–900.

16. Serop S, Vianna RN, Claeys M, De Laey JJ. Orbital myositis secondary to systemic lupus erythematosus. Acta Ophthalmol. 1994;72(4):520–3.

17. Squires RH Jr, Zwiener RJ, Kennedy RH. Orbital myositis and Crohn's disease. J Pediatr Gastroenterol Nutr. 1992;15(4):448–51.

18. Van de Mosselaer G, Van Deuren H, Dewolf-Peeters C, Missotten L. Pseudotumor orbitae and myasthenia gravis. A case report. Arch Ophthalmol. 1980;98(9):1621–2.

19. Young RS, Hodes BL, Cruse RP, Koch KL, Garovoy MR. Orbital pseudotumor and Crohn disease. J Pediatr. 1981;99(2):250–2.

20. Atabay C, Tyutyunikov A, Scalise D, Stolarski C, Hayes MB, Kennerdell JS, et al. Serum antibodies reactive with eye muscle membrane antigens are detected in patients with nonspecific orbital inflammation. Ophthalmology. 1995;102(1):145–53.

21. Smith JR, Rosenbaum JT. A role for methotrexate in the management of non-infectious orbital inflammatory disease. Br J Ophthalmol. 2001;85(10):1220–4.

22. Shah SS, Lowder CY, Schmitt MA, Wilke WS, Kosmorsky GS, Meisler DM. Low-dose methotrexate therapy for ocular inflammatory disease. Ophthalmology. 1992;99(9):1419–23.

23. Hatton MP, Rubin PA, Foster CS. Successful treatment of idiopathic orbital inflammation with mycophenolate mofetil. Am J Ophthalmol. 2005;140(5):916–8.

24. Zacharopoulos IP, Papadaki T, Manor RS, Briscoe D. Treatment of idiopathic orbital inflammatory disease with cyclosporine-A: a case presentation. Semin Ophthalmol. 2009;24(6):260–1.

25. Sanchez-Roman J, Varela-Aguilar JM, Bravo-Ferrer J, Sequeiros Madueno E, Fernandez de Bobadilla M. Idiopathic orbital myositis: treatment with cyclosporin. Ann Rheum Dis. 1993;52(1):84–5.

26. Diaz-Llopis M, Menezo JL. Idiopathic inflammatory orbital pseudotumor and low-dose cyclosporine. Am J Ophthalmol. 1989;107(5):547–8.

27. Schafranski MD. Idiopathic orbital inflammatory disease successfully treated with rituximab. Clin Rheumatol. 2009;28(2):225–6.

28. Ibrahim I, Barton A, Ibrahim A, Ho P. Idiopathic orbital inflammation successfully treated using rituximab in a patient with rheumatoid arthritis. J Rheumatol. 2012;39(7):1485–6.

29. Abell RG, Patrick A, Rooney KG, McKelvie PA, McNab AA. Complete resolution of idiopathic sclerosing orbital inflammation after treatment with rituximab. Ocul Immunol Inflamm. 2015;23(2):176–9.

30. On AV, Hirschbein MJ, Williams HJ, Karesh JW. CyberKnife radiosurgery and rituximab in the successful management of sclerosing idiopathic orbital inflammatory disease. Ophthal Plast Reconstr Surg. 2006;22(5):395–7.

31. Savino G, Battendieri R, Siniscalco A, Mandara E, Mule A, Petrone G, et al. Intraorbital injection of Rituximab in idiopathic orbital inflammatory syndrome: case reports. Rheumatol Int. 2015;35(1):183–8.

32. Garrity JA, Coleman AW, Matteson EL, Eggenberger ER, Waitzman DM. Treatment of recalcitrant idiopathic orbital inflammation (chronic orbital myositis) with infliximab. Am J Ophthalmol. 2004;138(6):925–30.

33. Wilson MW, Shergy WJ, Haik BG. Infliximab in the treatment of recalcitrant idiopathic orbital inflammation. Ophthal Plast Reconstr Surg. 2004;20(5):381–3.

34. Miquel T, Abad S, Badelon I, Vignal C, Warzocha U, Larroche C, et al. Successful treatment of idiopathic orbital inflammation with infliximab: an alternative to conventional steroid-sparing agents. Ophthal Plast Reconstr Surg. 2008;24(5):415–7.

35. Sahlin S, Lignell B, Williams M, Dastmalchi M, Orrego A. Treatment of idiopathic sclerosing inflammation of the orbit (myositis) with infliximab. Acta Ophthalmol. 2009;87(8):906–8.

36. Adams AB, Kazim M, Lehman TJ. Treatment of orbital myositis with adalimumab (Humira). J Rheumatol. 2005;32(7):1374–5.

37. Wilkin J, Dahl M, Detmar M, Drake L, Feinstein A, Odom R, et al. Standard classification of rosacea: report of the National Rosacea Society Expert Committee on the Classification and Staging of Rosacea. J Am Acad Dermatol. 2002;46(4):584–7.

38. Kroshinsky D, Glick SA. Pediatric rosacea. Dermatol Ther. 2006;19(4):196–201.

39. Del Rosso JQ, Thiboutot D, Gallo R, Webster G, Tanghetti E, Eichenfield L, et al. Consensus recommendations from the American Acne & Rosacea Society on the management of rosacea, part 1: a status report on the disease state, general measures, and adjunctive skin care. Cutis. 2013;92(5):234–40.

40. Gallo RL, Granstein RD, Kang S, Mannis M, Steinhoff M, Tan J, et al. Standard classification and pathophysiology of rosacea: the 2017 update by the National Rosacea Society Expert Committee. J Am Acad Dermatol. 2018;78(1):148–55.

41. Wilkin J, Dahl M, Detmar M, Drake L, Liang MH, Odom R, et al. Standard grading system for rosacea: report of the National Rosacea Society Expert Committee on the classification and staging of rosacea. J Am Acad Dermatol. 2004;50(6):907–12.

42. Parisi R, Yiu ZZN. The worldwide epidemiology of rosacea. Br J Dermatol. 2018;179(2):239–40.

43. Lacz NL, Schwartz RA. Rosacea in the pediatric population. Cutis. 2004;74(2):99–103.

44. Al-Dabagh A, Davis SA, McMichael AJ, Feldman SR. Rosacea in skin of color: not a rare diagnosis. Dermatol Online J. 2014;20(10):13030/qt1mv9r0ss.

45. Gonser LI, Gonser CE, Deuter C, Heister M, Zierhut M, Schaller M. Systemic therapy of ocular and cutaneous rosacea in children. J Eur Acad Dermatol Venereol. 2017;31(10):1732–8.

46. Marks R, Harcourt-Webster JN. Histopathology of rosacea. Arch Dermatol. 1969;100(6):683–91.

47. Vieira AC, Hofling-Lima AL, Mannis MJ. Ocular rosacea – a review. Arq Bras Oftalmol. 2012;75(5):363–9.

48. Cetinkaya A, Akova YA. Pediatric ocular acne rosacea: long-term treatment with systemic antibiotics. Am J Ophthalmol. 2006;142(5):816–21.

49. Chamaillard M, Mortemousque B, Boralevi F, Marques da Costa C, Aitali F, Taieb A, et al. Cutaneous and ocular signs of childhood rosacea. Arch Dermatol. 2008;144(2):167–71.

50. Tanzi EL, Weinberg JM. The ocular manifestations of rosacea. Cutis. 2001;68(2):112–4.

51. Reichenberg J. Perioral (periorificial) dermatitis. In: Dahl MV, Ofori AO, editors. UpToDate. Waltham: UpToDate. Accessed 24 Mar 2019.

52. Wladis EJ, Iglesias BV, Adam AP, Gosselin EJ. Molecular biologic assessment of cutaneous specimens of ocular rosacea. Ophthal Plast Reconstr Surg. 2012;28(4):246–50.

53. Buhl T, Sulk M, Nowak P, Buddenkotte J, McDonald I, Aubert J, et al. Molecular and morphological characterization of inflammatory infiltrate in rosacea reveals activation of Th1/Th17 pathways. J Invest Dermatol. 2015;135(9):2198–208.

54. Yamasaki K, Gallo RL. The molecular pathology of rosacea. J Dermatol Sci. 2009;55(2):77–81.

55. Yamasaki K, Gallo RL. Rosacea as a disease of cathelicidins and skin innate immunity. J Investig Dermatol Symp Proc. 2011;15(1):12–5.

56. Yamasaki K, Di Nardo A, Bardan A, Murakami M, Ohtake T, Coda A, et al. Increased serine protease activity and cathelicidin promotes skin inflammation in rosacea. Nat Med. 2007;13(8):975–80.

57. Wladis EJ, Carlson JA, Wang MS, Bhoiwala DP, Adam AP. Toll-like receptors and vascular markers in ocular rosacea. Ophthal Plast Reconstr Surg. 2013;29(4):290–3.

58. Yamasaki K, Kanada K, Macleod DT, Borkowski AW, Morizane S, Nakatsuji T, et al. TLR2 expression is increased in rosacea and stimulates enhanced serine protease production by keratinocytes. J Invest Dermatol. 2011;131(3):688–97.

59. Chang YS, Huang YC. Role of Demodex mite infestation in rosacea: a systematic review and meta-analysis. J Am Acad Dermatol. 2017;77(3):441–7.e6.

60. Bonnar E, Eustace P, Powell FC. The Demodex mite population in rosacea. J Am Acad Dermatol. 1993;28(3):443–8.

61. Utas S, Ozbakir O, Turasan A, Utas C. Helicobacter pylori eradication treatment reduces the severity of rosacea. J Am Acad Dermatol. 1999;40(3):433–5.

62. McClellan KJ, Noble S. Topical metronidazole. A review of its use in rosacea. Am J Clin Dermatol. 2000;1(3):191–9.

63. Liu RH, Smith MK, Basta SA, Farmer ER. Azelaic acid in the treatment of papulopustular rosacea: a systematic review of randomized controlled trials. Arch Dermatol. 2006;142(8):1047–52.

64. Del Rosso JQ, Bhatia N. Azelaic acid gel 15% in the management of papulopustular rosacea: a status report on available efficacy data and clinical application. Cutis. 2011;88(2):67–72.

65. Del Rosso JQ, Baldwin H, Webster G. American Acne & Rosacea Society rosacea medical management guidelines. J Drugs Dermatol. 2008;7(6):531–3.

66. van Zuuren EJ, Fedorowicz Z, Carter B, van der Linden MM, Charland L. Interventions for rosacea. Cochrane Database Syst Rev. 2015;(4):CD003262.

67. Bamford JT, Elliott BA, Haller IV. Tacrolimus effect on rosacea. J Am Acad Dermatol. 2004;50(1):107–8.

68. Breneman D, Savin R, VandePol C, Vamvakias G, Levy S, Leyden J. Double-blind, randomized, vehicle-controlled clinical trial of once-daily benzoyl peroxide/clindamycin topical gel in the treatment of patients with moderate to severe rosacea. Int J Dermatol. 2004;43(5):381–7.

69. Ozturkcan S, Ermertcan AT, Sahin MT, Afsar FS. Efficiency of benzoyl peroxide-erythromycin gel in comparison with metronidazole gel in the treatment of acne rosacea. J Dermatol. 2004;31(8):610–7.

70. Chang AL, Alora-Palli M, Lima XT, Chang TC, Cheng C, Chung CM, et al. A randomized, double-blind, placebo-controlled, pilot study to assess the efficacy and safety of clindamycin 1.2% and tretinoin 0.025% combination gel for the treatment of acne rosacea over 12 weeks. J Drugs Dermatol. 2012;11(3):333–9.

71. Ertl GA, Levine N, Kligman AM. A comparison of the efficacy of topical tretinoin and low-dose oral isotretinoin in rosacea. Arch Dermatol. 1994;130(3):319–24.

72. Fowler J Jr, Jackson M, Moore A, Jarratt M, Jones T, Meadows K, et al. Efficacy and safety of once-daily topical brimonidine tartrate gel 0.5% for the treatment of moderate to severe facial erythema of rosacea: results of two randomized, double-blind, and vehicle-controlled pivotal studies. J Drugs Dermatol. 2013;12(6):650–6.

14

73. Kim JH, Oh YS, Ji JH, Bak H, Ahn SK. Rosacea (erythematotelangiectatic type) effectively improved by topical xylometazoline. J Dermatol. 2011;38(5):510–3.

74. Del Rosso JQ. Management of facial erythema of rosacea: what is the role of topical alpha-adrenergic receptor agonist therapy? J Am Acad Dermatol. 2013;69(6 Suppl 1):S44–56.

75. Del Rosso JQ, Thiboutot D, Gallo R, Webster G, Tanghetti E, Eichenfield L, et al. Consensus recommendations from the American Acne & Rosacea Society on the management of rosacea, part 2: a status report on topical agents. Cutis. 2013;92(6):277–84.

76. Del Rosso JQ, Thiboutot D, Gallo R, Webster G, Tanghetti E, Eichenfield LF, et al. Consensus recommendations from the American Acne & Rosacea Society on the management of rosacea, part 3: a status report on systemic therapies. Cutis. 2014;93(1):18–28.

77. Bhatia ND, Del Rosso JQ. Optimal management of papulopustular rosacea: rationale for combination therapy. J Drugs Dermatol. 2012;11(7):838–44.

78. Schechter BA, Katz RS, Friedman LS. Efficacy of topical cyclosporine for the treatment of ocular rosacea. Adv Ther. 2009;26(6):651–9.

79. Wladis EJ. Intraductal meibomian gland probing in the management of ocular rosacea. Ophthal Plast Reconstr Surg. 2012;28(6):416–8.

80. Del Rosso JQ, Thiboutot D, Gallo R, Webster G, Tanghetti E, Eichenfield LF, et al. Consensus recommendations from the American Acne & Rosacea Society on the management of rosacea, part 5: a guide on the management of rosacea. Cutis. 2014;93(3):134–8.

81. Pelletier JL, Perez C, Jacob SE. Contact dermatitis in pediatrics. Pediatr Ann. 2016;45(8):e287–92.

82. Cohen DE, Heidary N. Treatment of irritant and allergic contact dermatitis. Dermatol Ther. 2004;17(4):334–40.

83. de Jongh CM, Khrenova L, Verberk MM, Calkoen F, van Dijk FJ, Voss H, et al. Loss-of-function polymorphisms in the filaggrin gene are associated with an increased susceptibility to chronic irritant contact dermatitis: a case-control study. Br J Dermatol. 2008;159(3):621–7.

84. Dhingra N, Shemer A, Correa da Rosa J, Rozenblit M, Fuentes-Duculan J, Gittler JK, et al. Molecular profiling of contact dermatitis skin identifies allergen-dependent differences in immune response. J Allergy Clin Immunol. 2014;134(2):362–72.

85. Liu J, Harberts E, Tammaro A, Girardi N, Filler RB, Fishelevich R, et al. IL-9 regulates allergen-specific Th1 responses in allergic contact dermatitis. J Invest Dermatol. 2014;134(7):1903–11.

86. Weston WL, Weston JA, Kinoshita J, Kloepfer S, Carreon L, Toth S, et al. Prevalence of positive epicutaneous tests among infants, children, and adolescents. Pediatrics. 1986;78(6):1070–4.

87. Bruckner AL, Weston WL, Morelli JG. Does sensitization to contact allergens begin in infancy? Pediatrics. 2000;105(1):e3.

88. Barros MA, Baptista A, Correia TM, Azevedo F. Patch testing in children: a study of 562 school-children. Contact Dermatitis. 1991;25(3):156–9.

89. Mortz CG, Lauritsen JM, Bindslev-Jensen C, Andersen KE. Contact allergy and allergic contact dermatitis in adolescents: prevalence measures and associations. The Odense Adolescence Cohort Study on Atopic Diseases and Dermatitis (TOACS). Acta Derm Venereol. 2002;82(5):352–8.

90. de Waard-van der Spek FB, Andersen KE, Darsow U, Mortz CG, Orton D, Worm M, et al. Allergic contact dermatitis in children: which factors are relevant? (review of the literature). Pediatr Allergy Immunol. 2013;24(4):321–9.

91. Fukuoka S, Arita R, Shirakawa R, Morishige N. Changes in meibomian gland morphology and ocular higher-order aberrations in eyes with chalazion. Clin Ophthalmol. 2017;11:1031–8.

92. Schalock PC. Common allergens in allergic contact dermatitis. In: Fowler J, editor. UpToDate. Waltham: UpToDate. Accessed 24 Mar 2019.

93. Goldenberg A, Silverberg N, Silverberg JI, Treat J, Jacob SE. Pediatric allergic contact dermatitis: lessons for better care. J Allergy Clin Immunol Pract. 2015;3(5):661–7; quiz 8.

94. Aquino M, Fonacier L. The role of contact dermatitis in patients with atopic dermatitis. J Allergy Clin Immunol Pract. 2014;2(4):382–7.

95. Kostner L, Anzengruber F, Guillod C, Recher M, Schmid-Grendelmeier P, Navarini AA. Allergic contact dermatitis. Immunol Allergy Clin N Am. 2017;37(1):141–52.

96. Fonacier L, Bernstein DI, Pacheco K, Holness DL, Blessing-Moore J, Khan D, et al. Contact dermatitis: a practice parameter-update 2015. J Allergy Clin Immunol Pract. 2015;3(3 Suppl):S1–39.

97. Wilkinson DS, Fregert S, Magnusson B, Bandmann HJ, Calnan CD, Cronin E, et al. Terminology of contact dermatitis. Acta Derm-Venereol. 1970;50(4):287–92.

98. Menne T, White I. Standardization in contact dermatitis. Contact Dermatitis. 2008;58(6):321.

99. Schalock PC, Dunnick CA, Nedorost S, Brod B, Warshaw E, Mowad C. American contact dermatitis society core allergen series. Dermatitis. 2013;24(1):7–9.

100. Gupta AK, Chow M. Pimecrolimus: a review. J Eur Acad Dermatol Venereol. 2003;17(5):493–503.

101. Katsarou A, Makris M, Papagiannaki K, Lagogianni E, Tagka A, Kalogeromitros D. Tacrolimus 0.1% vs mometasone furoate topical treatment in allergic contact hand eczema: a prospective randomized clinical study. Eur J Dermatol. 2012;22(2):192–6.

102. Margolis DJ, Abuabara K, Hoffstad OJ, Wan J, Raimondo D, Bilker WB. Association between malignancy and topical use of pimecrolimus. JAMA Dermatol. 2015;151(6):594–9.

103. Murphy PB HJ, Atwater AR. Allergic contact dermatitis. In: StatPearls [Internet]. 2018.

104. Scat Y, Liotet S, Carre F. [Epidemiological study of benign tumors and inflammatory pseudotumors of the eye and its adnexa]. J Fr Ophtalmol 1996;19(8–9):514–9.

105. Holds JBCW, Durairaj VD, Foster JA, Gausas RE, Harrison AR, Hartstein ME, Fante RG, Pelton RW. Acquired eyelid disorders. Section 7: orbit, eyelids, and lacrimal system. Basic Clin Sci Course Am Acad Ophthalmol. 2014:152–4.

106. Nemet AY, Vinker S, Kaiserman I. Associated morbidity of chalazia. Cornea. 2011;30(12):1376–81.

107. Liang L, Ding X, Tseng SC. High prevalence of demodex brevis infestation in chalazia. Am J Ophthalmol. 2014;157(2):342–8.e1.

108. Chen L, Chen X, Xiang Q, Zheng Y, Pi L, Liu Q, et al. Prevalence of low serum vitamin a levels in young children with chalazia in Southwest China. Am J Ophthalmol. 2014;157(5):1103–8.e2.

109. Puttgen KB. Juvenile xanthogranuloma (JXG). In: Levy ML, Corona R, editors. UpToDate. UpToDate, Waltham, MA. Accessed 24 Mar 2019.

110. Lenci LT KC, Clark TJ, Maltry AC, Syed NA, Allen RC, Shriver EM. Benign lesions of the external periocular tissues. 2017.

111. Ozer PA, Gurkan A. Eyelid nodule in a child: a chalazion or idiopathic facial aseptic granuloma? Eye (Lond). 2014;28(9):1146–7.

112. Bagheri A, Hasani HR, Karimian F, Abrishami M, Yazdani S. Effect of chalazion excision on refractive error and corneal topography. Eur J Ophthalmol. 2009;19(4):521–6.

113. Park YM, Lee JS. The effects of chalazion excision on corneal surface aberrations. Cont Lens Anterior Eye. 2014;37(5):342–5.

114. Santa Cruz CS, Culotta T, Cohen EJ, Rapuano CJ. Chalazion-induced hyperopia as a cause of decreased vision. Ophthalmic Surg Lasers. 1997;28(8):683–4.

115. Cottrell DG, Bosanquet RC, Fawcett IM. Chalazions: the frequency of spontaneous resolution. Br Med J (Clin Res Ed). 1983;287(6405):1595.

116. Perry HD, Serniuk RA. Conservative treatment of chalazia. Ophthalmology. 1980;87(3):218–21.

117. Garrett GW, Gillespie ME, Mannix BC. Adrenocorticosteroid injection vs. conservative therapy in the treatment of chalazia. Ann Ophthalmol. 1988;20(5):196–8.

118. Barbara M Mathes, Patrick C Alguire. Intralesional injection. In: Robert P Dellavalle, editor. UpToDate. UpToDate, Waltham. Accessed 24 Mar 2019.

119. Ahmad S, Baig MA, Khan MA, Khan IU, Janjua TA. Intralesional corticosteroid injection vs surgical treatment of chalazia in pigmented patients. J Coll Physicians Surg Pak. 2006;16(1):42–4.

120. Yagci A, Palamar M, Egrilmez S, Sahbazov C, Ozbek SS. Anterior segment ischemia and retinochoroidal vascular occlusion after intralesional steroid injection. Ophthal Plast Reconstr Surg. 2008;24(1):55–7.

121. Thomas EL, Laborde RP. Retinal and choroidal vascular occlusion following intralesional corticosteroid injection of a chalazion. Ophthalmology. 1986;93(3):405–7.

122. Aycinena AR, Achiron A, Paul M, Burgansky-Eliash Z. Incision and curettage versus steroid injection for the treatment of chalazia: a meta-analysis. Ophthal Plast Reconstr Surg. 2016;32(3):220–4.

123. Goawalla A, Lee V. A prospective randomized treatment study comparing three treatment options for chalazia: triamcinolone acetonide injections, incision and curettage and treatment with hot compresses. Clin Exp Ophthalmol. 2007;35(8):706–12.

124. Biuk D, Matic S, Barac J, Vukovic MJ, Biuk E, Matic M. Chalazion management--surgical treatment versus triamcinolon application. Coll Antropol. 2013;37(Suppl 1):247–50.

Ophthalmic Cancer and Masses

Contents

Tumors

Andrei P. Martin, Lauren A. Dalvin, Li-Anne S. Lim, and Carol L. Shields

Contents

© Springer Nature Switzerland AG 2021
R. Shinder (ed.), Pediatric Ophthalmology in the Emergency Room,
https://doi.org/10.1007/978-3-030-49950-1_15

15.1 Rhabdomyosarcoma

15.1.1 Introduction

Rhabdomyosarcoma (RMS) is a highly malignant tumor originating from pluripotent mesenchyme composed of striated muscle cells in various stages of development [1–5]. Rhabdomyosarcoma is the most common soft tissue sarcoma in the pediatric population [1–8], accounting for 5% of all childhood malignancies and 20% of all malignant soft tissue tumors of childhood [1]. Approximately 25%–35% of RMS originates from the head and neck region with 50% arising in the parameningeal area and 30% arising in the orbit [1, 4, 5]. There is a slight predilection for males. No known racial predilection has been established [1, 7]. Systemic associations include Li-Fraumeni syndrome, neurofibromatosis type I, familial cancer syndrome (p53 mutation), Noonan syndrome, Beckwith-Wiedemann syndrome, and Costello syndrome [1, 5].

15.1.2 Clinical Features

Rhabdomyosarcoma usually presents in the first decade of life at a mean age of 10 years [9]. Orbital RMS most commonly presents with unilateral proptosis (80–100%) that develops rapidly over weeks [1, 3–5]. Other presenting symptoms include globe displacement (80%), conjunctival and eyelid swelling (60%), ptosis (30–50%), and a palpable orbital mass (25%) most commonly in the superonasal orbit [1, 9]. In advanced cases, pain (10%) can be found [1]. In rare instances, RMS presents in the conjunctiva as a papillomatous, botryoid mass [10].

Clinically, orbital RMS presents as a unilateral, well-circumscribed, palpable mass (◘ Fig. 15.1a). In advanced orbital RMS, the mass can be irregular and ill-defined from pseudocapsule invasion. Secondary ocular complications include elevated intraocular pressure, exposure keratopathy, optic neuropathy, central retinal vein occlusion, and cen-

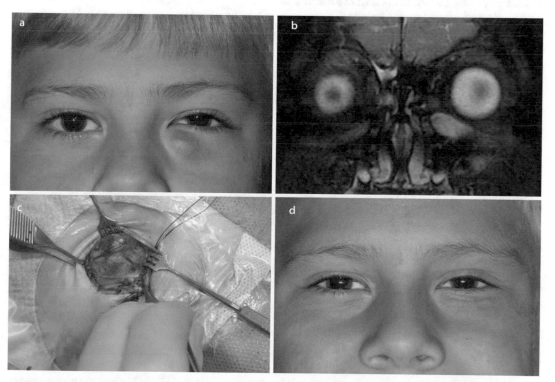

◘ **Fig. 15.1** Orbital rhabdomyosarcoma. **a** External examination disclosed an elevated reddish round mass located deep to the left lower lid. **b** T2-weighted coronal MRI image revealed a hyperintense inferomedial extra-conal mass. **c** External photograph of the surgical excision of the tumor that proved to be rhabdomyosarcoma. **d** External appearance 1 year after biopsy, chemotherapy, and radiotherapy

tral retinal artery occlusion [1]. Distant metastasis occurs in approximately 6% [9] and occurs hematogenously, most often to the lung, bone, and bone marrow [1 3–5, 7, 9].

15.1.3 Imaging

Neuroimaging is required to evaluate the extent of disease and rule out intracranial involvement. Computed tomography (CT) scan is superior for detecting bone involvement but exposes the child to radiation. Magnetic resonance imaging (MRI) does not involve radiation exposure, provides better spatial resolution and soft tissue detail, and more accurately detects intracranial spread [1–3, 5]. Orbital RMS is frequently located in the extraconal space but can be both intra- and extraconal. The mass is seen adjacent to the extraocular muscles without enlargement of the muscle belly [1, 3, 5]. Early orbital RMS does not invade bone, but larger, more advanced tumors can exhibit bone destruction and invade adjacent sinuses. Rhabdomyosarcoma appears isodense to muscle on CT, hypointense to fat on T1-weighted MRI, and hyperintense to muscle and fat on T2-weighted MRI and enhances with gadolinium contrast (◘ Fig. 15.1b). Systemic workup for metastasis can include nuclear bone scintigraphy positron emission tomography-computed tomography (PET-CT) and bone marrow biopsy. Bone scintigraphy is especially useful in the detection of osteoblastic spread, while PET-CT is used in the identification of bone and lymph node metastasis. Whole-body MRI is superior to PET-CT for recognition of distant spread [5].

> Radiologic Features of
> Rhabdomyosarcoma
> Rhabdomyosarcoma
> CT scan
> — Homogenous soft tissue mass isodense
>   to normal muscle

> MRI
> — T1: low to intermediate intensity, isointense to nearby muscle
> — T2: hyperintense
> — Post contrast: enhancing mass

15.1.4 Pathology

Tissue diagnosis is required prior to proceeding with treatment [7]. Orbital RMS can be classified into three histological subgroups: embryonal (50%–70%, botryoid subtype 5%), alveolar (20%–30%), and pleomorphic (5%–10%). The PAX3-FOXO1 fusion gene that occurs as a result of a stable reciprocal translocation of chromosome 2 and 13 is exclusive to alveolar RMS and is associated with a poorer prognosis [5].

15.1.5 Management and Prognosis

Orbital rhabdomyosarcoma is both a chemosensitive and radiosensitive tumor. Primary treatment includes incisional or excisional biopsy (◘ Fig. 15.1c) followed by adjuvant chemotherapy and/or radiotherapy. Staging according to the Intergroup Rhabdomyosarcoma Study Group (IRSG) classification (◘ Table 15.1) guides management (◘ Table 15.2) [1, 3, 5, 7]. Vincristine, actinomycin, cyclophosphamide, and doxorubicin are the most commonly used chemotherapeutic agents [1, 3, 5, 7]. Radiation treatment is usually at a dose of 36–50 Gy given over the course of 4–5 weeks. Patients should be monitored for radiation side effects including cataract, dry eye, orbital hypoplasia, ptosis, and radiation retinopathy. A multidisciplinary approach is required for optimal care. Prognosis for orbital RMS has improved over the years (◘ Fig. 15.1d) with overall survival of 92% at 5 years and 87% at 10 years for groups I, II, and III [5]. Orbital location, earlier diagnosis, favorable histopathology of embryonal type, and PAX3-FOXO1 fusion gene negative status are associated with a better prognosis.

Table 15.1 Intergroup rhabdomyosarcoma study group. Surgical-pathological grouping system [1]

Group	Definition
I	Localized tumor Completely resected with pathologically clear margins No regional lymph node involvement
Ia	Confined to muscle or organ of origin
Ib	Contiguous involvement outside the muscle or organ of origin
II	Localized tumor Residual disease and/or regional lymph node involvement
IIa	Microscopic residual disease No evidence of gross residual tumor or regional lymph node involvement
IIb	No microscopic residual disease Regional lymph node involvement
IIc	Microscopic residual disease Regional lymph node involvement
III	Localized tumor Incomplete resection with biopsy or gross residual disease
IV	Distant metastatic disease present

Information from Shields and Shields [1]

Table 15.2 Intergroup rhabdomyosarcoma study group. recommendations for treatment of orbital rhabdomyosarcoma [5]

Group	Radiation therapy	Chemotherapy
I	None	VA
II	36 Gy	VAC
III	45 Gy	VAC
IV	Intensive	Intensive

V = vincristine; A = actinomycin D; C = cyclophosphamide

Information from Jurdy et al. [5]

15.2 Leukemia

15.2.1 Introduction

Leukemia is a malignant neoplasm of the hematopoietic stem cells and is the most common childhood malignancy in the USA [11, 12]. In the pediatric population, acute lymphoblastic leukemia (ALL) accounts for 80% of all cases, while acute myeloblastic leukemia (AML) accounts for the remaining 20% [11]. Up to 69% of all patients with leukemia have ophthalmic involvement at some point in the course of the disease [12]. ALL is more common in non-Hispanic white males, while AML is more common in adult males of European descent [13].

15.2.2 Clinical Features

Acute lymphoblastic leukemia usually presents in the first decade of life between 2 and 5 years of age [13]. Leukemia can affect the eye primarily by direct infiltration or secondarily due to hyperviscosity or anemia. Primary ocular involvement can involve the anterior uvea, the orbit, and the optic nerve. In the anterior segment, leukemia can present with chemosis, iris mass, pseudohypopyon, or pseudouveitis. In the orbit, primary disease can present as a discrete mass known as a myeloid sarcoma or chloroma, which is composed of primitive granulocyte precursors. Chloroma is found in 3% of AML cases and is bilateral in approximately 60% [14]. The extraocular muscles as well as the lacrimal gland can be involved and mimic dacryoadenitis [15]. In the optic nerve, leukemic infiltration can present with acute vision loss and pain. Optic nerve infiltration can rapidly progress causing central retinal artery or vein occlusion, neovascular glaucoma, or retinal detachment. Secondary ocular involvement is most commonly seen as leukemic retinopathy (◘ Fig. 15.2) [11, 14], characterized by flame-shaped hemorrhages, often with white centers at the level of the nerve fiber layer, but can also present as hyphema or vitreous hemorrhage [11, 16].

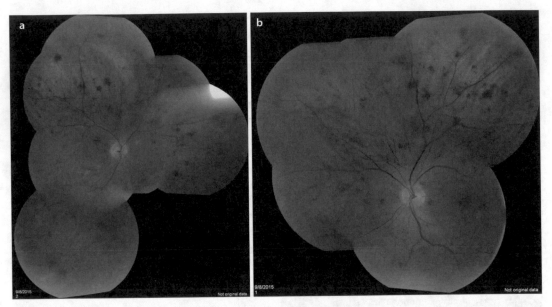

◘ Fig. 15.2 Leukemic retinopathy. Color fundus photograph of the right **a** and left **b** eye showing diffuse dot blot and flame-shaped retinal hemorrhages with hard exudates in the macula consistent with leukemic retinopathy

Vascular tortuosity, dilation, occlusion and perivascular sheathing can be present [16]. Leukemic retinopathy is the most common ophthalmic manifestation of leukemia [11, 14].

15.2.3 Imaging

Chloroma appears hypointense to isointense on T1-weighted MRI and isointense to hyperintense on T2-weighted MRI and shows enhancement with gadolinium contrast [11, 17]. Neuroimaging is required to rule out central nervous system disease.

> Radiologic Features of Orbital Chloroma
> Orbital Chloroma
> MRI
> — T1: hypointense to isointense
> — T2: isointense to hyperintense
> — Post contrast: enhancing mass

15.2.4 Pathology

Chloroma, appearing green on gross examination, is composed of immature white blood cells including myeloblasts, myelocytes, and promyelocytes [16]. In patients with leukemic retinopathy, histopathology shows evidence of retinal capillary endothelial loss similar to radiation retinopathy [12].

15.2.5 Management and Prognosis

Treatment of leukemia is led by a pediatric oncologist. Systemic chemotherapy and bone marrow transplantation are part of the treatment regimen; however, in cases where treatment of ocular leukemia is insufficient, adjuvant radiation is indicated and is useful for orbital and ocular leukemia, leukemic retinopathy, iris infiltration, and optic nerve head involvement [11, 12]. The presence of ocular, orbital, or CNS involvement indicates poor prognosis [12].

15.3 Metastatic Neuroblastoma

15.3.1 Introduction

Metastatic neuroblastoma is a rare neuroendocrine tumor that commonly originates from the adrenal glands [18] but can be found in other locations along the sympathetic chain

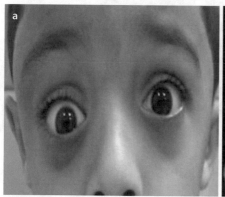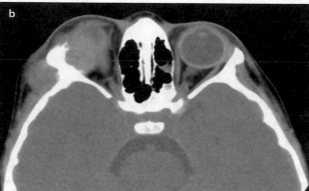

Fig. 15.3 Metastatic neuroblastoma. **a** External photograph of a 5-year-old male with painless right-sided proptosis, inferomedial globe dystopia, and decreased supraduction for 2 months from a superolat- eral periorbital mass. **b** Orbital CT scan showing an ill-defined lytic mass centered in the right zygoma with both intra- and extraorbital extension. (Photo courtesy of Dr. Roman Shinder)

in the neck, chest, abdomen, and pelvis [19]. Neuroblastoma is the most common extracranial solid tumor in children under 5-years-old and represents 7.5% of all cancers in children under 15 years of age [20]. The majority of cases present by 5 years of age and 90% occur before age 10 [20]. Metastatic neuroblastoma can involve the orbits in approximately 10%–20% of cases (■ Fig. 15.3a) [21]. There is a slight predilection for males. No known racial predilection has been established [20, 21].

15.3.2 Clinical Features

Metastatic neuroblastoma presents in a systemically unwell child at a mean age of 2.5 years [18]. The clinical features and rapid onset of this tumor resemble that of orbital RMS; however, the patients are usually younger and clinically ill. Neuroblastoma can present as a primary disease with opsoclonus or Horner's syndrome; as orbital metastatic disease manifesting with a classic triad of edema, ecchymosis, and proptosis; or as hypertensive retinopathy secondary to systemic hypertension [20, 21]. The classic "raccoon eyes" triad of proptosis, ecchymosis, and edema is common and arises from retrobulbar metastasis. In a study by Smith et al., in 14 cases of neuroblastoma, orbital metastasis was present in 6 (48%) [21]. Four patients presented bilaterally and two unilaterally. Common presenting signs included ptosis and ecchymosis, while proptosis and strabismus were less common [21].

15.3.3 Pathology

Histopathology of metastatic neuroblastoma is composed of embryonal neuroblasts arranged individually, as pseudorosettes, sheets, clumps, or cord-like groups within a sparse fibrous tissue stroma. The nucleus appears dark and vesicular with a high nuclear to cytoplasmic ratio [18].

15.3.4 Imaging

Metastatic orbital neuroblastoma has been known to mimic other orbital tumors such as RMS, hemangioma, and lymphangioma. Tumors mostly appear as a poorly defined mass in the posterolateral orbital wall, with bony destruction and intracranial extension on CT (■ Fig. 15.3b) [18]. On MRI, metastatic neuroblastoma shows low signal intensity on T1-weighted images, high signal intensity on T2-weighted images, and little to no enhancement on post-contrast images [19]. Further evaluation includes urinary catecholamine levels (elevated in 80%–90% of patients), chest X-ray to evaluate for a mediastinal mass, and bone marrow biopsy which frequently shows neuroblastoma cells [18].

Radiologic Features of Orbital Neuroblastoma

Orbital Neuroblastoma

MRI
- T1: hypointense
- T2: hyperintense
- Post contrast: little to no enhancement

15.3.5 Management and Prognosis

Management of metastatic orbital neuroblastoma includes intensive, multi-agent neoadjuvant chemotherapy followed by tumor resection [20]. The two most important clinical factors in predicting the outcome for neuroblastoma are the stage of disease and age at diagnosis. Metastatic neuroblastoma involving the orbits is categorized as stage IV disease according to the International Neuroblastoma Staging System [21], with a guarded 5-year survival of 50%.

15.4 Orbital Lymphangioma

15.4.1 Introduction

Lymphangioma (lymphovenous malformation) is a benign, hamartomatous, unencapsulated, vascular malformation typically diagnosed during early childhood [22–28], accounting for 25% of orbital vascular lesions and 4% of all orbital lesions [29]. There is a slight female predilection [25]. There is no known racial predilection or systemic association.

15.4.2 Clinical Features

Orbital lymphangioma is present from birth and largely remains asymptomatic or possibly unrecognized. These lesions commonly become clinically apparent following acute hemorrhage within the lesion, either spontaneous or secondary to trauma, or enlargement as a result of an upper respiratory tract infection [22–24, 26]. These events can cause a myriad of symptoms, including acute unilateral proptosis, pain, limitation of ocular movement, blepharoptosis, loss of vision, and globe displacement (◻ Fig. 15.4a). Orbital lymphangioma is a type 1 vascular malformation according to the International Orbital Society (◻ Table 15.3).

15.4.3 Imaging

On MRI, orbital lymphangioma appears as a multicystic, heterogeneous mass with fluid levels in the setting of acute or chronic intralesional hemorrhage [24].

15.4.4 Pathology

Histopathologically, lymphangioma is composed of multiple dilated sacs of irregular vascular channels with lymphocytes or lymphoid aggregates lined by a thin single layer of flattened endothelial cells (◻ Fig. 15.4b) [23–25].

15.4.5 Management and Prognosis

Management of orbital lymphangioma includes observation, drainage, debulking, complete excision, infusion of sclerosing agents, or a combination of sclerosing therapy and surgical excision. Treatment is guided by symptoms, risk of amblyopia, and cosmetic appearance. Sclerosing agents, including OK-432 (a biological product from *Streptococcus pyogenes*), Sotradecol (sodium tetradecyl sulfate), doxycycline, bleomycin, and sodium morrhuate, are administered by intralesional injection and result in significant reduction in tumor size [23–25, 30]. Complete surgical excision is technically difficult due to the poorly defined nature of the tumor (◻ Fig. 15.4c) and can be associated with complications including intraoperative hemorrhage and multiple recurrences [22–26, 30, 31]. Intraoperative use of fibrin glue can improve hemostasis and facilitate tumor exci-

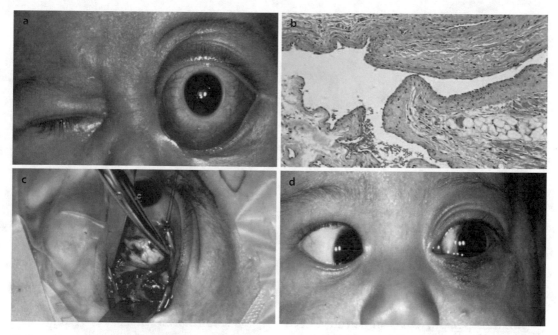

Fig. 15.4 Orbital lymphangioma. **a** External photograph of a 2-month-old child with proptosis and corneal exposure of the left eye secondary to orbital lymphangioma. **b** Histopathology showing irregular vascular channels and hemorrhage with organization (H&E, 10x). **c** Intraoperative photograph during excision. Consistent with lymphangioma. **d** External photograph of the same child 4 days after surgery

Table 15.3 Orbital vascular malformations [27]

No flow malformations (Type 1)	Lymphangiomas
Venous flow malformations (Type 2)	Primary varices Including: Distensible and nondistensible varieties Mixed forms with venous and no flow components (grouped here to emphasize the clinical importance of the venous relationship)
Arterial flow malformations (Type 3)	Secondary varices

Information from Harris [27]

sion [24, 30]. Medical therapy with oral sildenafil has been reported to be effective with collapse of the cystic spaces within the tumor [22]. Prognosis for orbital lymphangioma is variable depending on the size and location of the lesion (■ Fig. 15.4d).

15.5 Hemangioma of Infancy

Hemangioma of infancy is a benign, vascular tumor and is the most common vascular tumor of the pediatric population [32] occurring in 5%–10% of infants [32, 33]. Of all facial hemangioma, ocular hemangioma of infancy accounts for 24% [32]. In a survey of 1264 patients with orbital tumors by Shields et al., 213 (17%) had vascular tumors of which 36 (3%) were hemangioma of infancy [31]. Periocular hemangioma of infancy has a predilection for female gender and Caucasian race. Risk factors include multiple gestation pregnancy and premature birth [31, 32]. Systemic associations include PHACES syndrome (posterior fossa malformations, hemangiomas, arterial anomalies, cardiac defects, eye abnormalities, and sternal clefting), visceral hemangiomatosis (including subglottic hemangioma), Kasabach-Merritt syndrome, and Maffuci syndrome [31, 33, 34].

15.5.1 Clinical Features

Infantile hemangioma typically presents in infancy and is present at birth in 55% of cases [35, 36]. Periocular hemangioma of infancy typically appears as a small red lesion on the eyelid, which from the third month of life undergoes a phase of rapid proliferation and progressive enlargement [32]. This is followed by a slow involution phase over several months or years, characterized by a change in color from bright red to purplish gray. Approximately 30% completely regress by age 3 years and 76% by 7 years [33].

Infantile hemangioma can be categorized by the depth of skin involvement (superficial, deep, mixed) or by area of involvement (localized, segmental, indeterminate) [33]. Superficial hemangioma most often reaches its full size by 6–8 months of age while deep hemangioma can continue to grow until 12–14 months of age [32, 33]. Deep hemangioma can present with proptosis without any visible superficial hemangioma. In rare cases, hemangioma can also develop in other ocular locations such as the conjunctiva or iris [33].

Ocular sequelae of infantile hemangioma include amblyopia, cosmetic deformity, and orbitopathy. Large superonasal eyelid hemangioma tends to be more amblyogenic than those located in the central or temporal orbit, causing anisometropic astigmatic amblyopia or deprivation amblyopia [34].

15.5.2 Imaging

In the office, ultrasound is a quick noninvasive procedure that can characterize, localize, and determine the depth of the lesion without exposing the patient to radiation [33]. In addition, Doppler studies reveal the distinctive high flow pattern of hemangioma. When the diagnosis of hemangioma is uncertain, the gold standard imaging of choice is MRI with gadolinium contrast [33]. Hemangioma is seen as a well-circumscribed, densely lobulated mass with low-intensity septations and a pseudocapsule. On T1-weighted MRI, hemangioma is isointense to extraocular muscle and hyperintense in areas of thrombosis. On T2-weighted MRI, hemangioma is hyperintense to muscle. Post-contrast imaging shows gradual irregular enhancement with delayed washout [32].

Radiologic Features of Hemangioma of Infancy

Hemangioma of infancy

MRI

- T1: isointense signal to extraocular muscle with lobulated hypointense septations
- T2: hyperintense to muscle
- Post contrast: gradual enhancement with washout

15.5.3 Pathology

During the proliferative phase, infantile hemangioma is composed of densely packed endothelial cells with small vascular lumen forming capillaries that are separated by fibrous septations. During the involution phase, the regressing lesion displays increased fibrosis and hyalinization of capillary walls [32].

15.5.4 Management and Prognosis

All patients with infantile hemangioma should be referred to a pediatrician for systemic review and evaluation for visceral hemangiomas and other associations. Ocular management of infantile hemangioma is aimed at the prevention of amblyopia and cosmetic disfigurement. All patients should be assessed with cycloplegic refraction, and any refractive error and amblyopia should be treated. Close follow-up and observation of the lesion is an acceptable treatment plan, but in patients with potentially amblyogenic hemangioma of infancy, treatment is warranted. Systemic propranolol therapy is the treatment

15

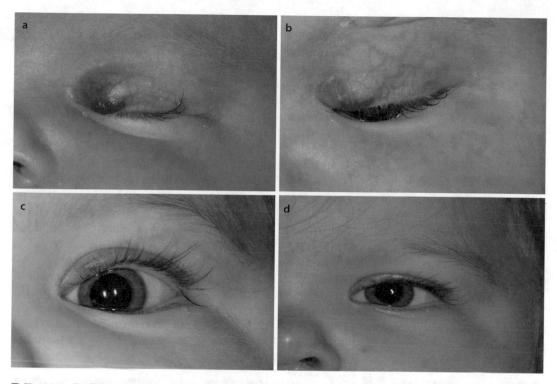

Fig. 15.5 Eyelid hemangioma of infancy. **a** External photograph of a hemangioma of infancy of the left upper eyelid. Regressing hemangioma at **b** 2, **c** 5, and **d** 10 months after initiating topical timolol therapy

of choice for infantile hemangioma (6) and requires a multidisciplinary team including a pediatrician and sometimes a pediatric cardiologist. Potential side effects include bradycardia, hypotension, bronchospasm, and hypoglycemia, making pretreatment assessment vital [37]. Oral propranolol given three times a day is usually titrated from a starting dose of 0.5 mg/kg/day up to 2 mg/kg/day over weeks with prompt clinical response seen as decrease in size, softening, and lightening in the color of the hemangioma [37]. Treatment is tapered and discontinued when response reaches a plateau or when the patient reaches 12 months of age [37]. For non-amblyogenic, superficial, and mixed hemangioma of infancy, treatment with topical beta-blockers has shown similar success with fewer systemic side effects. Topical 0.25% timolol gel applied twice daily over the hemangioma results in more than 50% decrease in lesion size after 2 months of treatment (■ Fig. 15.5) [38].

Systemic, intralesional, and topical corticosteroids have also been successful in the treatment of hemangioma of infancy. Steroids accelerate the regression of the lesion but can have significant systemic adverse effects including growth retardation, adrenal suppression, behavioral changes, and gastrointestinal upset [37, 39]. Intralesional steroids can cause local complications, including eyelid necrosis, central retinal artery occlusion, and ophthalmic artery occlusion [33]. Surgical resection has been largely surpassed by oral propranolol and topical timolol therapy. The prognosis for patients with infantile hemangioma is favorable, as the natural course of the disease is slow involution over many years.

15.6 Retinoblastoma

15.6.1 Introduction

Retinoblastoma (RB) is a neuroblastic tumor of embryonal retinal cells arising from the mutation of both copies of the *RB1* tumor suppressor gene located on the long arm of chromosome 13(13q14). As the most common malignant intraocular tumor in the pediatric population, it accounts for 11% of all cancers in infancy and 4% of all pediatric cancers with an incidence of 1 in 15,000 live births [40]. Risk factors for retinoblastoma include a known family history of the disease, 13q deletion syndrome, and maternal or paternal radiation exposure [40]. There is no known race or gender predilection [40–43].

15.6.2 Clinical Features

Retinoblastoma can occur as a result of an autosomal dominant hereditary germline mutation (40%) or a sporadic somatic mutation (60%) [40]. Germline RB has an earlier age of onset presenting in the first year of life and is more often bilateral or multifocal. These patients are at risk for pineoblastoma as well as secondary cancers, including osteogenic sarcoma, melanoma, breast cancer, and non-Hodgkins lymphoma [44]. In contrast, somatic RB occurs in older children age 1–3 years (mean 18 months), with 95% of tumors diagnosed before age 5 years [40, 41, 43, 45]. Tumors are usually unilateral and unifocal with no increased risk of secondary cancers. Presenting features of RB include leukocoria (56%) (◨ Fig. 15.6a), strabismus (24%), or poor vision (8%) [46]. Anterior segment findings of retinoblastoma include shallow anterior chamber, narrow or closed angles, elevated intraocular pressure, iris nodules or neovascularization, pseudohypopyon, or the presence of a whitish anterior chamber mass. Cataract or signs of inflammation are rare. On binocular indirect ophthalmoscopy, early RB presents as a round translucent thickening of the sensory retina (◨ Fig. 15.6b), with larger tumors, appearing as a round, opaque white or yellow retinal mass with fine intralesional blood vessels, a feeding retinal artery, and a

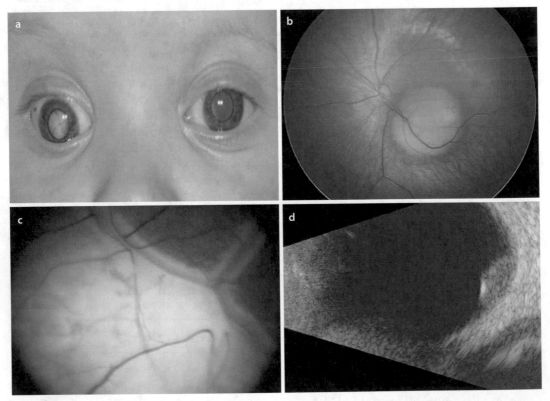

◨ **Fig. 15.6** Retinoblastoma. **a** External photograph of both eyes showing bilateral (right greater than left) leukocoria. **b** Retcam image of the left eye showing an elevated white intraocular mass along the inferior arcade of the left eye. **c** Retcam image of the right eye showing a creamy yellow intraocular mass occupying over 50% of the globe. **d** B-scan ultrasonography of the left eye showing a hypoechoic intraocular mass

draining vein (■ Fig. 15.6c). Lesions that reach 10 mm in diameter can present with calcifications that signify ischemia or necrosis [40]. Growth patterns exhibited by RB can be classified as endophytic, exophytic, or, rarely, a diffuse infiltrating type. Endophytic RB is characterized by the growth of RB within the retina and seeding into the vitreous cavity. Exophytic RB is characterized by growth deep within the retina into the subretinal space eventually leading to a retinal detachment [40]. Disc swelling can be seen secondary to raised intracranial pressure in the presence of pineoblastoma. External examination should also be performed to evaluate for lymphadenopathy and proptosis. Retinoblastoma is currently classified according to the International Classification of Retinoblastoma (ICRB) classification system (■ Table 15.4) [40, 44].

■ **Table 15.4** The international classification of retinoblastoma [47]

Group	Philadelphia version	CHLA version
A	RB ≤ 3mm[a]	RB ≤ 3 mm at least 3 mm from the foveola and 1.5 mm from the optic nerve No seeding
B	RB > 3mm[a] or Macular location (≤3 mm to the foveola) Juxtapapillary location (≤1.5 mm to the disc) Subretinal fluid ≤3 mm from margin	Retinal tumors of any size or location not included in group A No vitreous or subretinal seeding Small cuff of subretinal fluid ≤5 mm from tumor margin
C	RB with Subretinal seeds ≤3 mm from tumor Vitreous seeds ≤3 mm from tumor Both subretinal and vitreous seeds ≤3 mm from tumor	Discrete tumor of any size or location Focal vitreous and subretinal seeding that is local, fine, and limited (theoretically treatable with radioactive plaque) Up to one quadrant subretinal fluid

■ **Table 15.4** (continued)

Group	Philadelphia version	CHLA version
D	RB with Subretinal seeds >3 mm from tumor Vitreous seeds >3 mm from tumor Both subretinal and vitreous seeds >3 mm from tumor	Massive, nondiscrete endophytic or exophytic disease and/or Diffuse vitreous or subretinal seeding more extensive than Group C Retinal detachment >1 quadrant
E	Extensive RB occupying >50% globe or Neovascular glaucoma Opaque media from hemorrhage in the anterior chamber, vitreous or subretinal space Invasion of postlaminar optic nerve, choroid (>2 mm), sclera, orbit, anterior chamber	Massive RB with anatomic and functional destruction of the eye with one or more of the following: Neovascular glaucoma Massive intraocular hemorrhage Aseptic orbital cellulitis Tumor anterior to anterior vitreous face Tumor touching lens Diffuse infiltrating tumor Phthisis or pre-phthisis

Key: *RB* Retinoblastoma, *CHLA* Children's Hospital of Los Angeles
Information from Shields and Shields [47]
[a]Refers to 3 mm in basal dimension or thickness

15.6.3 Imaging

Indirect ophthalmoscopy by an experienced ocular oncologist is the most valuable tool to establish the diagnosis of RB. By ultrasonography, retinoblastoma is seen as a round intraocular mass with high internal echoes (■ Fig. 15.6d). Calcification is present in 95% of cases [40, 43], which differentiates RB from other intraocular tumors and Coats disease. On MRI, RB is hyperintense to vitreous on

T1-weighted imaging and hypointense to vitreous on T2-weighted imaging and shows marked heterogeneous enhancement post contrast. Studies should also evaluate for optic nerve involvement, extraocular extension, and pineoblastoma. Brain MRI should be repeated every 6 months until age 5 years to screen for pineoblastoma [40, 43]. Fluorescein angiography (FA) is an effective way to determine recurrences after treatment and can also identify ischemic retinopathy as well as anterior segment neovascularization. Ophthalmic vascular events following intra-arterial chemotherapy (IAC) such as vascular attenuations and vascular occlusions can also be seen on FA [48]. Features of active RB angiographically include prominent vessels in the arterial phase with leakage in the venous phase [40]. Optical coherence tomography (OCT) imaging can detect the presence of subretinal fluid, evaluate macular integrity, and identify microscopic RB not seen on ophthalmoscopy [40, 49]. Hand-held OCT can detect subclinical recurrences not readily identifiable on ultrasound or clinical examination [49]. Retcam™ photography utilizes a wide-angle camera for documentation and serial monitoring of RB. Retcam use in conjunction with FA is important for monitoring recurrences.

15.6.4 Pathology

Retinoblastoma appears as a mass of basophilic cells that contain round, oval, or spindle-shaped nuclei. Numerous mitotic figures and fragments of apoptotic nuclear debris are present. Characteristic tumor growth into the vitreous cavity or subretinal space with pseudorosette formation occurs when the RB tumor outgrows its blood supply leading to necrosis with associated calcification. Flexner-Wintersteiner rosettes represent early retinal differentiation and are a characteristic feature of retinoblastoma, while Homer-Wright rosettes indicate neuroblastic differentiation [40].

15.6.5 Management and Prognosis

As recent as two decades ago, retinoblastoma was managed with enucleation and external beam radiotherapy (EBRT). Both treatment modalities led to complications such as cosmetic deformity, bony hypoplasia, and risk of secondary tumors. More recently, safer, globe-saving treatment options including chemotherapy, brachytherapy, and IAC have become available [40, 41, 45, 50]. Goals in the treatment of RB are to save the life of the patient, preserve as much vision as possible, and minimize side effects of treatment, specifically secondary cancers. Retinoblastoma is a chemosensitive tumor, with systemic chemotherapy generally used as a primary treatment option, especially in patients with a germline mutation. The most common chemotherapeutic regimen used is carboplatin, etoposide, and vincristine (CEV) [40, 42–45], which is well tolerated by children and can be globe preserving in the majority of group A, B, C, and D patients. In a study by Shields et al., ocular salvage rates were 100%, 93%, 90%, and 47% for groups A, B, C, and D, respectively [40, 51]. Systemic chemotherapy not only treats RB but also offers systemic protection from the development of secondary cancers and metastasis. The most common cause of chemotherapy failure is recurrence of subretinal seeds and/or vitreous seeds [41]. One of the more recent innovations in RB treatment is intra-arterial chemotherapy, which allows for direct delivery of concentrated chemotherapeutic agents to the eye with minimal systemic absorption [40, 42, 45]. IAC can be used as primary treatment for unilateral or bilateral RB, for subsequent treatment of recurrence, or for management of vitreous or subretinal seeds. The route of delivery is through cannulation of the femoral artery, internal carotid artery, and ophthalmic artery. Melphalan, a nitrogen mustard alkylating agent, and topotecan, a topoisomerase I inhibitor, are the most common agents used in IAC. In a study by Shields et al., globe salvage rates after primary IAC were 100%, 100%,

94%, and 36% in patients with ICRB group B, C, D, and E tumors, respectively [42]. IAC success is determined by the tumor size and amount of vitreous and subretinal seeding present [40, 42, 45]. Advantages of IAC include lower systemic side-effects, higher concentration delivered to the tumor, and lower rates of hospitalization. The systemic chemoprotective effect of IAC is not known. Complications of IAC include periorbital edema, erythema, obstruction of ophthalmic and chorioretinal vessels, and systemic complications such as neutropenia [40, 42, 45]. Extensive vitreous seeds can be resistant to systemic chemotherapy and IAC but can respond to intravitreal chemotherapy using either topotecan or melphalan [40, 43]. Intravitreal chemotherapy in combination with IAC improved globe salvage rates in group D and E patients [52].

Focal therapies for early RB without retinal detachment or seeding include transpupillary thermotherapy (TTT) and cryotherapy [40, 42, 45]. Transpupillary thermotherapy is primarily used for early-stage RB and involves the application of heat directly to the tumor. Cryotherapy directly kills primary tumor cells, recurrent tumor cells, and small subretinal seeds through freezing treatment. Additionally, cryotherapy to the ora serrata prior to chemotherapy helps improve drug penetration to the tumor [40, 43].

In addition to being chemosensitive, RB is also radiosensitive. Brachytherapy with Iodine-125 can be used for primary localized tumors or localized recurrent and residual tumors. Plaque radiotherapy is customized to deliver a total dose of 35 Gy to the RB apex in 3–4 days and provides excellent tumor control in 96% of recurrent tumors and 90% of localized primary tumors [40, 41, 45]. Side effects from plaque radiation include cataract formation, scleral necrosis, radiation retinopathy, and papillopathy [40]. Even with all the globe-preserving advances in RB management, enucleation continues to be a life-saving option in RB treatment [40, 41, 43–50]. Indications for enucleation include failure of other therapies,

neovascular glaucoma, chronic retinal detachment, optic nerve invasion, or anterior chamber invasion [40, 43, 45]. During surgery it is optimal, especially in advanced cases, to acquire the longest possible optic nerve section and avoid globe perforation [40, 43]. Chemotherapy after enucleation should be performed in high-risk cases [40, 45, 50]. Genetic testing and counseling play an important role to identify at-risk family members and heritability patterns [43].

Retinoblastoma remains a therapeutic challenge. In developing regions such as Asia and Africa, mortality rate is 50% owing to late detection and advanced disease. In developed countries where health care is readily accessible and modern technology is available, the survival rate from this potentially fatal disease is greater than 95% [40, 41, 43, 45]. Early detection and access to healthcare lead to better prognosis.

15.7 Leukocoria

Leukocoria is an abnormal white pupillary reflex that can be physiologic when light reflects off the optic nerve or associated with a variety of ocular conditions, including congenital cataract (60%), retinoblastoma (18%), persistent fetal vasculature (PFV)(4.2%), Coats disease (4.2%), retinopathy of prematurity, ocular toxocariasis, and familial exudative vitreoretinopathy [40, 53]. In a clinical series of lesions simulating retinoblastoma (pseudo-retinoblastoma), Coats disease (40%) was the most frequent mimicker of RB, followed by PFV (28%), vitreous hemorrhage (5%), and ocular toxocariasis (4%) [53]. Clinical features, age at presentation, and characteristic imaging findings can differentiate these mimickers from retinoblastoma (◘ Table 15.5) [40, 53].

Coats disease is a primary retinal telangiectasia, commonly misdiagnosed as retinoblastoma. Coats disease presents at a later age compared to RB (5 years vs. 1.5 years), which is usually unilateral with a male gen-

Table 15.5 Differential diagnosis of retinoblastoma. features differentiating pseudoretinoblastoma from true retinoblastoma [53]

Feature	Retinoblastoma	Persistent fetal vasculature	Coats disease	Ocular toxocariasis
Family history	10% Familial	Mostly sporadic	Sporadic	Sporadic
Mean age of onset (years)	1.5	At birth	5	7.5
Gender	Male = female	Male = female	Mostly males	Male = female
Laterality	Unilateral or bilateral	Mostly unilateral	Mostly unilateral	Mostly unilateral
Leukocoria	Present in 90%	Present	Xanthocoria	Present
Intraocular mass	White intraretinal mass with a dilated feeding artery and a tortuous draining vein.	Traction of retinal vessels	Irregular dilation of retinal vessels with telangiectasia.	Traction of retinal vessels toward granuloma
Ultrasonography	Solid retinal mass with high-intensity echoes due to intratumoral calcification Retinal detachment	Microphthalmia Persistent hyaloid artery Retinal detachment No calcification No solid retinal mass	Retinal detachment Rarely, linear calcification at the level of retinal pigment epithelium	Solid retinal mass but lacks high-intensity internal echoes Retinal detachment No calcification

Information from Shields et al. [53]

der predilection [53]. Xanthocoria, yellow pupil, is the most common presenting feature of Coats disease and appears in 47% of patients (Fig. 15.7a) [40, 53]. Coats disease is characterized by irregular dilated capillaries, telangiectasia, and aneurysms on both sides of the circulation with associated retinal exudation, exudative retinal detachment (Fig. 15.7b), and retinal non-perfusion (Fig. 15.7c). Ultrasonography reveals retinal detachment without an intraocular mass (Fig. 15.7d).

Persistent fetal vasculature, formerly known as persistent hyperplastic primary vitreous (PHPV), is a unilateral, congenital malformation secondary to failure of regression of the primary vitreous. Persistent fetal vasculature manifests at birth with features that can include microphthalmia, leukocoria, cataract, Mittendorf's dot, persistent tunica vasculosa lentis, persistent hyaloid canal (Fig. 15.8a) with a hyaloid artery, and closed funnel reti-

nal detachment attached to the optic disc [40]. PFV can manifest as anterior, posterior, or combined anterior and posterior PFV, which is the most common subtype. Misdiagnosis is primarily due to the detection of leukocoria and is responsible for over 25% of pseudo-retinoblastoma [40]. On ultrasonography, PFV is seen as a persistent vestigial hyaloid with a hyaloid artery stemming from the disc, and rarely calcification (Fig. 15.8b) [40].

Retinopathy of prematurity (ROP) is a vascular proliferative retinopathy of premature low-birth-weight infants exposed to high and fluctuating levels of oxygen and accounts for 5% of pseudo-retinoblastoma [53]. Leukocoria is mainly due to retinal detachment or a retrolental fibrovascular mass (Fig. 15.9a) [40, 53]. Features of ROP include peripheral retinal neovascularization, vitreous traction, and retinal detachment (Fig. 15.9b). No calcification is seen on ultrasonography, and fluorescein angiography can display leakage

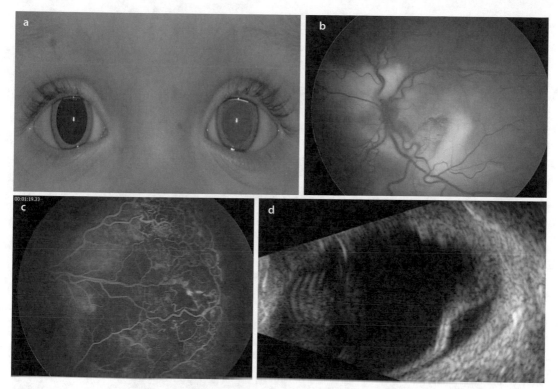

Fig. 15.7 Coats disease. **a** External photograph showing xanthocoria of the left eye. **b** Retcam retinal image of the left eye showing subretinal exudation and tortuous retinal vessels. **c** Fluorescein angiography of the left eye showing hyperfluorescence of the telangiec- tatic vessels with associated "light bulb" aneurysms and peripheral capillary non-perfusion. **d** B-scan ultraso- nography showing retinal detachment with subretinal fluid and absence of an intraocular mass

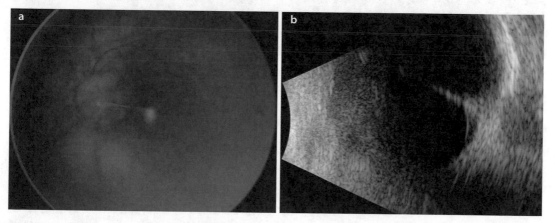

Fig. 15.8 Persistent fetal vasculature. **a** Retcam reti- nal image of the left eye showing a fibrovascular stalk stemming anteriorly from the optic disc to the lens. **b** B-scan ultrasonography showing a fibrovascular stalk with retinal traction and absence of calcification

due to neovascularization at the demarcation of the vascular and avascular retina.

Ocular toxocariasis is a parasitic infesta- tion caused by the nematode *Toxocari canis* or *Toxocara cati*, with domestic dogs and cats being the definitive hosts, respectively. Transmission occurs via the fecal-oral route by consumption of food or soil contaminated

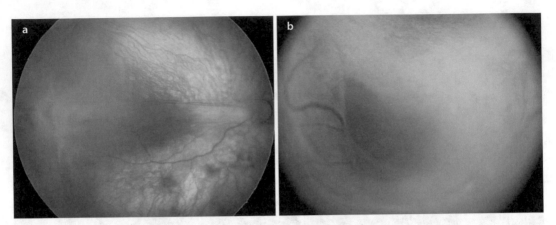

Fig. 15.9 Retinopathy of prematurity. **a** Retcam retinal image of the right eye showing stage 4A retinopathy of prematurity with partial retinal detachment and dragging of the retinal vessels. **b** Stage 5 retinopathy of prematurity showing total retinal detachment. (Photos courtesy of Dr. Antonio Capone, Jr. and Dr. Nathan Farley of Associated Retinal Consultants, William Beaumont Hospital, Royal Oak, MI)

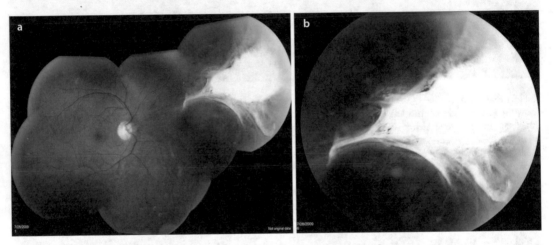

Fig. 15.10 Ocular toxocariasis. **a** Fundus photograph of the right eye showing a whitish-yellow peripheral retinal granuloma with retinal vessel dragging and absence of vitritis. **b** Focal elevated retinal granuloma with surrounding fibrovascular membrane and retinal pigment epithelium changes

by the feces of common host species. Leukocoria in ocular toxocariasis is secondary to the presence of a white, subretinal granulomatous mass, which can mimic exophytic retinoblastoma (Fig. 15.10a, b) [40]. On ultrasonography, an elevated intraocular mass can be present, but often without calcification.

Familial exudative vitreoretinopathy (FEVR) is an inherited abnormality of retinal development resulting in incomplete peripheral vascularization. FEVR is a bilateral, asymmetric condition that can present at any age with a mean age of presentation of 6 years old [40]. Leukocoria due to subretinal and intraretinal exudation can mimic RB. Features of FEVR include retinal traction, straightening of retinal vessels (Fig. 15.11a, b), and a characteristic non-vascularization of the retinal periphery (Fig. 15.11c). There is an absence of an intraocular mass on ultrasonography (Fig. 15.11d), and calcifications are not present on CT scan or MRI [40].

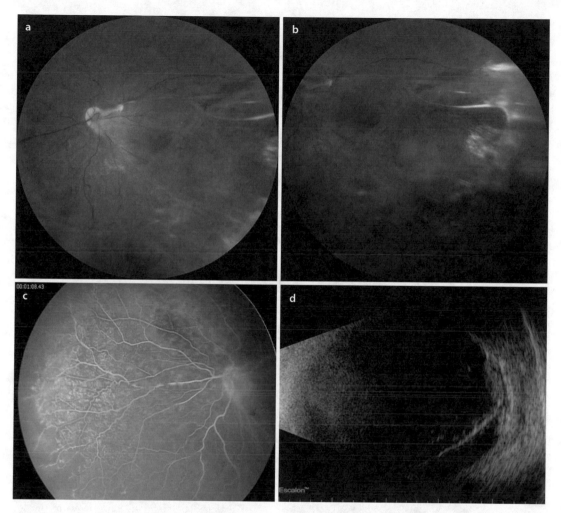

Fig. 15.11 Familial exudative vitreoretinopathy. **a** Fundus photograph of the left eye showing retinal traction and straightening of the retinal vessels. **b** Fundus photograph of the retinal periphery of the left eye showing retinal vessel straightening, macular dragging, and exudation. **c** Fluorescein angiography of the right eye showing peripheral avascular retina and retinal neovascularization. **d** B-scan ultrasonography showing retinal detachment with the absence of intraocular mass and calcifications

Case Presentation

A 14-month-old girl was referred to the ocular oncology clinic with bilateral leukocoria (■ Fig 15.12a) noted by her mother. On binocular indirect ophthalmoscopy, there was a creamy yellow intraocular mass with retinal detachment noted in both eyes. Examination under anesthesia was performed in the operating room. Retcam images were taken which confirmed the diagnosis of Group D retinoblastoma, right eye (■ Fig 15.12b), and Group E retinoblastoma, left eye. Ultrasonography and MRI revealed a calcified intraocular mass with extensive retinal detachment bilaterally (OU) (■ Fig 15.12c, d). FA and OCT showed total retinal detachment and iris neovascularization OU. The patient was treated with six cycles of systemic chemotherapy using the CEV regimen. On six-month follow-up, examination showed complete tumor regression in both eyes. Brain MRI every 6 months until age 5 was advised.

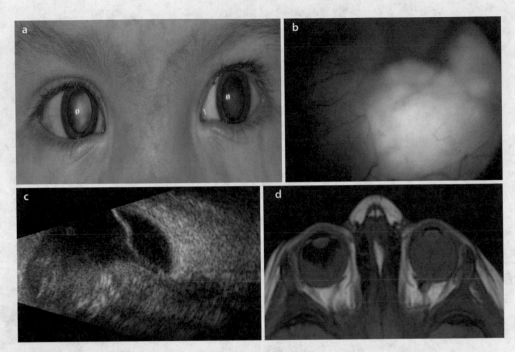

Fig. 15.12 Retinoblastoma. **a** External photograph showing bilateral (right greater than left) leukocoria from bilateral retinoblastoma. **b** Group D retinoblastoma of the left eye showing a creamy yellow intraocular mass. **c** B-scan ultrasonography showing a hyperechoic intraocular mass with extensive retinal detachment. **d** T1-weighted axial orbital MRI showing total retinal detachment in both eyes.

Key Points

- Pediatric ocular tumors can be intraocular or extraocular and can be threatening to life, vision, and cosmetic appearance.
- Prompt diagnosis and management are vital to preserving the patient's life, salvage the eye, and promote normal visual development.
- Orbital rhabdomyosarcoma, a tumor composed of striated muscle cells, is both chemosensitive and radiosensitive. Prognosis depends on the histopathologic subgroup.
- Leukemic retinopathy, clinically seen as retinal flame-shaped hemorrhages, is the most common ophthalmic manifestation of systemic leukemia.
- Neuroblastoma can present with the classic "raccoon eyes" triad of periorbital edema, ecchymosis, and proptosis, which is a sign of retrobulbar metastasis.
- Orbital lymphangioma, a benign vascular malformation present at birth, can remain asymptomatic and undiagnosed. Management is guided by risk for amblyopia, threatened visual function, and cosmetic appearance.
- Hemangioma of infancy can be treated with close observation or systemic beta-blocker therapy. Treatment is guided by risk for amblyopia or cosmetic concerns and is best handled by a multispecialty team.
- Retinoblastoma remains a therapeutic challenge but advances in modern sci-

15

ence have yielded a greater than 95% survival rate in developed countries. Early detection and access to equipped medical facilities lead to better prognosis.

- Detailed indirect ophthalmoscopy and multimodal imaging with ultrasonography, fluorescein angiography, optical coherence tomography, and magnetic resonance imaging can guide the ophthalmologist in differentiating retinoblastoma from pseudo-retinoblastoma.

❓ Review Questions (All Relate to the Same Patient)

1. A 2-year-old female with leukocoria in the right eye and strabismus was referred to you. Past medical history revealed that the child was born premature at 35 weeks gestation. The remainder of the history is unremarkable. On examination, a creamy yellow intraocular mass measuring approximately 6 × 6 mm is found in the macula along the inferotemporal arcade in the right eye. The vitreous is unremarkable. What is the most likely diagnosis?
   (a) Coats disease
   (b) Retinopathy of prematurity
   (c) Ocular toxocariasis
   (d) Retinoblastoma

2. Given your diagnosis, how will you manage the patient?
   (a) Refer to a pediatric infectious disease specialist to start albendazole treatment.
   (b) Do argon laser photocoagulation to prevent neovascularization.
   (c) Schedule examination under anesthesia with imaging, fluorescein angiography, OCT, and ultrasonography, advise genetic testing, and refer to pediatric oncology for chemotherapy.
   (d) Order a whole-body CT scan to look for systemic involvement.

3. Your colleague suggested that you perform a brain MRI every 6 months until your patient is 5 years old. What is the rationale behind this?
   (a) Monitoring for pineoblastoma and second cancers
   (b) Toxocara larvae can easily be monitored by MRI.
   (c) Evaluate the extent of retinal exudation and telangiectasia.
   (d) MRI can predict brain problems in premature babies.

✅ Answers
   1. (d)
   2. (c)
   3. (a)

References

Orbital Rhabdomyosarcoma

1. Shields J, Shields C. Rhabdomyosarcoma: review for the ophthalmologist. Surv Ophthalmol. 2003;48:39–57.
2. Koopman JH, van der Heiden-van der Loo M, van Dijk MR, Bijlsma WR. Incidence of primary malignant orbital tumours in the Netherlands. Eye. 2011;25:461–5.
3. Bravo-Ljubetic L, Peralta-Calvo J, Larranaga-Fragoso P, Pascual N, Pastora-Salvador N, et al. Clinical management of orbital rhabdomyosarcoma in a referral center in Spain. J Pediatr Ophthalmol Strabismus. 2016;53(2):119–26.
4. Boutroux H, Levy C, Mosseri V, Desjardins L, Plancher C, Helfre S, et al. Long-term evaluation of orbital rhabdomyosarcoma in children. Clin Exp Ophthalmol. 2014:1–8.
5. Jurdy L, Merks J, Pieters B, Mourits M, Kloos R, Strackee S, et al. Orbital rhabdomyosarcoma: a review. Saudi Journal of Ophthalmology. 2013;27:167–75.
6. Eade E, Tumuluri K, Do H, Rowe N, Smith J. Visual outcomes and late complications in paediatric orbital rhabdomyosarcoma. Clin Exp Ophthalmol. 2016:1–22.
7. Orbach D, Brisse H, Freneaux P, Husseini K, Aerts I, Desjardins L, et al. Effectiveness of chemotherapy in rhabdomyosarcoma: example of orbital primary. Expert Opin Pharmacother. 2003;4(12):2165–74.
8. Yazici B, Sabur H, Yazici Z. Orbital cavitary rhabdomyosarcoma: case report and literature review. Ophthal PLast Recontr Surg. 2014;20(1):e20–1.
9. Shields CL, Shields JA, Honavar SG, Demerci H. Clinical spectrum of primary ophthalmic rhabdomyosarcoma. Ophthalmology. 2001;108:2284–92.

10. Pennington JD, Welch RJ, Lally SE, Shields JA, Eagle RC, Shields CL. Botryoid rhabdomyosarcoma of the conjunctiva in a young boy. Middle East Afr J Ophthalmol. 2018;25(2):111–4.

Leukemia

11. Rao A, Neheedy J, Chen J, Robbins S, Ramkumar H. A clinical update and radiologic review of pediatric orbital and ocular tumors. J Oncol. 2013:1–22.

12. Sharma R, Grewal J, Gupta S, Murray P. Ophthalmic manifestations of acute leukemias: the ophthalmologist's role. Eye. 2004;18:663–72.

13. Rose-Inman H, Keuhl D. Acute leukemia. Emergency Medicince Clinics of North America. 2014;32(3):579–96.

14. Khaja W, Pgrebniak A, Bolling J. Combined orbital proptosis and exudative retinal detachment as initial manifestations of acute myeloid leukemia. J AAPOS. 2015;19:479–82.

15. Kiratli H, Balci K, Himmetoglu C, Uner A. Isolated extraocular muscle involvement as the ophthalmic manifestation of leukemia. Clin Exp Ophthalmol. 2009;37:609–13.

16. Reddy S, Jackson N, Menon B. Ocular involvement in leukemia – a study of 288 cases. Ophthalmologica. 2003;217:441–5.

17. Huang Y, Wang S, Chen S, Jou J. Bilateral acute proptosis as initial manifestation of acute myeloid leukemia. Orbit. 2015;34:5,248–52.

Metastatic Neuroblastoma

18. Garrity J, Henderson J, Cameron J. Henderson's orbital tumors. 4th ed: Lipincott Williams & Wilkins; 2007.

19. Papaionnou G, McHugh K. Neuroblastoma in childhood. Canccr Imaging. 2005;5(1):116–27.

20. Ahmed S, Goel S, Khandwala M, Agrawal A, Chang B, Simmons IG. Neuroblastoma with orbital metastasis: ophthalmic presentation and role of ophthalmologists. Eye. 2006;20:466–70.

21. Smith J, Diehl N, Smith B, Mohney B. Incidence, ocular manifestations, and survival in children with neuroblastoma: a population-based study. Am J Ophthalmol. 2010;149:677–82.

Lymphangioma

22. Gandhi N, Lin L, O'Hara M. Sildenafil for pediatric orbital lymphangioma. JAMA Ophthalmol. 2013;131(9):1228–30.

23. Jill R, Shiels W II, Foster J, Czyz C, Stacey A, Everman K, et al. Percutaneous drainage and ablation as first line therapy for macrocystic and microcystic orbital lymphatic malformations. Ophthal Plast Reconstr Surg. 2012;28:119–25.

24. Konal S, Leatherbarrow B. Orbital lymhangiomas: a review of management strategies. Curr Opin Ophthalmol. 2012;23:433–8.

25. Schwarz R, Ben Simon G, Cook T, Goldberg R. Sclerosing therapy as first line treatment for low flow vascular lesions of the orbit. Am J Ophthalmol. 2006;141:333–9.

26. Tunc M, Sadr E, Char D. Orbital lymphangiomas: an analysis of 26 patients. Br J Ophthalmol. 1999;83:76–80.

27. Harris G. Orbital vascular malformations: a consensus statement on terminology and its clinical implications. Am J Ophthalmol. 1999;127:453–5.

28. Ko F, DiBernardo C, Oak J, Miller N, Subramanian P. Confirmation of and differentiation among primary vascular lesions using ultrasonography. Ophthal Plast Reconstr Surg. 2011;27:431–5.

29. Shields JA, Shields CL, Scartozzi R. Survey of 1264 patients with orbital tumors and simulating lesions: the 2002 Montgomery lecture, part 1. Ophthalmology. 2004;111:997–1008.

30. Hayasaki A, Nakamura H, Hamasaki R, Makino K, Yan S, Morioka M, et al. Successful treatment of intraorbital lymphangioma with tissue fibrin glue. Surg Neurol. 2009;72:722–4.

31. Kahana A, Bohnsack B, Cho R, Maher C. Subtotal excision with adjunctive sclerosing therapy for the treatment of severe symptomatic orbital lymphangiomas. Arch Ophthalmol. 2011;129(8):1073–6.

Infantile Hemangioma of Infancy

32. Drolet B, Esterly N, Frieden I. Hemangiomas in children. N Engl J Med. 1999 July;341(3):1713–8.

33. Spence-Shishido A, Good W, Baselga E, Frieden I. Hemangiomas and the eye. Clin Dermatol. 2015;33:170–82.

34. Schwartz S, Blei F, Ceisler E, Steele M, Furlan L, Kodis S. Risk factors for amblyopia in children with hemangioma of infancy of the eyelids and orbit. J AAPOS. 2006;10:262–8.

35. Shields JA, Mashayekhi A, Kligman BE, et al. Vascular tumors of the conjunctiva in 140 cases. Ophthalmology. 2011;118:1747–53.

36. Shields JA, Shields CL. Vascular tumors and related lesions of the conjunctiva eyelid, conjunctival and orbital tumors: an atlas and textbook. 3rd ed. Philadephia: Lipincott Walters Kluwer; 2016. p. 349–66.

37. Missoi T, Lueder G, Gilbertson K, Bayliss S. Oral propranolol for treatment of periocular infantile hemangioma. Arch Ophthalmol. 2011;129(7):899–903.

38. Chambers C, Katowitz W, Katowitz J, Binebaum G. A controlled study of topical 0.25% timolol maleate get of the treatment of cutaneous infantile hemangioma of infancy. Ophthal Plast Reconstr Surg. 2012;28:103–6.

39. Levitt M, Coumou A, Groenveld L, Freling NJ, van der Horst C, Saeed P. Propranolol as first-line treatment in orbital infantile hemangiomas: a case series. Orbit. 2014;33(3):178–83.

Retinoblastoma and Leukocoria

40. Ramasubramanian A, Shields C. Retinoblastoma. 1st ed. New Delhi: Jaypee Brothers Medical Publishers; 2012.

41. Shields C. Forget-me-nots in the care of children with retinoblastoma. Semin Ophthalmol. 2008;23: 324–34.

42. Shields C, Manjandavida F, Lally S, Pierettia G, Arepalli S, Caywood E, et al. Intra-arterial chemotherapy for retinoblastoma in 70 eyes. Ophthalmology. 2014:1–8.

43. AlAli A, Kletke S, Gallie B, Lam W. Retinoblastoma for pediatric ophthalmologists. Asia-Pac J Ophthalmol. 2018;7:160–8.

44. Kleinerman R, Yu C, Little M, Abramson D, Seddon J, Tucker M. Variation of second cancer risk by family history of retinoblastoma among long term survivors. J Clin Oncol. 2012;30:950–7.

45. Shields DL, Shields JS. Retinoblastoma management: advance in enucleation, intravenous chemoreduction, and intra-arterial chemotherapy. Curr Opin Ophthalmol. 2010;21:203–12.

46. Abramson DH, Frank CM, Susman M, Whalen MP, Dunker IJ, Boyd NW. 3rd presenting signs of retinoblastoma. J Pediatr. 1998;132(3Pt 1):505–8.

47. Shields CL, Shields JA. Basic understanding of current classification and management of retinoblastoma. Curr Opin Ophthalmol. 2006;17.228–34.

48. Ancona-Lezama D, Dalvin LA, Lucio-Alvarez JA, Jabbour P, Shields CL. Ophthalmic vascular events after intra-arterial chemotherapy for retinoblastoma: real-world comparison between primary and secondary treatments. Retina. 2019;39(12):2264–72.

49. Gonzalez-Montpetit ME, Samara WA, Magrath GN, Shields CL. Detection of minimally visible recurrent retinoblastoma by hand-held spectral domain optical coherence tomography. J Pediatr Ophthalmol Strabismus. 2017;54:e6–8.

50. Abramson DH, Shields CL, Munier FL, Chantada GL. Treatment of retinoblastoma in 2015 agreement and disagreement. JAMA Ophthalmol. 2015;133(11):1341–7.

51. Shields CL, Mashayekhi A, Au AK. The international classification of retinoblastoma predicts chemoreduction success. Ophthalmol. 2006;224: 3376 2280.

52. Shields CL, Alset AE, Say EA, et al. Retinoblastoma control with primary intra-arterial chemotherapy: outcomes before and during the intravitreal chemotherapy era. J Pediatr Ophthalmol Strabismus. 2016;53(5):275–84.

53. Shields CL, Schoenberg E, Kocher K, et al. Lesions simulating retinoblastoma (pseudoretinoblastoma) in 604 cases. Ophthalmology. 2013;120:311–6.

Ophthalmic Plastics

Sana Ali Bautista and William Rocamora Katowitz

Contents

© Springer Nature Switzerland AG 2021
R. Shinder (ed.), *Pediatric Ophthalmology in the Emergency Room*,
https://doi.org/10.1007/978-3-030-49950-1_16

16.1 Introduction

Epiphora, or the overflow of tears, is a very common finding in the pediatric population. From an ophthalmic plastic perspective, epiphora can be caused by obstructive outflow mechanisms or hypersecretion secondary to eyelid/adnexal abnormalities. This chapter will largely focus on the most common causes of epiphora in the pediatric population, specifically congenital nasolacrimal obstruction and its associated pathologies and epiblepharon.

16.2 Anatomy: Lacrimal Drainage System

The nasolacrimal drainage system begins at the medial eyelid. The lacrimal drainage system consists of the lacrimal puncta, lacrimal canaliculi, lacrimal sac, and nasolacrimal duct [1] (◘ Fig. 16.1). The entire length of the drainage system from puncta to meatal opening of the nasolacrimal duct ranges from 25 mm in the newborn to about 35 mm in the adult.

Proper function of this system is essential in preventing epiphora as well as maintaining a healthy ocular surface. The lacrimal puncta (singular, punctum) are small openings located along the superior and inferior medial eyelid margin. The puncta lie in an elevated area of tissue known as the lacrimal papilla. The inferior punctum is approximately half a millimeter lateral to the superior punctum and lies 6.5 mm from the medial canthus. The size of the puncta is 0.2–0.3 mm in diameter and can stretch with punctal dilation [1]. Both puncta are inverted against the globe and are in complete contact with the globe upon eyelid closure. Each punctum drains into its corresponding canaliculus. The canaliculi are canals spanning 10 mm, located within the eyelid margin, medial to the puncta. Tears enter the puncta and travel into the vertical part of the canaliculus which is 2 mm in length and then into the horizontal canaliculus which traverses 8 mm medially, following the course of the lid margin. Next, the superior and inferior canaliculus combine to form a single common canaliculus just prior to the lacrimal sac in 90% of the population [2]. The common canaliculus drains via the internal punctum that enters the lateral surface of the upper one third of the lacrimal sac, in a slightly posterior and inferior location [1]. This angle of entrance forms the valve of Rosenmuller, a mucosal tissue fold preventing reflux. The lacrimal sac is approximately 10–15 mm in vertical length and is oval in shape. The lacrimal sac and the nasolacrimal duct are comprised of stratified columnar epithelium and contain mucus-secreting goblet cells unlike the more proximal portions of the nasolacrimal system. The upper portion of the sac is termed the fundus, while the lower portion is termed the body. The sac lies in a bony fossa between the anterior and posterior lacrimal crests, comprised of the maxillary and lacrimal bones, respectively. The sac spans 2–5 mm above the level of the medial canthal tendon and approximately 10 mm below. The lacrimal sac is anterior to the orbital septum, and there-

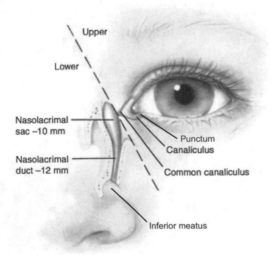

◘ **Fig. 16.1** Anatomy of the lacrimal outflow system. Canaliculi are approximately 10 mm in length. A 2 mm vertical portion widens from punctum into an ampulla where it joins the horizontal canaliculus to enter the sac at the common canaliculus. These structures constitute the upper lacrimal system. The lacrimal sac and duct are considered the lower lacrimal system. The nasolacrimal duct empties into the inferior meatus. [Reprinted by permission from Springer Nature Customer Service Centre GmbH: (Springer Publishing Company) [1]]

fore pathologic processes confined to the lacrimal sac are periorbital (preseptal) in nature. The location of the lacrimal sac relative to the medial canthal tendon aids in diagnosis of periorbital disease and will be discussed later in the chapter. The lacrimal sac is surrounded by periorbital fascia from the posterior lacrimal sac periosteum and receives attachments from the superior and deep limbs of the medial canthal tendon. The two portions of the medial canthal tendon straddle the sac before attaching to the anterior and posterior lacrimal crest (□ Fig. 16.2a). The contraction and relaxation of the orbicularis muscle, medial canthal tendon, and lacrimal sac fascial attachments during blinking results in negative pressure created within the lacrimal sac facilitating tear drainage from the ocular surface in a process termed the lacrimal pump (□ Fig. 16.2b). The sac continues and opens into the nasolacrimal duct, passing inferiorly, posteriorly, and laterally within a canal formed by the maxillary and lacrimal bones. This interosseous portion within the canal is 12 mm. The nasolacrimal duct opens into the inferior meatus of the nose, approximately 2.5 cm posterior to the naris, under the inferior turbinate at the valve of Hasner.

The most common cause of congenital nasolacrimal duct obstruction (CNLDO) is imperforation of the valve of Hasner. This mucosal fold of tissue remains imperforate in about 70% of newborns [2]; however, most resolve within the first month of life and spontaneous opening can continue in the first 6–12 months of life.

16.3 Congenital Nasolacrimal Duct Obstruction

Congenital nasolacrimal duct obstruction (CNLDO) occurs in approximately 5% of newborn infants. It is the most common cause of nasolacrimal duct obstruction in the pediatric age group. It is the most common cause of epiphora and periocular discharge in infants [3]. It is sporadic and occurs at similar rates in males and female. CNLDO can be unilateral or bilateral; however, unilaterality is present in 2/3 of cases. As aforementioned, the location of obstruction is most commonly at the distal valve of Hasner due to an imperforate membrane obstructing outflow [1]. Ninety percent of these cases spontaneously resolve by 12 months of age and most open spontaneously within 4–6 weeks of birth. The second most common cause of CNLDO is ductal stenosis [4]. Other less frequent causes of CNLDO include proximal lacrimal outflow agenesis or maldevelopment of the punctum and canaliculus. Proximal outflow obstruction can occur concurrently with distal obstruction. Risk factors associated with CNLDO at any level include newborns with midline facial anomalies, clefting syndromes, craniosynostoses, and Down syndrome [3]. Infants and children are at increased risk for nasolacrimal obstruction secondary to variation in structure and size of the immature nasolacrimal system. The inferior meatus is flatter and allows little space between the floor of the nose, lateral nasal wall, and inferior turbinate. The limited intranasal space may

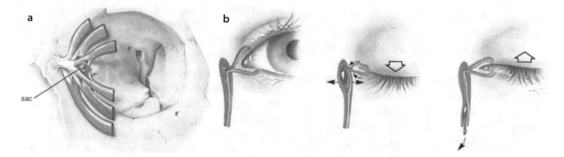

□ **Fig. 16.2** Lacrimal pump. A. Anatomic relationships of the medial canthal tendon and lacrimal sac. B. Stages of lacrimal pump cycle with blinking.

[Reprinted by permission from Springer Nature Customer Service Centre GmbH: (Springer Publishing Company) [1]]

cause impingement of the nasolacrimal duct opening by the inferior turbinate. This space increases with age. The lacrimal sac is also less developed and may impede outflow due to an improper pump mechanism. Congenital lacrimal sac mucocele also known as dacryocystocele and dacryocele forms when both the nasolacrimal duct and the internal punctum are closed in utero [5]. Congenital dacryoceles appear as medial canthal masses at birth. The fluid becomes purulent within days of birth, and neonatal dacryocystitis can occur which can be life-threatening.

Acquired nasolacrimal duct or canalicular obstructions can occur following trauma, viral conjunctivitis, acute dacryocystitis, and use of topical antiviral medications – however, this is out of the scope of this chapter.

16.3.1 Congenital Nasolacrimal Obstruction

16.3.1.1 History

Blockage of the valve of Hasner presents with symptoms such as chronic or intermittent tearing, mucoid or clear discharge, conjunctival injection, and sometimes eyelid edema. A parent may complain that his or her infant has recurrent "pink eye" which raises the suspicion of mucopurulent regurgitation onto the ocular surface causing conjunctivitis. Symptoms may be unilateral or bilateral. Intermittent tearing suggests a partial NLDO, while chronic tearing points to complete NLDO. Worsening with upper respiratory infection is also common. Although rare, preseptal cellulitis may be a complication of valve of Hasner obstruction. Tearing in the first 12 months of life is suspicious for CNLDO; however, there are other, more worrying causes that must initially be ruled out. A complete ophthalmologic examination including intraocular pressure, dilation, and refraction is important in a child with chronic tearing. The history is almost as vital as, if not more than, the examination. A detailed history is essential and should include questions regarding onset, duration, associated symptoms, past medical history, birth history, and

medications. CNLDO usually presents within the first 2 months of life in full-term infants. Some authors attribute this to tear production that approaches normal rate by 6 weeks of life [6]. Important associated symptoms such as blepharospasm, photophobia, strabismus, or nystagmus should cause concern for congenital glaucoma. Tearing is very common in congenital glaucoma and, if misdiagnosed, can lead to visually devastating outcomes. Significant itching or presence of tearing when outdoors suggests allergy. Other differential diagnoses include acute conjunctivitis and eyelid abnormalities such as entropion, epiblepharon, and trichiasis. Diagnosis is most often clinical for CNLDO, but certain signs can help elucidate the diagnosis.

16.3.1.2 Examination

A thorough ophthalmic exam should be performed in every child presenting with epiphora. Vision, pupil evaluation, extraocular motility, alignment, anterior segment, and dilated fundus examination with cycloplegic retinoscopy should be performed. Although less common than CNLDO, a comprehensive ocular exam can reveal congenital glaucoma which often presents with tearing in addition to photophobia and blepharospasm. If there is suspicion for glaucoma, it is necessary to perform an examination under anesthesia with measurement of intraocular pressure, gonioscopy, and careful eye examination. Failure to diagnose infantile glaucoma can lead to significant, irreversible vision loss.

Simple observation can help give many clues to the etiology of tearing. It is important to establish a relationship with both the parent and the child prior to examination in order to gain trust and cooperation [1]. Attention to the adnexal and eyelid structures is important. One of the most common causes of tearing from hypersecretion due to corneal irritation is from epiblepharon. This is different from a frank entropion where the eyelid margin is inwardly rotated. In epiblepharon the skin and orbicularis muscle override the lower (or upper) eyelid crease and push the eyelashes toward the eye. In more severe cases of epiblepharon, the eyelashes rub the cornea.

This finding is more common in children of Asian and Hispanic descent.

In older children, it may be possible to use a slit lamp biomicroscope for a better examination of the eyelids, puncta, and periorbita. Questions to consider include: Are the puncta absent (upper lacrimal system obstruction)? Are the lashes inverted toward the ocular surface? Is there any ocular surface or corneal abnormality (i.e., enlarged corneal diameter, conjunctivitis, keratitis)? Instillation of fluorescein onto the ocular surface and use of a Wood's lamp can show corneal abnormalities (i.e., abrasion, dryness, ulceration) which can lead to secondary hypersecretion. Are the eyelids in correct position? Eyelid abnormalities such as entropion and epiblepharon can irritate the cornea and are causes of secondary hypersecretion. The latter will be discussed later in the chapter. Craniofacial abnormalities including midfacial and eyelid abnormalities should be noted as they can be both associated with eyelid abnormalities and obstructive outflow.

The typical findings in a child with CNLDO include an increased tear lake, mucoid discharge, and eyelash crusting and mattering (■ Fig. 16.3) [1, 2]. Simple observation of a child with the help of a parent or caregiver may reveal periocular skin irritation and crusting. One of the most important and sensitive examination techniques which can also aid in diagnosis is palpation of the lacrimal sac area. This may be difficult in younger children but can be important in determining the location of nasolacrimal obstruction. Firm pressure is applied over the medial can-

thal area while the puncta are observed for reflux. Reflux of material onto the ocular surface implies a patent upper lacrimal system and obstruction distal to the lacrimal sac. However, if there is no reflux, it does not rule out a lower lacrimal system abnormality. Swelling in the medial canthal area is an important sign especially in neonates. Enlargement below the medial canthal tendon signifies either a dacryocele/dacryocystocele or, if erythematous with inflammatory signs, dacryocystitis. Swelling above the medial canthal tendon always requires further investigation as these may be neoplastic masses, frontal sinus encephaloceles, or anterior ethmoidal mucoceles [7].

16.3.1.3 Diagnosis
Dye Disappearance Test (DDT)

History and in-office examination can help rule out hypersecretory causes of tearing, but if there is still a concern regarding diagnosis, further testing may be required. In adults, irrigation of the nasolacrimal system can be performed; however, this is often not possible in the pediatric patient. A less invasive test of tear outflow can be performed termed the dye disappearance test (DDT). The dye disappearance test involves the instillation of fluorescein dye (dropper or wetting a fluorescein strip with topical anesthetic) into the lower fornices of both eyes. Excess dye is wiped from around the eye, and the ocular surface is observed after 5 minutes. The disappearance of dye from the ocular surface is observed using cobalt blue light on the slit lamp or Wood's lamp (■ Fig. 16.4). Obstruction of outflow is present if retained dye with increased tear meniscus is present at 5 minutes [8]. Disappearance of dye within 5 minutes indicates a patent nasolacrimal system. The DDT cannot localize the site of obstruction. It can also be difficult to assess the tear lake if the child begins to cry or becomes uncooperative after fluorescein instillation. The Jones dye tests are usually performed after the DDT in adults and can often localize obstruction to the upper or lower lacrimal system. However, like irrigation, these tests are not feasible in children.

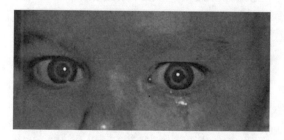

■ **Fig. 16.3** Clinical photograph in an infant showing left-sided epiphora due to congenital nasolacrimal duct obstruction. [Reprinted by permission from Springer Nature Customer Service Centre GmbH: (Springer Publishing Company) [1]]

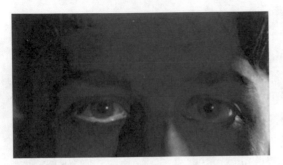

◘ Fig. 16.4 Fluorescein dye disappearance test. Positive fluorescein dye disappearance test with increased tear meniscus on the right side indicating outflow obstruction. The dye has disappeared from the left eye after 5 minutes of instillation. [Reprinted by permission from Springer Nature Customer Service Centre GmbH: (Springer Publishing Company) [1]]

Dacryocystography (DCG) and Dacryoscintigraphy (DSG)

Additional testing for outflow obstruction includes dacryocystography (DCG) and dacryoscintigraphy (DSG). These tests are reserved for selected patients or if there is an atypical history or examination. Dacryocystography (DCG) is a radiologic test that is helpful in determining anatomical abnormalities in the nasolacrimal system. It details the site of obstruction and is helpful in the setting of mucocele, stones, neoplasms, and fistulae [1]. Although helpful in adults, its use in children is limited because most of the aforementioned lacrimal pathologies are rare in the pediatric population. It also requires the use of general anesthesia in children. Orbital X-ray films are taken (AP and lateral) prior to examination. A radiopaque dye is then injected with a lacrimal cannula into the lower canaliculus of each eye. Serial anterior-posterior and oblique films are taken at 15 and 30 minutes after instillation [1]. DCG provides visualization of the lacrimal apparatus and sites of obstruction. DCG exposes the patient to radiation and thus further limits its use in the pediatric population.

Dacryoscintigraphy (DSG) is another diagnostic modality of tear outflow that is more practical in children. Unlike DCG, DSG does not require lacrimal injection of dye and therefore does not require general anesthesia

in young children. It also exposes the patient to much less radiation [9]. Patients are premedicated with potassium perchlorate (6 mg/kg) to prevent thyroidal uptake of the radioactive tracer, technetium-99 m pertechnetate. The patient is placed in front of a gamma camera such that both lateral canthi and the tip of the nose are visible in the camera's view. The parent can often hold the child's head in place for the test. Ten microliters of 100 µCi of technetium-99 m pertechnetate is then instilled into each eye. A gamma camera captures the emitted radiation from the tracer within the nasolacrimal system and creates a two-dimensional image. Sequential analogue images are taken four times per minute for 20 minutes. Flow into the sac usually occurs within 1 minute and into the duct within 2–3 minutes [1]. Delayed clearance can indicate a functional or anatomic obstruction. The patient can participate to help elucidate the cause of obstruction. Having the patient forcefully blink can increase the lacrimal pump force and overcome any functional obstruction. DSG can provide qualitative assessment of lacrimal outflow in select children and is often more practical than dacryocystography.

Imaging modalities such as computed tomography (CT) or magnetic resonance imaging (MRI) are usually not necessary for CNLDO. Dilation of the lacrimal sac can cause swelling inferior to the medial canthal tendon and is typical of dacryocele and therefore does not require imaging. However, if there is any questionable presentation, imaging is warranted. CT or MRI is necessary if a patient presents with swelling above the medial canthal tendon because imaging may show neoplasm, encephalocele, or ethmoidal mucocele. Imaging is also warranted in refractory dacryoceles. MRI is often preferred in the pediatric population due to the ionizing radiation and subsequent risk of secondary cancers when using CT. An exception is the presence of a canine maxillary tooth that may obstruct the lacrimal outflow at the level of the lacrimal duct and can only be fully appreciated with CT imaging [10].

16.3.1.4 **Management of CNLDO**

It is important to determine the specific cause of CNLDO prior to invasive therapy as treatment can vastly vary. In some cases, diagnosis and treatment are simultaneously accomplished. The initial treatment for CNLDO is conservative because spontaneous resolution can occur in 80% to 94.7% of cases within 12 months [11–15]. Conservative management consists of topical antibiotic eyedrop or ointment in conjunction with lacrimal sac Crigler massage (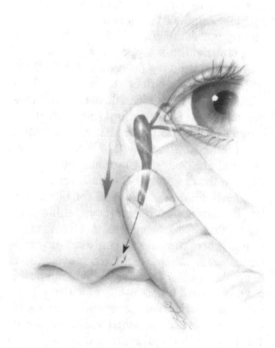 Fig. 16.5). The Crigler massage involves sliding the fingertip from a superior to inferior direction along the lacrimal crest, starting at the medial canthal tendon. Moderate pressure should be used over the sac and duct. Antibiotic ointment can be applied to the finger for lubrication during massage. Using dacryoscintigraphy, Foster and Katowitz demonstrated that the downward motion of the massage forces fluid down the obstructed duct [16]. Therefore, it is essen-

Fig. 16.5 In the Crigler massage, the fingertip should be placed over the medial canthal area and moderate pressure applied over the lacrimal as the fingertip is moved in an inferior direction. [Reprinted by permission from Springer Nature Customer Service Centre GmbH: (Springer Publishing Company) [1]]

tial to demonstrate proper massage technique to the caregivers. There have been no long-term effects associated with chronic (6–9 months) use of antibiotic ointments, erythromycin, or polymyxin B-bacitracin [17]. Polymyxin ointment is more prone to causing an allergic skin reaction than erythromycin; however, if the surrounding eyelid skin appears irritated and itches, the ointment should be stopped immediately.

Probing and Irrigation

If conservative measures fail, then the next step is probing the nasolacrimal duct. Initial probing has shown success rates of 96.4% when performed in patients younger than 13 months based on a large study by Katowitz and Welsh [11]. There is a decline in the success of probing as the child ages past 13 months. Therefore, the authors recommend that conservative measures be instituted until 12 months of age and, if unsuccessful, initial probing can be performed at approximately 1 year of age. In 2018, a large cohort study again reviewed the spontaneous resolution of patients with congenital NLDO and suggested that the optimal timing of initial surgical intervention may be between 9 months and 15 months of age [18]. Thus, while there is no accepted standard for the timing of surgery in infants, an initial intervention should be considered sometime around a child's first year of life. Success of probing also depends on the type and severity of the obstruction.

Probing can be performed in the office or operating room (OR) based on physician preference. An in-office probing is extremely painful and difficult in an awake, crying, and moving child. It carries the risk of false passage, infection, airway obstruction due to bleeding and edema, and ocular injury and should be considered only in newborns with unilateral dacryoceles.

Probing in the OR carries the risk of general anesthesia; however, it allows the surgeon to perform a complete diagnostic examination including inspection of the nasal passages and confirmation of diagnosis. Therapeutic probing can then be performed in a controlled setting and decreases the risk of damage to the fragile lacrimal system. If initial probing in the OR does not clear the obstruction, the surgeon may be able to perform infracture of the inferior turbinate with or without silicone intubation in the same procedure, decreasing the need for repeated anesthesia exposure.

In the OR, there should be an experienced pediatric anesthesiologist. The choice of endotracheal tube intubation (ETT) versus laryngeal masked airway (LMA) depends upon the risk of laryngospasm as well as need for intranasal access. LMA provides free access to the nose for retrieval of fluids during irrigation and ability to perform infracture of the inferior turbinate. LMA is advantageous in shorter procedures such as probing and irrigation and decreases the chance of laryngospasm because it does not manipulate the glottis or trachea and can be removed in a deep state easier than ETT. LMA maintains the airway and can be used for longer procedures should stenting or infracture become necessary. Laryngospasm is a life-threatening airway concern in the pediatric population and can also be minimized by decreasing secretions that stimulate the nose and throat. Small volume fluorescein irrigation (0.5 ml or less) and the use of nasal vasoconstrictors such as oxymetazoline 0.05% decrease the chance of irritation, while the latter also provides hemostasis.

After general anesthesia is achieved, the surgeon should first examine the lacrimal puncta. If they are both present on one side, probing and dilation of the upper puncta is warranted. Upper punctal probing is less manipulative to the upper lacrimal system as compared to inferior punctal probing which requires simultaneous manipulation of the lower eyelid. Probing and dilation must be performed carefully because aggressive dilation can lead to tearing of surrounding orbicularis oculi fibers. Forcing the probe can also create false passages. Significant dilation may cause loss of future canalicular stents, should they be needed. A blunt, 23-gauge lacrimal cannula is attached to a syringe containing several milliliters of diluted fluorescein solution. The cannula is used as a probe and is similar in diameter to the #0 or #00 Bowman lacrimal probe. The preferred cannula has a smooth tip with the port on the side and has a slight curve. As the cannula passes, the surgeon can feel for any strictures or stenosis in the upper puncta or canaliculi. If unable to pass, the surgeon should stop and use a smaller Bowman probe. The probe or cannula is passed down into the nasolacrimal duct until it meets resistance. The instrument should slide easily into the nasolacrimal duct and should not be forced. Dye is injected from the syringe to test the patency of the system which is confirmed when dye is suctioned from the inferior meatus. Inferior turbinate infracture is a procedure commonly performed by lacrimal surgeons to allow for less crowding of structures at the inferior meatus and the valve of Hasner, in an effort to improve tear drainage.

Nasolacrimal Stent Intubation

When upon probing the nasolacrimal system, a surgeon encounters mucosal or bony stenosis, a nasolacrimal stent may be placed. Most lacrimal surgeons consider this a secondary procedure after a failed probing; however, some authors support the placement of stents as a primary procedure for CNLDO [19]. Modern tear duct stents are made of silicone and can be bicanalicular or monocanalicular. The Crawford or Guibor stents are suaged to a metal probe that requires intranasal retrieval with a hook or hemostat. They also require being tied intranasally or being fixed to the nasal wall. Currently, bicanalicular stents are most often used for bicanalicular lacerations and dacryocystorhinostomy procedures. Monocanalicular stents represented a breakthrough in tear duct surgery as no endonasal securing procedure was needed. Monocanalicular Crawford or Ritleng probes may be used. When using a Ritleng stent, intranasal retrieval of the prolene thread guide of the stent is accomplished with a long hook. Both the monocanalicular and bicanalicular stents that are pushed into the nose offer the advantage of being able to treat nasolacrimal duct stenosis and have been compared in the literature [20]. Monocanalicular stents are preferred in most cases of ductal stenosis due to their many advantages. As aforementioned,

16

they do not require endonasal fixation which allows for faster surgery and decreased time under anesthesia. In addition to this, mono-canalicular stents have shown to be more successful, with lower rates of dislodgement, canalicular slitting, and premature removal in comparison with bicanalicular stenting [20]. The placement of a monocanalicular stent also does not require sedation for removal and is technically an easier procedure. A more recent variant of the Monoka stent that is pushed into the nose offers the advantage of not requiring intranasal retrieval, but is less effective in treating ductal stenosis and is indicated for mucosal obstructions in the tear system [21].

Complications of stenting should be explained prior to intubation. One of the most common complications of stenting is displacement of the silicone tubing up the duct and into the lacrimal sac. Since there is no endonasal fixation, the bicanalicular stent may be pulled at the medial canthus, pulling the knots of the tube into the lacrimal sac. This will be visible as a long loop of the tubing visible at the medial canthus and extending toward or lying on the globe. This can be managed by cutting the loop and pulling the knots out through the puncta. Monocanalicular stents can become unseated and sit loose in the eyelid. Less commonly monocanalicular stents can migrate into the nasolacrimal system causing inflammation and persistent symptoms including infection (dacryocystitis). Other complications of silicone stenting include pyogenic granuloma, conjunctival or corneal abrasion, and frank extrusion of tubing.

Canalicular slitting, or cheese wiring, of the canaliculi and puncta can occur with bicanalicular stenting especially if the loop is tied too tight initially. Slitting can also occur as a child's face and lacrimal system grow since the loop is a fixed length. The loop should be tied loosely enough to prevent canalicular slitting but also not so loose as to allow for extrusion.

Postoperative bleeding in the nose presenting as frank hemorrhage is uncommon but can be serious in a small child. If conservative measures such as oxymetolazine nasal spray, cold compresses, and head elevation do not work, nasal packing or cautery can be applied in a controlled setting.

Balloon Dacryoplasty

An alternative to stent placement is a procedure to widen the tear duct mucosa (and when possible soft bone). This procedure was developed from angioplasty technology and applied to tear duct surgery. It involves the intubation of the nasolacrimal system with a catheter that can expand when filled with saline with the use of a pressurized pump. Balloon dilation is applied to the lower portion of the nasolacrimal duct and again to the upper portion. Balloon dacryoplasty does not require stenting and therefore avoids the potential complications of stents such as stent prolapse, as well as the second OR procedure and anesthesia needed in many children for removal of the stent [22]. It is also technically easier than primary silicone intubation with similar success rates. A comparison of this procedure to stenting was found to be equally efficacious in a small series [23].

Dacryocystorhinostomy

If the lower tear system is unable to adequately transmit tears, a tear duct bypass may be needed. Ideally the upper system will transmit tears into the tear sac. If one or both puncta and canaliculi are patent, a connection of the tear sac can be made directly into the nose. This is a dacryocystorhinostomy (DCR), which involves making a window in the lacrimal sac fossa and opening the tear sac so tears may flow directly into the nose.

The decision to pursue DCR is undertaken after less invasive procedures have been attempted. The authors recommend less invasive procedures such as probing with possible infracture of the inferior turbinate, balloon dilation, and/or silicone stent intubation prior to DCR. Age does play a role in the decision to pursue DCR. Blood loss in the pediatric group is more significant the younger the patient. Intranasal passages are also much smaller which makes early surgery more challenging, requiring smaller instruments and endoscopes. DCR is usually not required in children less than 1 year of age; however, the authors have performed successful DCR in an infant as young as 2 weeks of age. The necessity of early DCR is uncommon and most often seen in cases with acute severe dacryocystitis in combination with osseous or craniofacial abnormalities.

This surgery classically has been accomplished via a medial canthal incision or lower eyelid crease incision. Kerrison rongeurs are used to create a window via bone removal of the lacrimal sac fossa bones. The lacrimal sac mucosa can then be directly anastomosed to the nasal mucosa in the form of sewn mucosal flaps. A lacrimal stent is helpful if placed to help prevent adhesions to the common canalicular opening and surgical rhinostomy.

With the advance of endoscopic endonasal surgery, the ability to perform DCR surgery without the need for a skin incision has evolved and is now considered as effective as the external approach [24].

Endoscopic formation of a rhinostomy can be performed with Kerrison rongeurs. Surgical instrumentation has evolved to allow for the use of high-powered drills, such as a diamond burr or more recently an ultrasonic bone aspirator as described by Murchison et al. [25]. This latter device is very effective in pediatric patients with a more crowded nasal anatomy.

Tear Duct Bypass Tube (Jones and Cox Tubes)

When the upper nasolacrimal system is unable to transmit tears, a connection must be made from the conjunctiva to the nose. This problem can be primary in the setting of agenesis of the lacrimal puncta and canaliculi or acquired due to nasolacrimal trauma or infection. A tube made of Pyrex glass (Jones or Cox) is inserted from the inferior-medial conjunctival cul-de-sac extending into the nose. Ideally, a surgical rhinostomy is created to allow the tube to be suspended by the conjunctiva and nasal mucosa.

16.3.1.5 Dacryocele/Dacryocystocele

Dacryocele, also known as dacryocystocele, is a type of CNLDO. It is an uncommon cause of CNLDO, but it requires prompt recogni-

tion and management. Congenital dacryocele occurs in utero from a distal blockage of the lacrimal sac causing it to distend and eventually kink off the connection to the canaliculus. It is also understood that the valve of Rosenmuller is a unidirectional valve and therefore would not drain the lacrimal sac via the canaliculi. The mucus secreted from the lacrimal sac accumulates and dilates the sac and duct. Amniotic fluid can also be trapped in the sac. Newborns present with a mass below the medial canthal tendon that may have a bluish hue (◘ Fig. 16.6). It can be misdiagnosed as a hemangioma due to the similar skin discoloration. Congenital dacryocele may also present with respiratory distress secondary to extension of the dilated duct into the nose or the concurrent presence of intranasal cysts. Neonates are obligatory nasal breathers, and therefore a nasal mass may cause difficulty with breathing and potentially be life-threatening [5]. A prompt recognition of the dacryocele is necessary because it is often complicated by dacryocystitis. Infection of the dacryocele contents leads to erythema, swelling, and systemic signs of illness in a neonate. Management of non-infected congenital dacryocele is initially conservative with gentle massage of the lacrimal sac in an attempt to clear the obstruction [26]. It is necessary to emphasize a gentle massage because vigorous massage may lead to lacrimal sac rupture and subsequent cellulitis. In addition to massage, warm compresses and topical antibiotics have also been used as conservative treatment for dacryocele. If the dacryo-

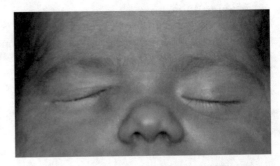

◘ **Fig. 16.6** Right-sided dacryocele. Clinical photograph in an infant showing a bluish subcutaneous mass just inferior to the medial canthal tendon

cele persists beyond 1 or 2 weeks, probing of the nasolacrimal system is indicated. This is unlike valve of Hasner obstruction but necessary due to the high risk of dacryocystitis. Probing can be done in office with observation or in the operating room under general anesthesia. Neonates are relatively immuno-compromised and are at high risk for sepsis and death if dacryocystitis is untreated [18]. Neonates with dacryoceles must be watched very closely in the first 2 weeks of life. Any sign of infection warrants the initiation of intravenous antibiotics and prompt surgery to relieve the obstruction. If the dacryocystitis is severe, it can cause cellulitis and even rupture the skin surface.

Intranasal cysts may block the distal end of the duct and have recently been associated as being present in most children with dacryoceles [18, 27]. These cysts can block the distal part of the duct and can be present in pediatric NLDO beyond the neonatal period. A suggestion of the presence of an intranasal cyst is failed nasolacrimal probing. In these situations, an examination under anesthesia with an endoscope may show the cyst. Levin et al. discovered associated intranasal cysts in 23 out of 24 patients with dacryoceles or dacryocystitis [27]. ◘ Table 16.1 summarizes an approach to the pediatric patient with dacryocystitis and dacryoceles.

16.3.2 Epiblepharon

Epiblepharon should always be considered as a cause of tearing in infants. It has been estimated that this eyelid malposition occurs in approximately 12.6% of Asians [28]. This condition can be congenital or acquired. It is most often caused by an overriding horizontal thin strip of eyelid skin and orbicularis oculi muscle causing the eyelashes to be directed vertically and should be differentiated from an entropion where the eyelid margin itself is rotated inward. The lower eyelid is often more involved than the upper. This is especially true in patients of Asian or Hispanic descent. When epiblepharon is diagnosed, it is important to assess the impact on the patient. Most of the time, epiblepharon is asymptomatic in children and can be observed. In obtaining a history, the frequency of tearing and eye rubbing should alert the physician to the severity of epiblepharon. Similar to other eyelid malpositions, misdirection of lashes may cause ocular surface symptoms ranging from mild to severe including epiphora, foreign body sensation, photophobia, and blepharospasm [29].

On exam, visual acuity should be measured. In an infant, preferential gaze testing should be tested to screen for amblyopia. A patient who has unilateral symptoms should raise the concern for deprivation amblyopia

◘ Table 16.1 Age-related management of pediatric dacryocystitis and dacryocele

Is there an infected tear system	Age <6 months	Age >6 months	Notes
Yes (dacryocystitis)	Consider admission and IV antibiotics	Oral antibiotics (only if afebrile) with close follow-up	Consider surgery with persistent fevers and symptoms
No (unilateral dacryocele)	Office probing with close observation for respiratory distress	Consider surgery given risk for dacryocystitis	Beware of the presence of an intranasal cyst
No (bilateral dacryocele)	Do not probe in the office. Promptly schedule for surgery given the risk of respiratory distress and dacryocystitis	Do not probe in the office. Promptly schedule for surgery given the risk of respiratory distress and dacryocystitis	Beware of the presence of an intranasal cyst

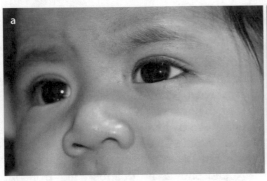

Fig. 16.7 Lower eyelid epiblepharon. **a** Clinical photograph of a 6-month-old with lower eyelid epiblepharon. **b** Clinical photograph of that same patient 6 months after bilateral lower eyelid epiblepharon repair using the technique described in **Fig. 16.8

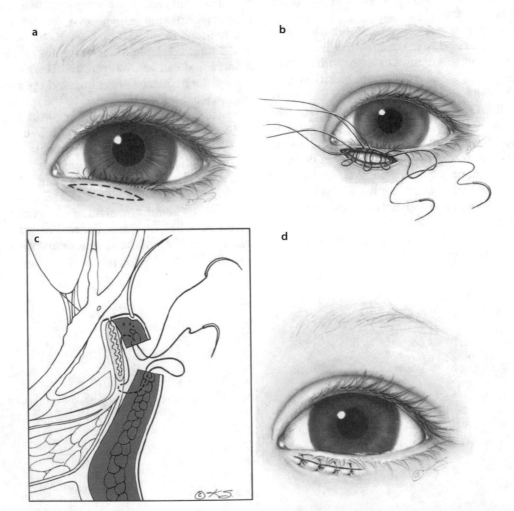

Fig. 16.8 Repair of epiblepharon. **a** The ellipse of skin and orbicularis oculi are marked for excision on the lid. **b** Orbicularis and lower eyelid retractors along the inferior aspect of the incision are sutured to the tarsus and orbicularis along the superior edge of the incision using a double-armed suture. **c** Diagrammatic representation of suture placement in sagittal section. **d** The skin is closed with absorbable suture. [Reprinted by permission from Springer Nature Customer Service Centre GmbH: (Springer Publishing Company) [1]]

due to symptomatic epiblepharon. A corneal exam followed by fluorescein staining is critical to assess the clinical impact of the lashes rubbing on the cornea. ■ Figure 16.7 depicts a pediatric patient with lower eyelid epiblepharon before and after surgical repair. No corneal staining or the presence of scant punctate epithelial erosions can be managed with observation and/or lubricants. Confluent epithelial erosions, corneal abrasion, or rarely corneal ulceration would warrant surgical repair. In most cases surgery can be avoided, but should be considered if medical management has failed, especially if a child has evidence of vision compromise from the epiblepharon.

If surgery is needed in the lower eyelid, a surgical repair involves an incision just below the eyelashes (subciliary incision). The lower eyelid retractors should be dissected and advanced onto the tarsus to rotate the eyelashes anteriorly. Care must be made to not be overaggressive which can induce an ectropion. A small ellipse of skin and orbicularis can be removed and the skin closed with a running gut suture. This technique is summarized in ■ Fig. 16.8a–d. An upper eyelid surgical repair of epiblepharon may require a skin crease incision to debulk and remove skin and orbicularis oculi as needed.

Case Presentation

A 2-week-old male presented to the emergency department, brought in by his mother with complaints of redness and swelling under the infant's left eyelid as well as increasing discharge from the left eye for 2 days. The mother reported he was born with a "bump" under his left eyelid. She expressed concern that he was not feeding well and had a fever. On examination, there was an erythematous mass overlying the left medial lower eyelid with associated preseptal cellulitis (■ Fig. 16.9a). There were no signs of respiratory distress. Maxillofacial CT was ordered sec-

ondary to severity and globe displacement. The neonate was urgently brought to the operating room, and intravenous antibiotics were started. Nasal endoscopy revealed a cyst at the level of the inferior turbinate. A microdebrider was used to remove the cyst as well as irrigate and aspirate the purulent material which was sent for culture. The intranasal cyst was marsupialized, and patency of the nasolacrimal system was confirmed with fluorescein dye instillation. The dacryocystitis resolved and the patient showed marked improvement (■ Fig. 16.9b).

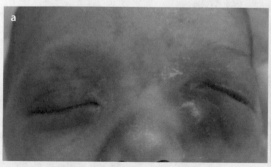 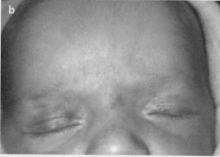

■ Fig. 16.9 Acute dacryocystitis. a Clinical photograph showing significant periorbital edema and erythema centered at the left lacrimal sac fossa. b Clinical photograph showing marked improvement 1 week after antibiotic and surgical therapy

Key Points

- Surgical interventions in infants under the age of 12 should be reserved for cases of dacryoceles or dacryocystitis or when a patient is already under general anesthesia for a different surgery.
- Most cases of congenital nasolacrimal duct obstruction resolve by the age of 12 months.
- During nasolacrimal duct probing, if ductal stenosis is encountered, consider placing a stent or performing a balloon dacryoplasty concurrently.
- Dacryocystorhinostomy can be reserved for cases in which more conservative interventions have failed.
- Epiblepharon can often be managed with ocular lubricants alone without the need for surgery.

❓ Review Questions

1. A 6-month-old presents with unilateral tearing and discharge. There is no lacrimal sac mass or expressible mucus with massage. What is the best treatment for this child?
   - (a) An in-office probing
   - (b) A probing under general anesthesia
   - (c) No intervention since this will likely get better by age 1
   - (d) Tear duct massage and topical antibiotics until the symptoms improve up to 12 months of age

2. A 24-month-old female has persistent right-sided tearing without discharge after the placement of a monocanalicular stent at age 13 months. The stent was kept in place for 3 months and was removed in the office. The child has remained symptomatic despite surgery 8 months ago. In-office dye disappearance testing is 2+ on the right and 0 on the left. What is the best treatment for this child?
   - (a) Observation only. The child can grow out of this problem and is not at risk for dacryocystitis since she has had surgery already.
   - (b) In-office probing and stenting.
   - (c) Given the persistent symptoms, consider a repeat probing and stent, or balloon dacryoplasty or dacryo-cystorhinostomy.
   - (d) Jones or Cox tube placement since a probing with stent has failed.

3. A 4-month-old girl of Korean descent present with tearing and no discharge. Handheld slit lamp reveals bilateral lower eyelid epiblepharon with the central and medial lashes touching the cornea. You perform a dye disappearance test and see only trace dye pooling in the eyelid after 5 minutes. The corneas do not stain with fluorescein. What is the best approach for this patient?
   - (a) Take this child to the operating room, and perform lower eyelid retractor advancements to repair the lower eyelid epiblepharon.
   - (b) Start this child on a topical antibiotic ointment.
   - (c) Since there is no corneal staining, you can start this child on a moderately viscous artificial tear four times a day.
   - (d) Prescribe a very viscous artificial tear (for severe dry eye) to be applied every 3 hours.

✓ Answers

1. (d)
2. (c)
3. (c)

References

1. Katowitz JA, Katowitz WR. Pediatric oculoplastic surgery. 2nd ed. Cham: Springer International Publishing; 2018.
2. Cassady JV. Developmental anatomy of nasolacrimal duct. Arch Ophthalmol. 1952;47(2):141–58.
3. Nelson LB, Calhoun JH, Menduke H. Medical management of congenital nasolacrimal duct obstruction. Ophthalmology. 1985;92(9):1187–90.
4. Nasolacrimal duct obstruction, congenital [Internet]. Bacterial Conjunctivitis – EyeWiki. 2018 [cited 2019 Feb 11]. Available from: http://eyewiki.aao.org/Nasolacrimal_Duct_Obstruction,_Congenital.
5. Nerad JA, Carter KD, Alford M. Oculoplastic and reconstructive surgery. St. Louis: Mosby Elsevier; 2008.

16

6. Nelson LB. Treatment of congenital nasolacrimal duct obstruction. J Pediatr Ophthalmol Strabismus. 2016;53(5):246–50.

7. Guerry D, Kendig EL. Congenital impatency of the nasolacrimal duct. Arch Ophthalmol. 1948; 39(2):193–204.

8. Salvin JH, Schnall B. Refractive corrections in infants. Journal of Pediatric Ophthalmology & Strabismus. 2012;49(4):198–200.

9. Heyman S, Katowitz JA. Dacryoscintigraphy. In: Pediatric nuclear medicine. New York: Springer; 1985. p. 233–43.

10. Fayet B, Racy E, Bordonné C, Katowitz WR, Katowitz J, Brémond-Gignac D. Complex bony congenital nasolacrimal duct obstruction caused by an adjacent canine tooth bud. Ophthal Plast Reconstr Surg. 2019;35(1):23 4.

11. Katowitz JA, Welsh MG. Timing of initial probing and irrigation in congenital nasolacrimal duct obstruction. Ophthalmology. 1987;94(6):698–705.

12. Peterson RA, Robb RM. The natural course of congenital obstruction of the nasolacrimal duct. J Pediatr Ophthalmol Strabismus. 1978;15:246.

13. Nelson LB, Calhoun JH, Menduke FI. Medical management of congenital nasolacrimal duct obstruction. Ophthalmology. 1985;92:1187.

14. Price HW. Dacryostenosis. J Pediatr. 1947;30(3):302–5.

15. Paul TO. Medical management of congenital nasolacrimal duct obstruction. J Pediatr Ophthalmol Strabismus. 1985;22:68–70.

16. Foster JA, Katowitz JA, Heyman S. Results of dacryoscintigraphy in passage of congenitally blocked nasolacrimal duct. Ophthal Plast Reconstr Surg. 1996;12:27–32.

17. Crigler LW. The treatment on congenital dacryocystitis. JAMA. 1923;81:23.

18. Payesse E, Coats D, Bernstein J, Go C, de Jong A. Management and complications of congenital dacryocele with concurrent intranasal mucocele. J AAPOS. 2000;4(1):46–53.

19. Engel JM, Hicuje-Schmidt C, Khammar A, Ostfeld BM, Vyas A, Ticho BH. Monocanalicular silastic intubation for the initial correction of congenital nasolacrimal duct obstruction. J AAPOS. 2007;11(2):183–6.

20. Kominek P, Cervenka S, Pniak T, Zelenik K, Tomášková H, Matoušek P. Monocanalicular versus bicanalicular intubation in the treatment of congenital nasolacrimal duct obstruction. Graefes Arch Clin Exp Ophthalmol. 2011;249:1729–33.

21. Fayet B, Katowitz WR, Racy E, Ruban J, Katowitz JA. Pushed monocanalicular intubation: an alternative stenting system for the management of congenital nasolacrimal duct obstructions. J AAPOS. 2012;16(5):468–72.

22. Ali M. Chapter 16. Minimal invasive lacrimal surgeries: balloon dacryoplasty. In: Lacrimal drainage surgery. New Delhi: Jaypee Brothers Medical Publishers; 2014. p. 79–85.

23. Goldstein SM, Goldstein JB, Katowitz JA. Comparison of monocanalicular stenting and balloon dacryoplasty in secondary treatment of congenital nasolacrimal duct obstruction after failed primary probing. Ophthal Plast Reconstr Surg. 2004;20(5):352–7.

24. Fayet B, Katowitz WR, Racy E, Ruban JM, Katowitz JA. Endoscopic dacryocystorhinostomy: the keys to surgical success. Ophthal Plast Reconstr Surg. 2014;30(1):69–71.

25. Murchison AP, et al. The ultrasonic bone aspirator in transnasal endoscopic dacryocystorhinostomy. Ophthal Plast Reconstr Surg. 2013;29(1):25–9.

26. Schnall BM, Christian CJ. Conservative treatment of congenital dacryocele. J Pediatr Ophthalmol Strabismus. 1996;33:219–21.

27. Levin AV, Wygnanski-Jaffe T, Forte V, Buckwalter JA, Buncic JR. Nasal endoscopy in the treatment of congenital lacrimal sac mucoceles. Int J Pediatr Otorhinolaryngol. 2003;67(3):255–61.

28. Kim JS, Jin SW, Hur MC, Kwon YH, Ryu WY, Jeong WJ, Ahn HB. The clinical characteristics and surgical outcomes of epiblepharon in Korean children: a 9-year experience. J Ophthalmol. 2014;2014:156501, 5 pages. https://doi.org/10.1155/2014/156501.

29. Sundar G, Young SM, Tara S, Tan AM, Amrith S. Epiblepharon in east Asian patients: the Singapore experience. Ophthalmology. 2010;117(1):184–9.

Headache, Visual Loss and Papilledema

Valerie I. Elmalem, Duaa Sharfi, and Daniel Wang

Contents

© Springer Nature Switzerland AG 2021
R. Shinder (ed.), *Pediatric Ophthalmology in the Emergency Room*,
https://doi.org/10.1007/978-3-030-49950-1_17

17.1 Introduction

This chapter describes the workup of visual loss and the various presentations and diagnostic criteria for headaches in the pediatric population. The provider will learn examination techniques to differentiate between objective and nonorganic visual loss. The material will also enable healthcare providers to recognize signs of underlying conditions that manifest as headaches and efficiently treat chronic headache disorders.

17.2 Nonphysiologic Visual Loss

Nonphysiologic visual loss, or nonorganic visual loss (NOVL), manifests as a decrease in visual acuity or color vision, photopsias, or visual field defect that cannot be explained by a physiologic process [1]. It falls on a wide spectrum of conditions that include conversion disorder, malingering, and factitious disorder. When there is underlying pathology but the visual loss is exaggerated, it is called functional overlay. These patients present unique challenges for the provider and caretakers.

17.2.1 Etiology

NOVL is a diagnosis of exclusion, obtained with a meticulous history and neuro-ophthalmic physical examination that cannot identify an organic cause. A patient with NOVL may be a malingerer who will present with exaggerated symptoms of vision change and the intention of attaining a secondary gain [2]. NOVL may also present in a patient with an underlying factitious disorder who develops subconscious symptoms [2].

The patient may present with complaints of monocular or binocular change in vision. The degree of symptoms may vary from blurriness to complete visual loss. Visual field defects most commonly include generalized constriction, tunnel vision, or, less commonly, homonymous hemianopia.

NOVL is often associated with a high prevalence of a concurrent psychiatric disorder such as depression, anxiety, or panic disorder. Nevertheless, it is important to recognize that organic disorder may still coexist and the burden of differentiating between functional overlay and malingering is on the provider, often resulting in extensive testing [3].

Nonorganic visual loss is often triggered by a psychosocial stressor. Consider:
- Physical or sexual abuse
- Bullying
- Unstable family structure
- Academic difficulties
- Change in environment

17.2.2 Epidemiology

Incidence in school-aged children is reportedly 1.75%, with a higher predominance in adolescents [4]. It is more common in females than males. Several studies note an earlier age of presentation among female patients, with age of onset at 8–9.4 years old compared to onset at age 10 years old in males [5–7]. Children are more likely to present with symmetric bilateral symptoms. Several underlying psychosocial stressors may be present in patients with NOVL including physical or sexual abuse, bullying, unstable family structure, academic difficulties, and change in environment [4].

17.2.3 Diagnosis

The provider must maintain a high level of suspicion and pay attention to visual behavior. If the patient can easily navigate his or her environment and the visual loss seems out of proportion to visual behavior and examination findings, evaluation for nonorganic visual loss should be performed. Comprehensive dilated ophthalmic and neurologic examination will often reveal inconsistent findings that will lead to a diagnosis of NOVL. The caretaker may provide history of a recent psychological stressor that preceded the symptoms. Visual acuity recorded may be inconsistent when tested multiple times. The goal of the examination is to demonstrate better than reported visual acuity and normal or inconsistent objective ophthalmic examination findings.

When testing visual acuity in mild to moderate NOVL (with reported Snellen visual acuity of 20/100 or better), it is usually necessary to start from the bottom of the eye chart and to provide constant encouragement for the patient to try to identify at least one letter on the line being tested. One may also test stereo acuity in which the patient wears 3-D glasses and identifies objects that are in three dimension (◘ Figure 17.1a). In order to successfully perform the stereo test, the patient must have good visual acuity *in both eyes* and the eyes must be well aligned. Patients with true monocular severe visual loss will not be able to see in three dimension on the stereo test. In the presence of acute monocular severe visual loss (20/400 or worse) and an otherwise normal-appearing anterior and posterior segment of the eye, one would suspect retrobulbar optic nerve pathology, and a relative afferent pupillary defect (RAPD) should be present (◘ Figure 17.1b). If absent, the provider may test each eye separately with the optokinetic nystagmus (OKN) drum or strip, which should produce jerk nystagmus if visual acuity is 20/400 or better (◘ Figure 17.1c). If the patient claims light perception or no light perception vision, the provider can hold a portable mirror and gently rotate it. If the visual acuity is good enough to make out the shape of their face, the provider will notice the patient's eye moving to follow the facial reflection (◘ Figure 17.1d).

Visual field testing may be helpful in establishing a diagnosis; however, younger children will not be able to comprehend or cooperate with the test. Visual field testing may be suitable for adolescents and will demonstrate a few classic findings highly suggestive of NOVL. These findings include tunnel as opposed to funnel visual field [4]. The visual field should expand as the target moves further back (corresponding to the degree of visual field) (◘ Fig. 17.2).

17.2.4 Management

Reassurance to the child and the parents is an important approach to treatment [8, 9]. The provider may state that there is no sign of permanent damage to the eye and that the child will likely improve with time. There must be an attempt to address the inciting social stressor. It is discouraged to confront the patient with inconsistencies in examination findings or to belittle his or her symptoms. Regular follow-up appointments are important to document improvement and continue evaluation for coexisting organic etiologies.

17.2.5 Prognosis

Prognosis is favorable for most patients as normalization of vision is expected with time. While most patients do not harbor an underlying psychiatric diagnosis, some may benefit from further evaluation and management by a psychiatrist [4].

17.3 Migraine

Migraine is the most common subtype of chronic primary headache in the pediatric population [10, 11]. When untreated, it can have a significant effect on quality of life leading to decreased school attendance and decline in academic performance and socialization [12].

17.3.1 Pathophysiology

There are several proposed theories explaining the pathophysiology behind migraines. While the consensus is that the mechanism is multifactorial, the exact etiology remains unclear.

One theory is that is it caused by the activation of the trigeminovascular system with the release of pro-inflammatory mediators like vasoactive intestinal peptide (VIP), substance P, and calcitonin gene-related peptide in the synapses of trigeminal nerve branches

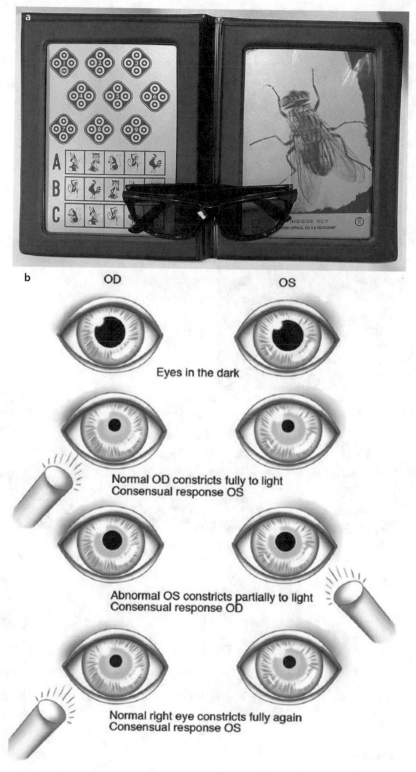

◻ Fig. 17.1 Examination techniques for nonorganic visual loss. **a** Titmus stereo acuity test. **b** Testing for a relative afferent pupillary defect (Adapted with permission from ▶ https://neupsykey.com/neuro-ophthalmology-9/#c010_f001). **c** Optokinetic nystagmus (OKN) drum. **d** Mirror test. (Reproduced with permission from the American Academy of Ophthalmology. © 2020 American Academy of Ophthalmology)

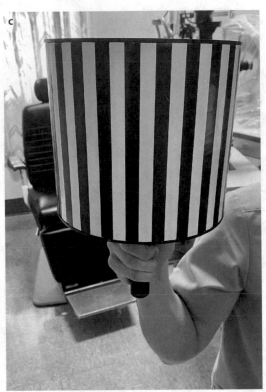

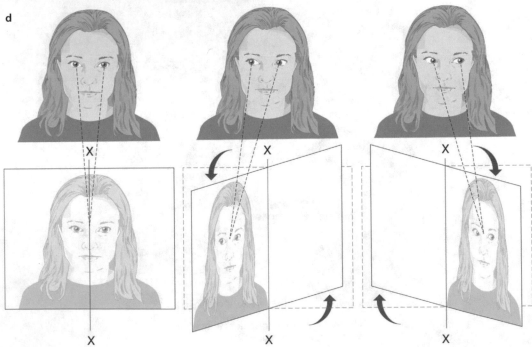

■ **Fig. 17.1** (continued)

17

surrounding cerebral and meningeal vessels [10, 13]. This subsequently leads to vasodilation and disruption of the blood-brain barrier that further stimulates the trigeminovascular system. Another proposed mechanism behind migraines is explained by aberrant central catecholaminergic system leading to cortical hyperexcitability [10]. Low magnesium levels have also been associated with abnormal afferent transmission of pain [10].

For migraine with aura, another theory describes a pattern of hyperperfusion followed by hypoperfusion occurring at the level of the brainstem, mediated by alternating neuronal activation and suppression, or *cortical spreading depression*. This process of neurogenic inflammation leads to nociceptor activation and cortical blood flow disruption [10, 14].

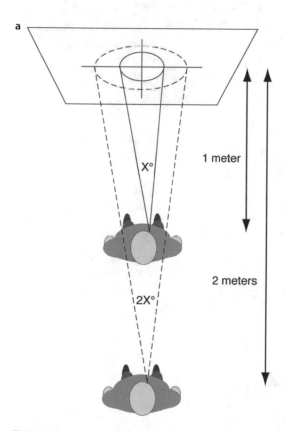

Fig. 17.2 Visual field patterns in nonorganic visual loss. **a** Tangent screen with tunnel vision. One should expect the visual field to expand when tested further away from the screen. If it remains the same, this is not physiologic. (Reproduced with permission from the American Academy of Ophthalmology. © 2020 American Academy of Ophthalmology). **b** Normal Humphrey visual field. **c** Humphrey visual field with generalized constriction. (Adapted with permission from the American Academy of Ophthalmology. © 2020 American Academy of Ophthalmology). **d** Humphrey visual field clover leaf pattern (unreliable) (Adapted with permission from the American Academy of Ophthalmology. © 2020 American Academy of Ophthalmology). **e** Goldmann visual field spiral with intersecting isopter lines. (Adapted with permission from the American Academy of Ophthalmology. © 2020 American Academy of Ophthalmology)

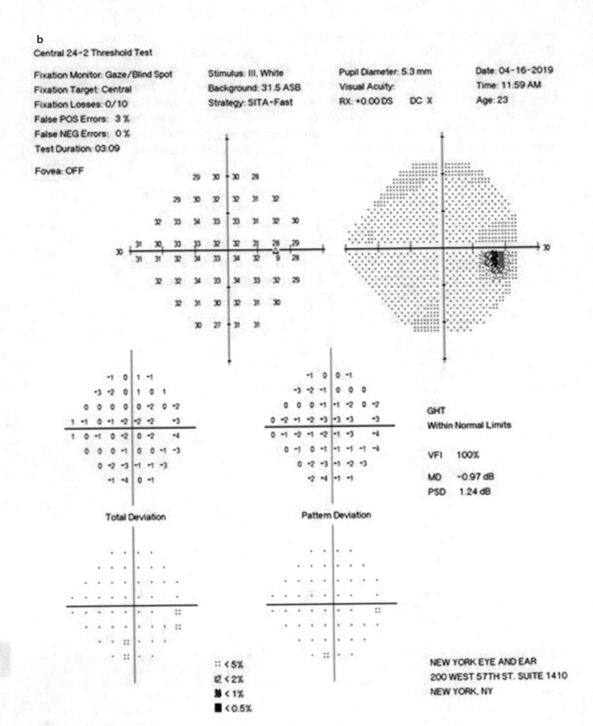

b

Central 24-2 Threshold Test

Fixation Monitor: Gaze/Blind Spot
Fixation Target: Central
Fixation Losses: 0/10
False POS Errors: 3 %
False NEG Errors: 0 %
Test Duration: 03:09

Fovea: OFF

Stimulus: III, White
Background: 31.5 ASB
Strategy: SITA-Fast

Pupil Diameter: 5.3 mm
Visual Acuity:
RX: +0.00 DS   DC X

Date: 04-16-2019
Time: 11:59 AM
Age: 23

Total Deviation

Pattern Deviation

GHT
Within Normal Limits

VFI   100%

MD   -0.97 dB
PSD   1.24 dB

:: < 5%
▨ < 2%
▨ < 1%
■ < 0.5%

NEW YORK EYE AND EAR
200 WEST 57TH ST. SUITE 1410
NEW YORK, NY

◻ Fig. 17.2 (continued)

17

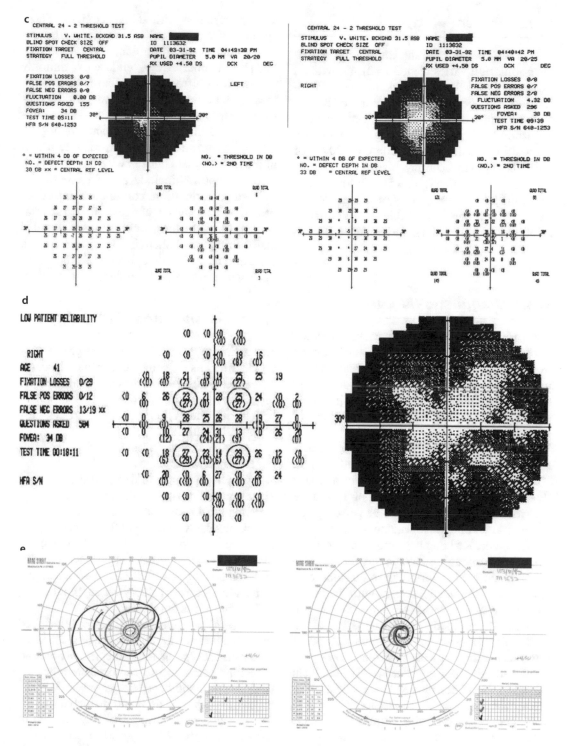

■ **Fig. 17.2** (continued)

17.3.2 Epidemiology

The prevalence of migraine among the pediatric population varies from 3 to 21.4% with an increasing prevalence from childhood to adolescence [15]. Female predominance of 2.5:1 is noted from adolescence and lasts through adulthood. Migraine may have a genetic predisposition with approximately 70% of patients reporting family history in at least one family member [10, 15]. Children with migraine have worse quality of life and higher rates of comorbid anxiety, depression, ADHD, sleep disorders, and epilepsy [10, 11, 15, 16].

17.3.3 Diagnostic Workup

A thorough history and physical examination is often sufficient to establish a clinical diagnosis of migraine. Physical examination including a neurologic examination is not expected to reveal any focal neurological deficits or signs leading to a secondary cause of headache.

In certain cases, laboratory workup, neuroimaging, or an electroencephalographic study may be required to evaluate for a seizure disorder or a secondary cause of headache. Neuroimaging should always be performed if there is any concern for a structural etiology of headache. Red flag warning signs requiring urgent neuroimaging include any focal neurologic deficit lasting longer than 60 minutes, a change in headache pattern with increased frequency and severity of headache, or the presence of papilledema. Examination of the optic disc is essential in evaluation of all patients presenting with headache.

Based on the International Headache Society (IHS) International Classification of Headache Disorders 3rd edition (ICHD-3), a diagnosis of migraine requires ≥5 separate episodes of headache lasting from 4 to 72 hours when untreated. These headaches must be associated with at least two of the following characteristics: unilateral location, pulsatile in nature, aggravation by activity, and interference with daily activities. These episodes are commonly associated with nausea, vomiting, photophobia, and phonophobia [17]. Unlike adults, children commonly present with bifrontal pain that is difficult to localize and associated with vague premonitory symptoms such as fatigue, sleep difficulty, mood changes, and hyperactivity [18]. Cranial autonomic symptoms may be found in the majority of children with migraine [19]. These symptoms include at least one of the following: lacrimation, conjunctival injection, ptosis, miosis, nasal congestion, periorbital edema, facial flushing, or sweating. A detailed history may be challenging to obtain from a child and may require exclusion of other etiologies with appropriate supplementary testing.

17.3.4 Classification of Migraine

According to the ICHD-3 [20], migraine may be classified as episodic or chronic. *Episodic migraines* are recurrent attacks, while *chronic migraines* are ≥15 headaches per month, 8 of which fit the criteria for migraine, for ≥3 months' duration.

Migraine is also classified as *migraine without aura* and *migraine with aura*.

Aura is a prodromal sensation, often a visual, somatic, or less commonly an olfactory manifestation that precedes a migraine attack or seizure episode [20]. The visual phenomenon lasts less than 1 hour, must be completely reversible, and may have positive features (bright scintillations, flashing lights) or negative features (blurry vision, blind spots, or homonymous hemianopia).

Migraine without aura, previously referred to as "common migraine" for being the most common subtype of migraine, usually lacks a preceding activation of the brainstem or cortical function and hence does not have preceding symptoms such as visual disturbance.

Migraine with aura, previously referred to as "classic migraine," or *typical aura with headache*, has a biphasic pattern that begins with an aura and is followed by a headache. Children may not be able to adequately describe these auras. Encouraging them to

17

draw these experiences may prove to be helpful in making a diagnosis. Another subtype of migraine with aura includes *typical aura without headache* in which patients experience the aura with a mild or no distinct headache within the subsequent hour.

Hemiplegic migraine is associated with fully reversible motor weakness, with or without speech, visual, or sensory symptoms. *Retinal vasospasm, also called "retinal migraine",* is associated with fully reversible monocular visual phenomena, usually described as acute visual loss in a similar pattern of amaurosis fugax. Retinal vasospasm is more common in patients with migraine, but is not associated with cortical spreading depression.

17.3.5 Management

Management of migraine is divided into abortive and preventative treatment. The following recommendations are largely based on adult studies as there is limited data for high-quality randomized controlled studies in the pediatric population [21–23]. A crucial element of management is proper education of the patient and family. A headache diary suitable for children may help identify and avoid precipitating triggers and help monitor efficiency of treatment. Triggers may include stress, menstrual cycle, irregular meals, poor sleeping patterns, or specific foods or odors [24].

Once prodromal symptoms or headache starts, the patient should be encouraged to rest in a dark, quiet room.

During an acute attack, the earlier the intervention is given the more likely it is to be effective. In mild to moderate headaches, the first drug of choice is an analgesic, preferably acetaminophen or nonsteroidal anti-inflammatory drugs (NSAIDs). Acetaminophen pediatric dosage is 15 mg/kg every 2–4 hours not exceeding 1000 mg per dose or three doses per day. Ibuprofen pediatric dosage is 10 mg/kg every 4–6 hours not exceeding 40 mg/kg per day. If migraines are accompanied by significant nausea or vomiting, an antiemetic agent may be considered. Alternatively, analgesics and antiemetics may be administered in suppository form.

In moderate to severe attacks, or in mild attacks that are refractory to analgesics, migraine-specific agents like triptans should be considered separately or in combination with an NSAID. Sumatriptan is often the first choice and can be started at the smallest dose of 25 mg orally or 5 mg nasal spray. While there is no consensus on when to transition to adult dosing, many physicians will treat children over the age of 10 who weigh ≥ 50 kg with adult dosage of sumatriptan. For children who are unable to swallow pills, oral disintegrating formulations of rizatriptan, zolmitriptan, and almotriptan may be used. Ergotamine drugs have been largely replaced by sumatriptan for abortive treatment due to their side effect profile and potential to worsen nausea, vomiting, and symptoms related to vasospasm. The efficacy of valproate has not been well established in children. Opioids, benzodiazepines, and barbiturates are habit-forming drugs with significant side effects and should not be used to treat migraine in children.

Preventative treatment should be considered in patients with frequent and disabling migraines, or with failure or adverse side effects of acute therapy [25]. Preventative medications such as cyproheptadine, amitriptyline, propranolol, topiramate, and riboflavin may be started at the lowest dose and titrated until therapeutic effects are attained or maximum dose is reached. A trial period of 1–3 months should be considered before switching to another agent.

17.3.6 Prognosis

Long-term follow-up studies have demonstrated that the majority of pediatric patients improve with time and comprehensive headache management as the frequency or severity of their headaches decreases with age [26–28]. The most important prognostic factors include medical and psychiatric comorbidities.

17.4 Cluster Headache

Cluster headaches are debilitatingly painful and often a source of great distress. It commonly presents with unilateral stabbing or throbbing pain, maximally noted around the orbits, and is associated with transient autonomic symptoms such as lacrimation, ptosis, and rhinorrhea. The headache occurs in a "cluster" of episodes throughout the day lasting 5–180 minutes. This type of headache rarely occurs in the pediatric population but has a fairly typical presentation similar to those in adult patients [20, 29].

17.4.1 Pathophysiology

There are several postulated theories regarding the pathophysiology of cluster headaches; however, it remains incompletely understood. The unilateral boring orbital pain is suggestive of the involvement of ipsilateral trigeminovascular complex and the trigeminal-autonomic reflex pathway. The reflexive autonomic symptoms support the activation of the ipsilateral parasympathetic nerves [30].

17.4.2 Epidemiology

Cluster headache is a rare subgroup of chronic headaches. The prevalence of cluster headache in the general population is <1%, while the prevalence of childhood onset is 0.1%. It is more common in males than females with the ratio of 4.3:1. With age, childhood-onset cluster headache can go into spontaneous remission or become less frequent with prolonged periods of remission between attacks [31, 32].

17.4.3 Diagnostic Workup

Cluster headache is largely a clinical diagnosis made with a meticulous and detailed headache history. Cluster headache can be confused with migraine or sinusitis. Correct diagnosis can be made with targeted history, physical examination, and appropriate imaging when indicated to rule out potentially life-threatening conditions.

ICHD-3 diagnostic criteria allow practitioners to reliably differentiate cluster headaches from other headache disorders. Cluster headache presents with unilateral orbital or periorbital severe pain that lasts a few minutes to 180 minutes when treated. Acute attacks may occur several times a day to every other day. These episodes are accompanied by a sense of restlessness and the following autonomic signs: lacrimation, nasal congestion, rhinorrhea, miosis, ptosis, conjunctival injection, or facial perspiration. These attacks occur steadily for weeks to months followed by a period of remission.

Patients commonly present to the emergency department with an acute attack and to the clinic in between attacks. A thorough physical examination will show visual acuity that is unchanged from baseline, usually a normal pupillary reaction, confrontation visual fields, extraocular movements, color vision, and dilated funduscopic examination. If a patient presents with active symptoms, the slit lamp examination may reveal unilateral conjunctival injection, tearing, and less likely ptosis and miosis. Assessment of the cranial nerves should always be done and is expected to be normal. Imaging is not routinely obtained unless the patient presents with "red flags" or if the constellation of symptoms are not supportive of a diagnosis of benign cluster headaches. "Red flags" can include neurological findings, increased frequency or severity of headache, focal neurological symptoms, meningeal signs, systemic symptoms, or nighttime awakening.

Visual field testing can assess for scattered visual field loss or homonymous visual field defects; however, the required cooperation may be limited in the pediatric population.

17.4.4 Classification of Cluster Headaches

The ICHD-3 classifies cluster headaches as *episodic* or *chronic*. *Episodic* cluster headaches present with at least two attacks lasting a week to a year and separated by a period of remission ≥3 months. *Chronic* cluster headaches present with attacks that occur for a period of ≥1 year without a remission period or one lasting <3 months.

17.4.5 Management

Treating cluster headaches in pediatric patients is aimed at improving their quality of life. The duration of treatment greatly varies as these patients tend to experience remission with age. Certain behavior modifications such as adequate sleep, hydration, and exercise have been associated with decreased headache frequency and severity. Common triggers such as exposure to tobacco as well as certain food and beverages have been implicated in the onset of cluster headaches and should be avoided. As for treatment of acute episodes, oxygen therapy is the recommended initial approach [33, 34]. Considering oxygen therapy may not be readily available at home, many practitioners will treat with subcutaneous or intranasal triptan (off-label) to provide relief as it has been shown to have good efficacy in adults and tolerability in adolescents [34].

17.4.6 Prognosis

Cluster headaches can be extremely debilitating when not properly managed and have been associated with higher risk of depression and lower quality of life. There are a limited number of long-term studies available evaluating the evolution of cluster headaches from childhood to adulthood. A few studies demonstrate that episodes may increase in frequency or remain the same, and complete resolution with age rarely occurs [35–37].

17.5 Photophobia and Post-Traumatic Headache

Photophobia is a common and disabling condition noted in many patients with ocular or neurologic disorders such as uveitis, blepharospasm, chronic headaches, or post-traumatic

brain injury. Excessively bright light leads to discomfort or pain, and the patient subsequently adopts an aversion to light and reports "seeing better" in dim lighting. Symptoms are perpetuated by the patient wearing dark sunglasses to avoid photophobia resulting in dark adaptation and a more intense photophobia response when the sunglasses are removed.

17.5.1 Association with Headache Syndromes

Chronic headache syndromes such as tension headaches, cluster headaches, and migraines are a common cause of photophobia [38]. According to the ICHD-3 (◼ Table 17.1), a major diagnostic criterion for migraine is photophobia and may be reported by patients during or between attacks [38]. Different light stimuli such as flickering light, fluorescent light, or bright sunlight have been implicated in triggering migraine attacks [39] (◼ Table 17.2).

17.5.2 Post-Traumatic Photophobia

Post-traumatic photophobia commonly occurs in the acute and subacute phase (7–19 days) of a traumatic brain injury (TBI) [40]. The development of photophobia after TBI may be accounted for by the injury of intracranial structures and inflammation of the trigeminal nociceptive pathway [41]. TBI is associated with many post-traumatic chronic pain conditions, headache being the most common (prevalence 58%). More specifically, there is a higher risk of developing migraine-like headache after TBI [42, 43]. Given the intimate relationship between migraine and photophobia, the prevalence of photophobia in TBI patients is not surprising [42, 43].

17.5.3 Treatment

Chronic photophobia in children can be addressed with FL-41 filtered lenses, which are rose-tinted. These lenses filter out certain

■ **Table 17.1** International Classification of Headache Disorders-3 (2018) ► https://ichd-3.org/

Part I: The primary headaches	Part II: The secondary headaches	Part III: Neuropathies and facial pains and other headaches	Part IV: Appendix
1. Migraine	5. Headache attributed to trauma or injury to the head and/or neck	13. Painful lesions of the cranial nerves and other facial pain	A1. Migraine
2. Tension-type headache (TTH)	6. Headache attributed to cranial or cervical vascular disorder	14. Other headache disorders	A2. Tension-type headache (alternative criteria)
3. Trigeminal autonomic cephalgias (TACs)	7. Headache attributed to nonvascular intracranial disorder		A3. Trigeminal autonomic cephalgias (TACs)
4. Other primary headache disorders	8. Headache attributed to a substance or its withdrawal		A4. Other primary headache disorders
	9. Headache attributed to infection		A5. Headache attributed to trauma or injury to the head and/or neck
	10. Headache attributed to disorder of homeostasis		A6. Headache attributed to cranial and/or cervical vascular disorder
	11. Headache or facial pain attributed to disorder of the cranium, neck, eyes, ears, nose, sinuses, teeth, mouth, or other facial or cervical structure		A7. Headache attributed to nonvascular intracranial disorder
	12. Headache attributed to psychiatric disorder		A8. Headache attributed to substance or its withdrawal
			A9. Headache attributed to infection
			A10. Headache attributed to disorder of homeostasis
			A11. Headache or facial pain attributed to disorder of the cranium, neck, eyes, ears, nose, sinuses, teeth, mouth, or other facial or cervical structure
			A12. Headache attributed to psychiatric disorder

17

◻ Table 17.2 Common headache syndromes and their clinical features

Common headache syndromes	Headache characteristics	Duration	Associated symptoms
Migraine	Unilateral throbbing pain	4–72 hours	Phonophobia, photophobia, nausea, vomiting, aggravated by activity
Tension-type headache (TTH)	Bilateral, band-like squeezing pain	30 minutes to 7 days	Phonophobia or photophobia, tenderness of pericranial muscles
Paroxysmal hemicrania	Unilateral paroxysmal severe pain	2–30 minutes	Ipsilateral cranial autonomic symptoms (ipsilateral conjunctival injection, lacrimation, miosis or ptosis, nasal congestion, eyelid edema, facial sweating)
Cluster headache (CH)	Unilateral electric or stabbing pain	Clusters lasting 15 180 minutes for period of 1–3 months	Ipsilateral cranial autonomic symptoms
Short-lasting unilateral neuralgiform headache	Unilateral frequent attacks	1 second to 10 minutes	Ipsilateral conjunctival injection and lacrimation
Headache secondary to vascular disorder	Acute and severe	Continued	Often accompanied by focal neurological deficits
Headache attributed to a substance exposure or withdrawal	Unilateral or bilateral	Substance exposure: immediately within hours Substance withdrawal: weeks to hours	
Headache secondary to infection	Systemic infection: diffuse, moderate-severe intensity Meningoencephalitis: holocranial vs. nuchal	Remits with infection In minority of cases headache persists >3 months after resolution of infection	Fever, nausea/vomiting, lethargy, and convulsions

wavelengths of blue and green present in fluorescent lighting, which are thought to be particularly bothersome for patients with migraine and TBI.

Wearing FL-41 filtered lenses reduces light sensitivity, frequency and severity of migraine (by over half in children), and improves contrast perception [42–44].

17.6 Papilledema

17.6.1 Definition

Papilledema refers to swelling of the optic nerve secondary to elevated intracranial pressure (ICP) (◻ Fig. 17.3). Profound, permanent vision loss may occur secondary to irreversible

▫ Fig. 17.3 Frisen grading system for papilledema. **a** Grade 0, no disc edema; **b** Grade 1, mild papilledema with a C-shaped nerve fiber layer disc edema sparing the temporal disc; **c** Grade 2, mild to moderate papilledema with 360 degree edema; **d** Grade 3, moderate to severe papilledema with obscuration of vessels as they leave the disc; **e** Grade 4, severe papilledema with obscuration of major vessels on the disc; **f** Grade 5, severe papilledema with most major vessels obscured and marked disc elevation. (Reproduced with permission from the American Academy of Ophthalmology. © 2020 American Academy of Ophthalmology)

damage to the optic nerves. The underlying etiologies for elevated ICP that may result in papilledema in children are numerous but are classified into two main categories: idiopathic and secondary causes of elevated ICP [45].

17.6.2 Clinical Presentation

Elevated ICP may present with a variety of different symptoms. Commonly, patients will present with headaches, pulsatile tinnitus, horizontal diplopia, and transient visual obscurations (TVOs) [45]. Additionally, nausea and associated vomiting may also be observed. Headaches due to elevated ICP are typically present upon awakening, refractive to pain medication, and worse in the supine position. Diplopia is typically horizontal, reflecting the presence of a unilateral or bilateral sixth nerve palsy. Transient visual obscurations consist of blackouts or blur-outs of vision lasting a few seconds and are often prompted by positional changes such as bending over or with Valsalva pressure. Visual acuity is usually normal in patients with papilledema, but may drastically worsen in chronic cases. Blind spot enlargement is classically appreciated in papilledema; however, rapid progressive visual field loss and even blindness may ensue within a period of weeks to months.

17.6.3 Diagnosis

Diagnosis of papilledema requires direct examination of the optic nerve to determine the presence of disc swelling. Once established and elevated ICP is suspected, an evaluation of the etiology begins. Neuroimaging with both magnetic resonance imaging (MRI) of the brain and orbits and magnetic resonance venography (MRV) are often advocated. MRI permits the evaluation of secondary causes of elevated ICP such as intracranial masses or hydrocephalus. MRV allows for the assessment of occult cerebral venous thrombosis, an etiology that is occasionally not readily appreciated on standard MRI sequences. Elevation of ICP is confirmed through lumbar puncture. CSF cytology and chemistry studies performed during the study may also elucidate infectious, inflammatory, neoplastic, and secondary causes of elevated ICP. An opening pressure greater than 28 cmH_2O is considered elevated for children, although greater than 25 cm H20 is considered elevated in those not sedated during lumbar puncture and in non-obese children [45].

17.6.4 Etiology

Causes of papilledema in children and required workup:
- *Idiopathic intracranial hypertension:* obtain history of recent weight gain/obesity, use of steroids, oral contraceptives, acne treatment, or tetracycline antibiotics; negative neuroimaging, lumbar puncture with opening pressure ≥ 28 cmH_2O and normal CSF content
- *Intracranial tumor:* MRI brain with and without contrast
- *Cerebral venous sinus thrombosis:* obtain history of blood clots, recent head trauma, sinusitis, or otitis media; MRV head without contrast, lumbar puncture with opening pressure
- *Hydrocephalus:* MRI brain with evaluation of cerebrospinal fluid dynamics
- *Meningitis:* vital signs, lumbar puncture with opening pressure and CSF studies with gram stain and culture

17.6.4.1 Idiopathic Intracranial Hypertension or Pseudotumor Cerebri Syndrome

Primary pseudotumor cerebri syndrome, also known as idiopathic intracranial hypertension (IIH), is a condition characterized by signs and symptoms of increased intracranial pressure with no recognizable cause and normal brain parenchyma. Aplastic anemia and iron deficiency have been linked to idiopathic intracranial hypertension. Weight gain and obesity are strongly associated with IIH. These patients demonstrate the signs and symptoms of elevated ICP, but lack any localizing finding on neurological examination and have otherwise normal neurodiagnostic studies with the exception of increased CSF pressure confirmed on lumbar puncture. IIH is described in further detail in the next section.

17.6.4.2 Secondary Causes of Papilledema

Secondary ICP elevation with papilledema may be caused and may be a presenting sign of a myriad of etiologies including but not limited to space-occupying tumor, hydrocephalus, an abnormality of the cerebral spinal fluid outflow tract, dural venous sinus thrombosis, meningitis, iatrogenically induced by medication, or in association with a systemic disorder. A thorough medical history may provide diagnostic clues to the etiology. History of blood clots, recent head trauma, sinusitis, or otitis media may be suggestive of dural venous sinus thrombosis. Fever, malaise, or neck stiffness may suggest meningitis.

17.6.5 Treatment

Treatment and management of papilledema is often guided by the degree of visual impairment at the time of presentation. An interdisciplinary approach with an ophthalmologist should be implemented to closely monitor and prevent significant visual morbidity from papilledema. For secondary causes of papilledema, the underlying etiology must be addressed as directed. In primary papilledema, treatment is directed at lowering ICP via medications such as diuretics (acetazolamide, topiramate, or furosemide). Surgical approaches are often undertaken when presentation at initial diagnosis is severe.

17.7 Idiopathic Intracranial Hypertension

17.7.1 Definition

Idiopathic intracranial hypertension (IIH), otherwise known as pseudotumor cerebri syndrome (PTCS), encompasses a constellation of symptoms due to elevated intracranial pressure (ICP) of unclear etiology [45]. Although most typically observed in obese women of childbearing age, the pediatric population may be affected as well [46, 47]. PTCS is classically regarded as either primary or secondary. Primary PTCS has an uncertain etiology and no identifiable cause, while secondary PTCS may be associated with a number of medical conditions and medications [45].

17.7.2 Epidemiology

There are an estimated 0.9 per 100,000 cases of PTCS in both the general pediatric and adult populations [47–49]. Female sex and obesity are more strongly associated with PTCS in older rather than younger pediatric patients [48–50]. In addition to weight, height and linear growth acceleration appear to play a role [51].

17.7.3 Pathophysiology

The pathophysiology of pediatric IIH is complex, but is fundamentally related to abnormal cerebral spinal fluid (CSF) dynamics, either impaired CSF outflow, aberrant CSF production, or a combination [52]. In primary PTCS, distinct driving factors derived by age, sex, and weight contribute [53]. The current theory is that there is an interplay and multifaceted relationship between obesity, pubertal status, sex, and age, which may be acting to influence CSF production or outflow [53]. In early and late adolescence, adiposity is clearly associated with primary PTCS; however, in younger children, factors other than obesity seem to contribute to the disease [54].

Secondary IIH is a clinical diagnosis that is linked to one or more of a variety of identifiable causes, including venous sinus thrombosis, various medications, and medical conditions other than obesity [53]. More common causes of secondary IIH in the pediatric population include withdrawal from chronic corticosteroids, exposure to tetracycline-related antibiotics, vitamin A and retinoid usage, and synthetic growth hormone exposure [55].

17.7.4 Clinical Presentation

Papilledema is the hallmark ophthalmologic finding of IIH, although rare cases may occur without papilledema. Common clinical symptoms may include headache, nausea, vomiting, tinnitus, neck stiffness, transient visual obscurations, decreased vision, and diplopia [46]. Children with PTCS have a higher frequency of ocular motility dysfunction compared with adults, with a sixth nerve palsy being the most common, affecting as many as 40% of patients [46–56].

17.7.5 Diagnosis

Assessment for the presence or absence of papilledema is the first critical step in diagnosis of PTCS. A careful examination of the optic nerve head is necessary; but orbital ultrasound and optical coherence tomography (OCT) imaging may be useful adjunctive tests [54]. The diagnosis of PTCS requires the presence of normal brain parenchyma on contrast-enhanced neuroimaging [54]. The primary role of MRI is to exclude other causes of elevated ICP such as hydrocephalus, mass, other structural lesions, and abnormal meningeal enhancement. Common radiological signs include flattening of the posterior sclera, enhancement of the prelam-

inar optic nerve, and an empty sella [58, 59]. A MR venogram is not always necessary, but should be considered for patients with high suspicion for cerebral venous sinus thrombosis. Venous imaging should be considered for atypical presentations/populations such as males and thin females [54]. Lumbar puncture is necessary to document an elevated ICP and to ensure a normal CSF composition. In adults and nonobese children with sedation, an ICP greater than 25 cmH$_2$0 is the criterion for abnormal elevation. For obese children who receive sedation, opening pressure greater than 28 cmH$_2$O is considered elevated [57]. CSF composition should be normal.

17.7.6 Treatment

Goals of treatment are aimed at preventing permanent vision loss and relieving symptoms associated with elevated ICP. Two mainstays of treatment are focused on medications to lower ICP and directed weight loss [54]. PTCS does not always require treatment, and medical treatment is usually started when the patient begins to experience visual deficits [60]. Carbonic anhydrase inhibitors such as acetazolamide reduce CSF production and provide effective management in PTCS. Alternative therapies such as furosemide, topiramate, and spironolactone are less commonly used. When associated with obesity or being overweight, weight loss becomes an important part in the treatment and management of PTCS. Based on studies in adults, patients are advised to lose 6–10% of body weight to manage the disease acutely and prevent its recurrence [61, 62]. Weight loss goals should however be balanced with the consideration that many pediatric patients are still growing and that specific goals should depend on the patient's age, body mass index, and comorbidities [54]. Nonconservative, surgical interventions are reserved for only severe cases where patients have demonstrated progressive vision loss despite maximal medical therapy, or in cases of severe visual loss at the time of presentation. Optic nerve sheath fenestration is indicated when vision impairment is the primary concern, while CSF shunting (lumboperitoneal or ventriculoperitoneal) is preferred for children with refractory headaches, severe visual impairment, and papilledema unresponsive to standard medical treatment [60].

While long-term prognosis is not definitively determined with certainty, recurrence rates for pediatric IIH are cited to be around 40%, with recurrences being common after stopping treatment [63]. Pubertal age carries a worse prognosis for visual outcome than other ages [64].

Case Presentation

A 9-year-old boy presents with subacute visual loss in the right eye over the last month. He has no past medical or ocular history. General examination reveals a well-nourished boy in no acute distress with a flat affect. Visual acuity is light perception in the right eye and 20/25 in the left eye. Pupils are equal and there is no relative afferent pupillary defect (RAPD). Confrontation visual field is full in the left eye, and the patient is unable to identify fingers in the right eye. The mirror test shows eye movement with movement of the mirror for both eyes. He is able to identify the three-dimensional animals and all the circles on the Titmus stereoacuity test. Examination of the anterior and posterior segment of the eye is unremarkable. A conversation with the mother outside the examination room confirms declining grades in school over the last few months and a few trips to the school principal for fights with a boy at school. The mother is advised that there is evidence of nonorganic visual loss (no RAPD and normal eye examination, positive mirror test, normal Titmus stereoacuity) and the patient should receive counseling regarding possible bullying at school. The vision should improve over time once the underlying cause is addressed.

Case Presentation

A 12-year-old girl presents with headache for the last 3 to 4 months. Height and weight are 5 foot 2 inches and 230 pounds, respectively. Past medical history is significant for eczematous dermatitis and acne. Medications include triamcinolone 1% topical ointment, isotretinoin, and minocycline. Best corrected visual acuity is 20/20 in both eyes, color vision is full, and confrontation visual fields are full. Pupils are equal and there is no relative afferent pupillary defect. Formal Humphrey visual field shows enlargement of the blind spot and mild peripheral constriction in both eyes. Eye examination reveals normal anterior segment and grade 3 papilledema in both eyes. Brain MRI with and without contrast and MRV are unremarkable. Lumbar puncture opening pressure is 32 cmH$_2$O in the lateral decubitus position, and CSF contents are unremarkable. She is advised to stop taking triamcinolone, isotretinoin, and minocycline. She is treated with acetazolamide 500 mg PO twice daily and referred to neuro-ophthalmology for careful monitoring. She is counseled to follow a low-salt diet and lose 6% of her body weight (about 14 pounds). She is advised that if her papilledema does not improve and she has progressive visual loss despite medical treatment (including weight loss, stopping the offending medications, and treatment with acetazolamide), she may require surgical management of pseudotumor cerebri.

17

Key Points

- Nonorganic visual loss is a conversion disorder in which the visual loss is not physiologic or the examination findings do not coincide with the reported severity of visual loss.
- Nonorganic visual loss is often triggered by a psychosocial stressor including physical or sexual abuse, bullying, unstable family structure, academic difficulties, or change in environment.
- Migraine is the most common headache syndrome in children and can have comorbid anxiety, depression, ADHD, sleep disorders, and epilepsy.
- Papilledema causes peripheral constriction of the visual field and the central visual acuity is usually preserved until significant damage to the optic nerve occurs.
- Workup of papilledema should include urgent MRI to exclude other causes of elevated ICP such as hydrocephalus, mass, other structural lesions, and abnormal meningeal enhancement, especially in children who have a normal BMI and rapid onset of symptoms.

Review Questions

1. All of the following are tests for nonorganic visual loss except
   (a) Mirror test
   (b) Tangent screen
   (c) Goldmann visual field test
   (d) Optical coherence tomography

2. Which of the following features of headache warrant urgent neuroimaging?
   (a) Scintillating scotoma in the right visual field lasting 15 minutes
   (b) Focal neurologic deficit lasting 3 hours followed by headache
   (c) Headache associated with photophobia
   (d) Homonymous hemianopia lasting 20 minutes followed by headache

3. Which of the following is a treatment for severe papilledema associated with rapid onset of significant visual loss in idiopathic intracranial hypertension?
   (a) Weight loss of 6–10% body weight at presentation
   (b) Acetazolamide
   (c) Optic nerve sheath fenestration
   (d) Topiramate

✅ Answers

1. (d)
2. (b)
3. (c)

References

1. American Psychiatric Association: Diagnostic and Statistical Manual of Mental Disorders, 5th edition. Arlington, VA: American Psychiatric Association, 2013.
2. Thompson HS. Functional visual loss. Am J Ophthalmol. 1985;100:209–13.
3. Scott JA, Egan RA. Prevalence of organic neuro-ophthalmologic disease in patients with functional visual loss. Am J Ophthalmol. 2003;135:670–5.
4. Lim SA, Siatkowski RM, Farris BK. Functional visual loss in adults and children patient characteristics, management, and outcomes. Ophthalmology. 2005;112:1821–8.
5. Catalano RA, Simon JW, Krohel GB, Rosenberg PN. Functional visual loss. Ophthalmology. 1986;93:385–90.
6. Barnard NA. Visual conversion reaction in children. Ophthalmic Physiol Opt. 1989;9:372.
7. Bain KE, Beatty S, Lloyd C. Non-organic visual loss in children. Eye (Lond). 2000;14(Pt 5):770–2.
8. Van Balen AT, Slijper FE. Psychogenic amblyopia in children. J Pediatr Ophthalmol Strabismus. 1978;15:164–7.
9. Yasuna ER. Hysterical amblyopia in children. Am J Dis Child. 1963;106:558–63.
10. Strickland N, Dong Y. Head pain in pediatrics. In: Suen J, Petersen E, editors. Diagnosis and management of head and face pain. Cham: Springer; 2018.
11. Termine C, Ozge A, Antonaci F, Natriashvili S, Guidetti V, Wöber-Bingöl C. Overview of diagnosis and management of paediatric headache. Part II: therapeutic management. J Headache Pain. 2011;12(1):25–34. https://doi.org/10.1007/s10194-010-0256-6. Epub 2010 Dec 18. Review. PubMed PMID: 21170567; PubMed Central PMCID: PMC3072476.

12. Kernick D, Reinhold D, Campbell JL. Impact of headache on young people in a school population. Br J Gen Pract. 2009;59(566):678–81.

13. Kaube H, Katsarava Z, Przywara S, et al. Acute migraine headache: possible sensitization of neurons in the spinal trigeminal nucleus? Neurology. 2002;58:1234.

14. Leão AA. Pial circulation and spreading depression of activity in cerebral cortex. J Neurophysiol. 1944;7:391.

15. Bellini B, Cescut A, Saulle C, et al. Headache and comorbidity in children and adolescents. J Headache Pain. 2013;14(1) https://doi.org/10.1186/1129-2377-14-79.

16. Wöber-Bingöl Ç. Acute treatment for primary headache disorders in children. In: Mitsikostas D, Paemeleire K, editors. Pharmacological management of headaches, Headache. Cham: Springer; 2016.

17. Elser JM, Woody RC. Migraine headache in the infant and young child. Headache. 1990;30:366.

18. Dooley JM, Pearlman EM. The clinical spectrum of migraine in children. Pediatr Ann. 2010;39:408.

19. Gelfand AA, Reider AC, Goadsby PJ. Cranial autonomic symptoms in pediatric migraine are the rule, not the exception. Neurology. 2013;81(5):431–6. https://doi.org/10.1212/WNL.0b013e31829d872a.

20. Headache Classification Committee of the International Headache Society (IHS). The international classification of headache disorders, 3rd edition. Cephalalgia. 2018;38:1.

21. Lewis D, Ashwal S, Hershey A, et al. Practice parameter: pharmacological treatment of migraine headache in children and adolescents: report of the American Academy of Neurology Quality Standards Subcommittee and the Practice Committee of the Child Neurology Society. Neurology. 2004;63:2215.

22. El-Chammas K, Keyes J, Thompson N, et al. Pharmacologic treatment of pediatric headaches: a meta-analysis. JAMA Pediatr. 2013;167:250.

23. O'Brien HL, Kabbouche MA, Hershey AD. Treating pediatric migraine: an expert opinion. Expert Opin Pharmacother. 2012;13:959.

24. Metsähonkala L, Sillanpää M, Tuominen J. Headache diary in the diagnosis of childhood migraine. Headache. 1997;37:240.

25. Shamliyan TA, Kane RL, Ramakrishnan R, Taylor FR. Episodic migraines in children: limited evidence on preventive pharmacological treatments. J Child Neurol. 2013;28:1320.

26. Bille B. Migraine in childhood and its prognosis. Cephalalgia. 1981;1:71.

27. Cologno D, Torelli P, Manzoni GC. Migraine with aura: a review of 81 patients at 10-20 years' follow-up. Cephalalgia. 1998;18:690.

28. Bille B. A 40-year follow-up of school children with migraine. Cephalalgia. 1997;17:488.

29. Maytal J, Lipton RB, Solomon S, Shinnar S. Childhood onset cluster headaches. Headache. 1992;32:275–9. https://doi.org/10.1111/j.1526-4610.1992.hed3206275.x.

30. Wei DY, Yuan Ong JJ, Goadsby PJ. Cluster headache: epidemiology, pathophysiology, clinical features, and diagnosis. Ann Indian Acad Neurol. 2018;21(Suppl 1):S3–8. https://doi.org/10.4103/aian.AIAN_349_17. Review. PubMed PMID: 29720812; PubMed Central PMCID: PMC5909131.

31. Russell MB. Epidemiology and genetics of cluster headache. Lancet Neurol. 2004;3:279.

32. Fischera M, Marziniak M, Gralow I, Evers S. The incidence and prevalence of cluster headache: a meta-analysis of population-based studies. Cephalalgia. 2008;28:614.

33. Nesbitt AD, Goadsby PJ. Cluster headache. BMJ. 2012;344:e2407.

34. Cohen AS, Burns B, Goadsby PJ. High-flow oxygen for treatment of cluster headache: a randomized trial. JAMA. 2009;302(22):2451–7. https://doi.org/10.1001/jama.2009.1855.

35. Lampl C. Childhood-onset cluster headache. Pediatr Neurol. 2002;27:138–40. https://doi.org/10.1016/S0887-8994(02)00406-X.

36. Antonaci F, Alfei E, Piazza F, De Cillis I, Balottin U. Therapy-resistant cluster headache in childhood: case report and literature review. Cephalalgia. 2010;30:233–8.

37. Arruda MA, Bonamico L, Stella C, Bordini CA, Bigal ME. Cluster headache in children and adolescents: ten years of follow-up in three pediatric cases. Cephalalgia. 2011;31:1409–14. https://doi.org/10.1177/0333102411418015.

38. Drummond PD. A quantitative assessment of photophobia in migraine and tension headache. Headache. 1986;26:465–9.

39. Vanagaite J, Pareja JA, Storen O, White LR, Sand T, Stovner LJ. Light-induced discomfort and pain in migraine. Cephalalgia. 1997;17:733–41.

40. Vincent AJ, Spierings EL, Messinger HB. A controlled study of visual symptoms and eye strain factors in chronic headache. Headache. 29(8):523–7.

41. Waddell PA, Gronwall DM. Sensitivity to light and sound following minor head injury. Acta Neurol Scand. 1984;69:270–6.

42. Digre KB, Brennan KC. Shedding light on photophobia. J Neuroophthalmol. 2012;32(1):68–81. https://doi.org/10.1097/WNO.0b013e3182474548.

43. Nampiaparampil DE. Prevalence of chronic pain after traumatic brain injury: a systematic review. JAMA. 2008;300:711–9.

44. Good PA, Taylor RH, Mortimer MJ. The use of tinted glasses in childhood migraine. Headache. 1991;31:533–6.

45. Friedman DI, Liu GT, Digre KB. Revised diagnostic criteria for the pseudotumor cerebri syndrome in adults and children. Neurology. 2013;81:1–7.

46. Rangwala LM, Liu GT. Pediatric idiopathic intracranial hypertension. Surv Ophthalmol. 2007;52:597–617.

47. Phillips PH. Pediatric pseudotumor cerebri. Int Ophthalmol Clin. 2012;52:51–9.

48. Gordon K. Pediatric pseudotumor cerebri: Descriptive epidemiology. Can J Neurol Sci. 1997;24:219–21.

49. Bursztyn LL, Sharan S, Walsh L, et al. Has rising pediatric obesity increased the incidence of idiopathic intracranial hypertension in children? Can J Ophthalmol. 2014;49:87–91.

50. Balcer LJ, Liu GT, Forman S, et al. Idiopathic intracranial hypertension: relation of age and obesity in children. Neurology. 1999;52:870–2.

51. Sheldon CA, Paley GL, Xiao R, et al. Pediatric idiopathic intracranial hypertension: age, gender, and anthropometric features at diagnosis in a large, retrospective, multisite cohort. Ophthalmology. 2016;123:2424–31.

52. Mollan SP, Ali F, Hassan-Smith G, et al. Evolving evidence in adult idiopathic intracranial hypertension: pathophysiology and management. J Neurol Neurosurg Psychiatry. 2016;87:982–92.

53. Sheldon C, Paley GL, Beres SJ, McCormack S, Liu GT. Pediatric pseudotumor cerebri syndrome: diagnosis, classification and underlying pathophysiology. Semin Pediatr Neurol. 2017;24 https://doi.org/10.1016/j.spen.2017.04.002.

54. Brara SM, Koebnick C, Porter AH, Langer-Gould A. Pediatric idiopathic intracranial hypertension and extreme childhood obesity. J Pediatr. 2012;161:602–7.

55. Paley GL, Sheldon CA, Burrows EK, et al. Overweight and obesity in pediatric secondary pseudotumor cerebri syndrome e1. Am J Ophthalmol. 2015;159:344–52.

56. Phillips PH, Repka MX, Lambert SR. Pseudotumor cerebri in children. J AAPOS. 1998;2:33–8.

57. Avery RA, Shah SS, Licht DJ, et al. Reference range for cerebrospinal fluid opening pressure in children. N Engl J Med. 2010;363:891–3.

58. Brodsky MC, Vaphiades M. Magnetic resonance imaging in pseudotumor cerebri. Ophthalmology. 1998;105:1686–93.

59. Görkem SB, Doganay S, Canpolat M, Koc G, Dogan MS, Per H, Coskun A. MR imaging findings in children with pseudotumor cerebri and comparison with healthy controls. Childs Nerv Syst. 2015;31:373–80.

60. Dipasquale V, Di Rosa G, Savasta S, Merlo O, Concolino D, Arrigo T. Management of pediatric pseudotumor cerebri syndrome. J Pediatr Neurol. 2015;13:058–61.

61. Wong R, Madill SA, Pandey P, Riordan-Eva P. Idiopathic intracranial hypertension: the association between weight loss and the requirement for systemic treatment. BMC Ophthalmol. 2007;7:15.

62. Ko MW, Chang SC, Ridha MA, et al. Weight gain and recurrence in idiopathic intracranial hypertension: a case-control study. Neurology. 2011;76:1564–7.

63. Kesler A, Fattal-Valevski A. Idiopathic intracranial hypertension in the pediatric population. J Child Neurol. 2002;17:745–8.

64. Stiebel-Kalish H, Kalish Y, Lusky M, et al. Puberty as a risk factor for less favorable visual outcome in idiopathic intracranial hypertension. Am J Ophthalmol. 2006;142:279–83.